# Treating the Body in Medicine and Religion

Modern medicine has produced many wonderful technological breakthroughs that have extended the limits of the frail human body. However, much of the focus of this medical research has been on the physical, often reducing the human being to a biological machine to be examined, understood, and controlled. This book begins by asking whether the modern medical milieu has overly objectified the body, unwittingly or not, and whether current studies in bioethics are up to the task of restoring a fuller understanding of the human person. In response, various authors here suggest that a more theological/religious approach would be helpful or perhaps even necessary.

Presenting specific perspectives from Judaism, Christianity, and Islam, the book is divided into three parts: "Understanding the Body," "Respecting the Body," and "The Body at the End of Life." A panel of expert contributors – including philosophers, physicians, and theologians and scholars of religion – answers key questions such as: What is the relationship between body and soul? What are our obligations toward human bodies? How should medicine respond to suffering and death? The resulting text is an interdisciplinary treatise on how medicine can best function in our societies.

Offering a new way to approach the medical humanities, this book will be of keen interest to any scholars with an interest in contemporary religious perspectives on medicine and the body.

**John J. Fitzgerald** is Associate Professor of Theology and Religious Studies at St. John's University, U.S.A. He specializes in ethics, with particular attention to fundamental and health care issues. He has published one other book, *The Seductiveness of Virtue: Abraham Joshua Heschel and John Paul II on Morality and Personal Fulfillment* (Bloomsbury T&T Clark, 2017), and written multiple articles on ethics and religion in academic journals.

**Ashley John Moyse** is the McDonald Postdoctoral Fellow in Christian Ethics and Public Life at Christ Church, University of Oxford. He is a theologian with enduring interest in moral and political theology and particular interest in bioethics and medical humanities. His research has been presented and published internationally, including his book *Reading Karl Barth, Interrupting Moral Technique, Transforming Biomedical Ethics* (Palgrave Macmillan, 2015).

# Routledge Studies in Religion

For more information about this series, please visit: www.routledge.com/religion/series/SE0669

# Treating the Body in Medicine and Religion

Jewish, Christian, and Islamic
Perspectives

Edited by John J. Fitzgerald
and Ashley John Moyse

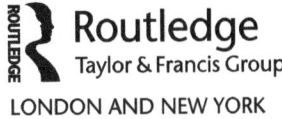
Routledge
Taylor & Francis Group

LONDON AND NEW YORK

First published 2019 by Routledge

2 Park Square, Milton Park, Abingdon, Oxon, OX14 4RN
605 Third Avenue, New York, NY 10017

*Routledge is an imprint of the Taylor & Francis Group, an informa business*

First issued in paperback 2020

*British Library Cataloguing-in-Publication Data*
A catalogue record for this book is available from the British Library

*Library of Congress Cataloging-in-Publication Data*
Names: Fitzgerald, John J., editor. | Moyse, Ashley John,
  1977– editor.
Title: Treating the body in medicine and religion : Jewish, Christian,
  and Islamic perspectives / edited by John J. Fitzgerald and Ashley
  John Moyse.
Description: Milton Park, Abingdon, Oxon ; New York, NY :
  Routledge, 2018. | Series: Routledge studies in religion | Includes
  bibliographical references and index.
Identifiers: LCCN 2018014366 | ISBN 9781138484856 (hardback :
  alk. paper) | ISBN 9781351050876 (ebook)
Subjects: LCSH: Medical ethics. | Medicine—Religious aspects. |
  Bioethics.
Classification: LCC R725.55 .T74 2018 | DDC 174.2—dc23
LC record available at https://lccn.loc.gov/2018014366

ISBN: 978-1-138-48485-6 (hbk)
ISBN: 978-0-367-78631-1 (pbk)

Typeset in Sabon
by Apex CoVantage, LLC

In memory of H. Tristram Engelhardt, Jr.

1941–2018

An outstanding and kind-hearted influence on so many
of those who engage in theological dialogue

# Contents

# Notes on contributors

Timothy James Carey, Ph.D., received his doctorate in Comparative Theology at Boston College in Chestnut Hill, Massachusetts, where he studied Muslim-Christian relations in sub-Saharan Africa. His current research examines the respective Sunni Muslim and African Catholic responses to the HIV/AIDS pandemic in Nairobi, Kenya, as a case study for practical interreligious dialogue. He has lectured internationally on issues related to theological bioethics and has published in the *Dharmaram Journal of Theology* and *Theology & Sexuality*. A former Fellow at the Boisi Center for the Study of Constitutional Democracy, Carey is the author of *Muslim and Catholic Responses to HIV and AIDS in Kenya* (Lexington Books, 2018).

Elliot N. Dorff, Ph.D., is Rector and Distinguished Service Professor of Philosophy at American Jewish University in Los Angeles, California, and Visiting Professor at UCLA School of Law. He is Chair of the Conservative Movement's Committee on Jewish Law and Standards, and he has chaired the Society of Jewish Ethics; the Academy of Jewish Philosophy; the Academy of Judaic, Christian, and Islamic Studies; and the Jewish Law Association, of which he was Honorary President between 2012 and 2016. He has served on three federal commissions on issues of health care, sexual ethics, and research on human subjects, respectively, and he is now a member of the State of California's Ethics Committee governing stem cell research within the state. He has written thirteen books and over 200 articles on Jewish ethics, law, and theology, and he has edited or co-edited another fourteen books on those subjects, including the *Oxford Handbook of Jewish Ethics and Morality* (Oxford University Press, 2013).

H. Tristram Engelhardt, Jr., Ph.D., M.D. (1941–2018) was Professor in the Department of Philosophy at Rice University and Professor Emeritus at Baylor College of Medicine in Houston, Texas. He was Senior Editor of two journals published by Oxford University Press (the *Journal of Medicine and Philosophy* and *Christian Bioethics*) and Senior Editor of two book series published by Springer (*Philosophy and Medicine* and

*Philosophical Studies in Contemporary Culture*). He was also the author of more than five hundred publications, as well as editor of over thirty volumes. His books include *The Foundations of Bioethics* (Oxford, rev. ed., 1996) and *The Foundations of Christian Bioethics* (Scrivener, 2000). He was the father of three daughters and has thirteen grandchildren. His recent honors included the receipt of the Lifetime Achievement Award from the American Society for Bioethics and Humanities.

**John J. Fitzgerald**, J.D., Ph.D., is Associate Professor in the Department of Theology and Religious Studies at St. John's University in Queens, New York. He specializes in ethics, with particular attention to fundamental and health care issues. He is the author of *The Seductiveness of Virtue: Abraham Joshua Heschel and John Paul II on Morality and Personal Fulfillment* (Bloomsbury T&T Clark, 2017) and has published articles in the *Notre Dame Journal of Law, Ethics, and Public Policy*; the *Proceedings of the American Catholic Philosophical Association*; *Studies in Christian Ethics*; the *Journal of Catholic Social Thought*; the *Journal of Spirituality in Mental Health*; the *Journal of Moral Theology*; and *Christian Bioethics*.

**Cortney Hughes Rinker**, Ph.D. is Associate Professor in the Department of Sociology and Anthropology at George Mason University in Fairfax, Virginia, where she is also a faculty affiliate of Women and Gender Studies and a member of the steering committee for the Ali Vural Ak Center for Global Islamic Studies. Her areas of interest are medical anthropology, Islam, pain management, end-of-life care, reproductive health, ethics, technology, and public policy, and she conducts ethnographic research in the Washington, DC area, and in Morocco. She is the author of *Islam, Development, and Urban Women's Reproductive Practices* (Routledge, 2013), and co-editor (with Sheena Nahm) of *Applied Anthropology: Unexpected Spaces, Topics, and Methods* (Routledge, 2016). She has published articles in *Medical Anthropology Quarterly, Arab Studies Journal, Medical Anthropology, Practicing Anthropology, Interdisciplinary Journal of Research on Religion, Journal of Telemedicine and e-Health*, and *Southern Anthropologist* and has a chapter in the edited volume *Anthropology of the Middle East and North Africa: Into the New Millennium* (Indiana University Press, 2013). She currently serves as the co-editor of *Anthropology & Aging*, the official journal of the Association for Anthropology, Gerontology, and the Life Course.

**D. Gareth Jones**, M.D, D.Sc., CNZM (Companion of the New Zealand Order of Merit), FAS (Fellow of the Anatomical Society, UK), FRSB (Fellow of the Royal Society of Biology, UK), is Emeritus Professor of Anatomy at the University of Otago in Dunedin, New Zealand. His past positions at the University include Headship of the Department of

Anatomy, Director of the Bioethics Centre, and Deputy Vice-Chancellor (Academic and International). He served for a number of years on the Advisory Committee on Assisted Reproductive Technology (ACART) and has chaired the Ethics Committee of the Royal New Zealand Plunket Society for many years. His published books include *The Peril and Promise of Medical Technology* (Peter Lang, 2013), *Speaking for the Dead: The Human Body in Biology and Medicine* (Ashgate, 2nd ed., 2009, with Maja I. Whitaker) and *Medical Ethics* (Oxford University Press, 4th ed., 2005, with Alastair Campbell and Grant Gillett).

**Ingrid Mattson,** Ph.D., is a scholar of Islamic Studies, an expert in interfaith relations, and a Muslim religious leader. Since 2012, she has held the London and Windsor Community Chair in Islamic Studies at Huron University College in London, Canada. Previously she was Professor of Islamic Studies and Director of the Center for Christian-Muslim Relations at Hartford Seminary (Connecticut), where she developed and directed the first accredited graduate program for Muslim chaplains in America. Her writings focus on Qur'anic Studies, theological ethics, and interfaith engagement. Mattson is past president of the Islamic Society of North America (Washington, DC and Plainfield, IN), is a Senior Fellow of the Royal Aal al-Bayt Institute for Islamic Thought (Amman, Jordan), and has served on many boards, including the Interfaith Taskforce of the White House Office of Faith-Based and Neighborhood Partnerships. Some of her work can be found on her website: ingridmattson.org.

**Jacek L. Mostwin,** M.D., D. Phil., is Professor of Urology at the Johns Hopkins School of Medicine in Baltimore, Maryland. With Rene Genadry, he is co-author of *A Woman's Guide to Urinary Incontinence* (Johns Hopkins University Press, 2008). He has been a member of the Johns Hopkins Hospital Ethics Committee since 1992, serving as co-chairman from 2007 to 2013. He teaches medical ethics in the School of Medicine and is a member of the Harvard Macy Medical Educators faculty and the International Medical Committee of Lourdes. From 1996 to 2012, he was medical director of the annual Lourdes pilgrimage of the Federal Association of the Order of Malta. He maintains an active medical practice at Johns Hopkins and is also currently a Visiting Scholar at the Oxford Center for Life-Writing at Oxford University, studying biographies and memoirs of patients and practitioners.

**Ashley John Moyse,** Ph.D., is the McDonald Postdoctoral Fellow in Christian Ethics and Public Life at Christ Church, University of Oxford. He was previously the John Templeton Foundation Postdoctoral Fellow in Theology and Science at Regent College, Vancouver. His research has been presented and published internationally, including his monograph *Reading Karl Barth, Interrupting Moral Technique, Transforming Biomedical*

*Ethics* (Palgrave Macmillan, 2015). He has co-edited and contributed to *Correlating Sobornost: Karl Barth in Conversation with the Russian Orthodox Tradition* (Fortress, 2015) and *Kenotic Ecclesiology: Select Writings of Donald M. MacKinnon* (Fortress, 2015). Finally, he is the co-editor and advisor for *Dispatches: Turning Points in Theology and Global Crises*, a book series with Fortress Press.

**Autumn Alcott Ridenour**, Ph.D., is Assistant Professor in the Department of Religious and Theological Studies at Merrimack College in North Andover, Massachusetts. Her primary interests are in the areas of theological, philosophical, and social ethics, with attention to history and systematic theology. She is the author of *Sabbath Rest as Vocation: Aging Toward Death* (T&T Clark, 2018) and has published articles in *Christian Bioethics*, the *Journal of the Society of Christian Ethics*, and the *Hastings Center Report*, as well as several book chapters for edited volumes.

**Noam Stadlan**, M.D., is Vice-Chairman of the Department of Neurosurgery at NorthShore University HealthSystem in Skokie, Illinois, and Assistant Professor in the Division of Neurosurgery of the Pritzker School of Medicine at the University of Chicago. His focus is on Jewish medical ethics, in particular the definition of death. He has published articles in medical journals (*The Spine Journal* and *Neurosurgery*) and journals of Jewish interest (*Ḥakirah* and *Meorot*), authored two book chapters on surgical technique, and written a chapter on defining death in the twenty-first century in *Halakhic Realities: Collected Essays on Brain Death* (Maggid, 2015). He served as chairman of the ethics committee of the Neurological and Orthopedic Institute of Chicago and currently is chairman of the Professional Conduct and Ethics Committee of the North American Spine Society. In his free time, he is studying for a Master of Science degree in Medical Ethics at New York Medical College.

**Matthew S. Vest**, Ph.D., is an Instructor in Bioethics and Assistant Director of Education Programs at the Ohio State University Division of Bioethics. He completed a Fellowship in Bioethics at OSU in 2014 and teaches both undergraduate and graduate courses at OSU. Prior to joining the OSU Division of Bioethics, he taught moral philosophy, rhetoric, and various humanities courses for twelve years on the secondary and post-secondary levels. Vest has published reviews and articles on topics ranging from pedagogy, ethical decision making, enhancement, and more.

**Susan E. Zinner**, J.D., M.H.A., M.S.J., is Professor in the School of Public and Environmental Affairs at Indiana University Northwest in Gary, Indiana. She is the author of a dozen peer-reviewed articles and book chapters in edited book collections and scholarly journals, including the *Cambridge Quarterly of Health Care Ethics*, *The Journal of Public*

*Integrity, Legal Perspectives in Bioethics*, and the *American Journal of Hospice and Palliative Medicine*. She has taught graduate and under-graduate law, bioethics, and public administration courses since 1998 and speaks on these subjects at national and international conferences.

# Foreword

Everybody is the same. Or is it that everybody is different? Or to say the same thing, only differently: Every body is the same. Every body is different. Each of the two previous sentences carries the other one within it. To say that "every body is the same" is to name the fact that there are multiple different bodies that are declared the same by virtue of the fact that they share similar features. To say that "every body is different" is to say that each different body shares the same quality of a body, such that they can be brought under the same term, *difference*. Of course, to point to these oddities of language is to note at the same time that this is not just a problem of language, but it is a problem of bodies, which always participate in various multiple forms of being.

Yet strangely enough, the Western mindset seems to think that bodies are just the clay material onto which culture and religious meaning and value are applied as a veneer. This tendency to think that all bodies are the same is at the heart of the Western medical-scientific enterprise, which is bent on simplicity. Science, like all our drives to know (as per Aristotle), is an endeavor to say what is truly the same in multiple different instances, what single theory can explain them. When it comes to electrons, it in fact does not matter which specific electron we claim to be within a spatial field of an atom. Yet, when it comes to the human body, the specificity of which body we mean really does *matter*. The physician is always concerned with this particular body sitting before her, not the body in general and not the corpse upon which she learned.

In our ethics, we modern Westerners also have the generalizing tendency to say that bodies are in fact the same, morally speaking. If they are, then we can say what is owed, ethically speaking, to everybody, to every body. That is the claim of universal justice in the late modern West, to bracket all culture and proclaim that we are all the same and we all should be treated the same. Thus, many social scientific researchers set out to show that both religious thinking on some aspect of the body and ethics turn out to have a similar secular analog. However, just when we think we have made some progress toward a universal ethics – an ethics that treats every body the same – some quirky spiritualist or religionist will make a claim on the body, claiming that this body is different because it has been circumcised or baptized. We Western, secular, scientific practitioners of medicine are told, "Hold on! This particular body is different. This particular body has been marked with a cultural difference that says that this body, despite what it looks like, is in actuality different." Can such a physician strike the same pose to every body, if every body is different? Can such a physician, if he is male, strike the same pose to the female Muslim body as he can strike to the corpse upon which he learned anatomy? Though it may be difficult for us to believe, to proclaim the universal sameness of all bodies is to do violence against the proclamation of Muslims about the difference of the female Muslim body.

The authors of the present volume are also grappling with questions of sameness and difference when it comes to embodiment. Western, secular, scientific medicine is often assumed to be the normative stance toward the body. But to say that all bodies are the same, or to say that all religions are manifestations of the same thing we call spirituality, is to ignore the particular ways that bodies are marked with meaning by different religions. Hoping to draw attention to our sameness as embodied creatures, the authors within this volume point toward a kind of dignity inherent in every body and acknowledge various points of agreement between cultures in our approach to the body. Yet, at the same time, these authors are aware that religious and cultural differences *matter*; they really change the way we understand and treat the matter of the body, and thus the difference made by religion ought to matter to medicine. Every essay in this book takes seriously the matter of the body, whether the author may call our attention to similarities and/or differences. When at the end of *The Anticipatory Corpse*, I asked the question (or did I make a statement?), "Might it not be that only theology can save medicine?" I meant that we must look to those pre-modern traditions of embodiment (that we name to be religions) to see if we can once again engage the living body, a body alive in its cultural significance. To that end, the volume is a very good start.

Jeffrey P. Bishop

# Acknowledgments

The editors would like to convey their sincere gratitude to the organizers of the Third Annual Conference on Medicine and Religion (2014), which was the initial impetus for this project, and to all who expressed interest in participating in the present collection. Special thanks are also due to Ryan Nash for his invaluable assistance in finding other key contributors; Jeffrey Bishop, Charlie Camosy, Jonathan Crane, Farr Curlin, Celia Deane-Drummond, and Abdulaziz Sachedina for their willingness to carefully review the entirety of this work and contribute our foreword and five endorsements, respectively; and Jack Boothroyd, Kevin Kelsey, and Joshua Wells at Routledge for their guidance through the editorial process.

To our contributors: you each have labored diligently to prepare thoughtful and engaging essays. We are thankful for your participation in this anthology and for your patience. The volume's strength and incisive commentary on the body in medicine and religion is due to your attention to curiosities and crises within the practice and science of medicine. We trust this volume will ensure your works are widely read.

Ashley: I would like to thank my colleagues at Christ Church, University of Oxford who have kindly welcomed me into a new academic home and to the McDonald Centre for Theology, Ethics, and Public Life. To my former colleagues at Regent College, especially to Jens Zimmerman and Ross Hastings: your collaboration and collegiality is appreciated immensely. I am grateful for the time and space to be able to pursue projects such as this one, among others, which were made possible in part through the support of a grant from the John Templeton Foundation. Finally, to my family: it is a joy to share life and adventure with you all – Aime, Theodore, and Seamus.

John: I'm grateful to the Department of Theology and Religious Studies at St. John's University for granting me teaching reductions to work on this manuscript and other projects, to Ashley for his seasoned editorial advice over the past few years, to Elliot Dorff for reviewing my chapter and providing thorough suggestions regarding the material on Maimonides, to Celia Deane-Drummond for offering some additional helpful feedback on my chapter, and to my family for their love and support.

# Introduction

*John J. Fitzgerald and Ashley John Moyse*[1]

The institution of medicine exists to attend to the limitations and frailties of physical bodies. Yet the advent of new technologies and knowledge at the boundaries of scientific endeavor and clinical practice – including genetics, regenerative medicine, and the like – presents new possibilities for the human body on display for modern medicine. But these also include the possibility for a problem – specifically, the reduction of the patient to a mere body to be studied, known, and mastered in the modern medical milieu.

The objectifying of the body in medicine has been the subject of recent research, notably Jeffrey Bishop's *The Anticipatory Corpse: Medicine, Power, and the Care of the Dying*. Bishop has argued that the metaphysics of modern medicine is reduced to efficient causation, which concerns itself with *how* the body moves. Building upon Michel Foucault's work, he traces how medical preoccupations since the Enlightenment have moved from living bodies to dead matter. This move is bolstered by the modern sciences, which claim the body as an object to observe and control. Thus, as Bishop discerns, the dead body is the ideal body, for by it we come to know of the parts and learn how to animate them – albeit with no particular *telos*. Accordingly, for Bishop, the ontology prevailing in modern medicine is one *reduced to mere mechanics*. With an interest in knowing *how* the body functions and how to maintain such function, health professionals and scientists may have distanced themselves, wittingly or otherwise, from the subject of study.

Bishop suggests that without an alternative narrative that can challenge the hegemony of the prevailing ontology, we may be unable to resist the dominance of objectification, mechanization, and control. But as Notre Dame theologian Gerald McKenny has argued, contemporary philosophical bioethics may not be up to this task.[2] Perhaps this is why Bishop concludes his book with the provocative phrase, "Might it not be that only theology can save medicine?"[3] Here he calls medical practitioners to see, once again, the human being before them – and in so doing he wonders whether theology might provide the catechetical formation required to save the physician encumbered by modern preoccupations with knowing and doing.

*The Anticipatory Corpse* has been widely lauded as a landmark publication in medical humanities. It is one that raises various concerns regarding a deficient approach to the human person in the contemporary medical context, although they are not the sole impetus for the present anthology. Biomedical advances and a diminishing understanding of how to wield modern powers over or at the service of the human body have brought biomedical professionals to confront many pressing inquiries: What is the relationship between body and soul and between individual persons and the community? To whom does the body belong? What are our obligations toward human bodies? How should medicine respond to suffering and death? The answers provided to date have been diverse, conflicting, and in flux, and the attention given to these matters in recent edited collections has been lacking.

Nevertheless, the aforementioned questions and concerns were explored at the Third Annual Conference on Medicine and Religion, co-sponsored by the University of Chicago, Texas Medical Center, and Saint Louis University in March 2014. There academics and physicians alike labored to respond, offering diverse perspectives informed by Judaism, Christianity (including Catholicism, Orthodoxy, and Protestantism), and Islam. This volume, nurtured after the conference, draws from many who presented at the conference along with other scholars, who together offer engaged and thoughtful answers to such questions as those above. Through its special focus on the three Abrahamic religions and its distinctive inclusion of scholars from various disciplines, this anthology aims to help philosophers, theologians, health care professionals, and others reach more informed and even self-transformative conclusions about the meaning, value, responsibilities, and goals of our bodily existence.

The following reflections are divided into three parts: "Understanding the Body," "Respecting the Body," and "The Body at the End of Life." Entrance into these sections is preceded by a prologue, "Which Medicine? Whose Religion?" Written by the late distinguished bioethics scholar H. Tristram Engelhardt, Jr., this essay serves as a challenge to not only the readers of this volume but also its contributors. We are each one cautioned regarding the difficulties of theological dialogue on medicine. This admonition relates quite closely to the principal vision of *Christian Bioethics*, the journal Engelhardt founded to engage in non-ecumenical dialogue on questions that arise from the science and practice of medicine. Here the reader is reminded that there is not one monolithic tradition from which one might speak as a Christian. One might also be advised that in addition to the diversity of Christian voices, a panoply of religions is also at work to understand the problems and pains of human beings, which are further attended to by the numerous modes of medicine, including Western, Chinese, and so on. Accordingly, a given dialogue – for instance, between Orthodox monks and Southern Baptist Protestant pastors – faces the obstacles of different fundamental assumptions about science, medicine, and religion. That said, Engelhardt is quick to add that he does not mean to discourage such dialogue, as long as it does not simply reduce religion to a means to some secular goal and takes differences seriously, for indeed it can lead to a fuller understanding of them.

With these initial remarks duly noted, since any coherent discussion of the human body must be prefaced with some examination of its nature, the first part ("Understanding the Body") addresses philosophical and theological anthropologies. The section opens with Ashley John Moyse's essay, "Responsibility for the Broken Body: Exploring the Invitation to Respond to the Presence of the Other," which takes its cue from Bishop and serves as a call to those engaged in the practice of medicine to respond to the presence of the human body. This invitation is goaded by the theological significance of the human body; in the words of E. L. Mascall, "Christianity has consistently claimed to be concerned with body and soul at once." Moyse grounds such concern with the indivisible body and soul in his reading of Swiss Reformed theologian Karl Barth. Here he draws us toward Barth's relational anthropology, in which we discover a particular responsibility toward the body and soul of the Other. Subsequently, Moyse proposes that a complementary anthropology might benefit medicine. Yet the aim is not to pursue a theological intervention that colonizes medicine. Rather, the aim here is to proclaim the theological such that the physician, for example, might learn to encounter her patient in the fullness of his being and by a posture of responsibility grounded by love.

Sharing concerns about approaches that divorce the body from the soul, Matthew S. Vest, in his "Embodied Soul and Ensouled Body: Reflections on Ravaisson and Theological Methodology," offers the nineteenth-century French philosopher Félix Ravaisson's alternative view of the human person. Ravaisson's account is grounded in habit, "a spontaneous disposition or tendency that emerges amidst change" and that is manifested as an "*idea* becomes *being*" in the body. This notion of habit explains that our souls can achieve a kind of moral maturity that is at the same time rooted in our corporal functions. In fact, habit is both a "law of the limbs" and a "law of grace" and even discloses "God within us." Thus, in place of a rigid mind-body dualism, habit serves as a phenomenological paradigm to reveal a robust ontology of material things, including the human body. Vest highlights the medical implications of such a paradigm; physicians should attend not simply to the bodily needs of their patients but also to their moral and spiritual health. The remainder of his piece explores the possibility of common ground between Ravaisson's thought and Eastern Christian ascetic theology (including that of Gregory the Theologian and Maximus the Confessor, who are venerated in the Catholic and Orthodox traditions): namely, their emphasis on self-development toward the good of loving union with the divine.

Turning to non-Christian thought, Elliot N. Dorff contributes a chapter on Jewish anthropology. In "Judaism on the Body and the Practice of Medicine," he demonstrates that the Bible and the classical Rabbis of the Mishnah, Talmud, and Midrash confirm that our body and soul are integrated. Accordingly, doctors should consider the moral and religious background of a patient in determining the causes of and appropriate responses to a given medical issue. Other basic anthropological assumptions in Jewish thought with health care applications include the following: our bodies are on loan from God (so we must take care of them), all of us (including those with disabilities) are created in the image of the divine, and our bodies are mortal. Dorff moves on to consider how taking care of a patient's body is a communal effort that involves patients, physicians, and family members and to acknowledge the limits of medicine in curing disease and the corresponding role of hospice care. He concludes with a biblical command that encapsulates the foregoing considerations: "Choose life."

The final essay of the first section explores the Islamic understanding of embodiment. "'The Believer is Never Impure': Islam and Understanding the Embodied Person," by Ingrid Mattson, presents Islam as a religion that gives substantial attention to the human body. But such regard can introduce significant challenges for the practice of medicine. For example, Mattson presents Islamic law, which requires purity for the performance of ritual acts. Such acts are rendered *prima facie* invalid by the expulsion of bodily excretions. This understanding could instill a sense of repulsion at persons in a certain state of impurity or uncleanness – for instance, due to certain medical conditions. But as Mattson explains, the Prophet Muhammad declares that "the believer is never impure" fundamentally; in fact, the dominant Muslim tradition has extended this recognition to all of humanity. Her essay puts forth distinctive insights that echo those from previous chapters. For example, while she states that traditional Islamic discourses posit "a degree of dualism between body and soul," she affirms that they still value the body, which has legitimate needs that ought to be satisfied and which is an essential component of the person even after death. Regarding medicine in particular, Islamic traditions suggest that we should seek the remedy that God has ordained for each illness, and they promote a "holistic approach" to healing that sees the person's body, mind, and soul as closely related.

While the first part of this book touches on the provision of care for ourselves and others, the second part ("Respecting the Body") focuses on this issue more thoroughly. Jacek L. Mostwin's essay, "Reverence for the Body: An Ethical Principle Grounded in Human Experience," inaugurates this section and centers Albert Schweitzer's principle of Reverence for Life directly within the setting in which medical work takes place: the body. Much of medicine, such as bedside nursing, surgery, the care of wounds, and the feeding and clothing of the disabled or infirm, involves encounters with the body in a dimension beyond language. As Mostwin points out, in these milieus the profession is able to express what it knows through action without speech. Accordingly, his argument proposes that Reverence for the Body may be considered a fundamental ethical principle that arises from encountering the body of others and that can be learned from experience. Such a principle also has a long history in the broadly construed Christian tradition, as well as other religious worldviews, and can elevate the concept of the body from a purely material dimension to one that is transcendent. In the end, Mostwin boldly suggests that Reverence for the Body offers the potential for enhancing global discussion on bioethical principles irrespective of religion, law, or language.

Picking up from Mostwin's expansive interreligious engagement, John J. Fitzgerald focuses specifically on two medieval philosopher-theologians in "Healthy Legacies? Moses Maimonides and Thomas Aquinas on Caring for Others and Ourselves." Here Fitzgerald contends that these thinkers raise some key considerations that can still inform medical ethicists and others today. For instance, Maimonides (also a physician) holds that health care professionals are obliged to restore what their patients have lost (as per Deut. 22:2), affirms that we must be concerned for the welfare of animals, and provides various practical guidelines for safeguarding our own health – many of which are consistent with contemporary research. Aquinas also maintains that actions that have good and bad effects can be permissible as long as any bad ones are not intended, outlines a number of noteworthy arguments against suicide, but also says that we should love our lives in "due measure." Furthermore, both authors call attention to the goodness of visiting the sick, suggest that caring for ourselves is a moral task, and demonstrate that moderation in food and drink is conducive to other virtuous conduct and to our physical and emotional well-being. Fitzgerald also attends to some of the more questionable claims of these figures, and he concludes with some reflections on the benefits of engaging in comparative ethics and interreligious dialogue, both in general and in a Jewish-Catholic-medical context.

Next, this collection returns to a consideration of Islam with Cortney Hughes Rinker's "Islam, Medicine, and Practice: The Manifestation of Islamic Moral Values in Everyday Aspects of the U.S. Health Care System." Drawing from her interviews with Sunni Muslim imams, physicians, and patients, Hughes Rinker posits that certain fundamental Western medical practices embodied in American health care are "sites of religious meaning-making" for Muslim participants in her research. For instance, the system of scheduling and keeping appointments corresponds with the Prophet Muhammad's insistence on fulfilling one's promises. The importance of specializing in a particular area and providing referrals to others outside of one's expertise is also reflected in Islam, which boasts a tradition of specialty medicine going back to medieval times. Furthermore, the sanitization of hands and instruments can resonate with those who are concerned with maintaining cleanliness prior to religious rituals. Each of these practices involves care for the bodies under the doctor's watch and thereby echoes the primacy of respect in Islamic teachings. Hughes Rinker does not rule out the possibility of differences between predominant Islamic values and Western medical practices, nor does she deny that values in other religious traditions can also overlap with these practices, but she does suggest that – contrary to certain contemporary narratives in a post-September-11 world – Islam is not fundamentally opposed to innovation or Western values.

The second section closes with Timothy James Carey's essay, "A Shared Common Good: Catholic and Muslim Bioethical Approaches to HIV/AIDS in Kenya," which directs us once again to a comparative and interreligious approach. More specifically, the ethico-legal principle of *maṣlaḥa* (as developed in the work of the fourteenth-century Sunni Maliki legal scholar Abū Isḥāq Ibrāhīm al-Shāṭibī) closely parallels the notion of the common good in contemporary Catholic social thought, and both concepts call for attention to the bodily needs of the hungry, the thirsty, and the sick. At the same time, Carey grants that there may be certain differences in emphasis between Catholic and Muslim approaches; for instance, the latter highlight God's omnipotence in curing disease (while not denying humans' responsibility for their actions). He continues by examining Catholic and Muslim responses to HIV/AIDS in Kenya and points to collaborative efforts between leaders of both religions. The author concludes by highlighting the complementarity of universal principles and particular contexts and emphasizing that a theologically oriented bioethics can be an "avenue for interreligious dialogue and mutual self-discovery in the face of such a debilitating disease."

These deliberations on the challenge of HIV/AIDS lead naturally to the third and final part of this collection, "The Body at the End of Life." The lead essay by Susan E. Zinner, "In the Land of Pain: Why Daudet and Hitchens Are Still Relevant," examines the autobiographical works of the nineteenth-century French novelist Alphonse Daudet (influenced by his Catholic upbringing) and the late British-American writer Christopher Hitchens (an avowed anti-theist), in particular the records of their respective terminal illnesses. As Zinner explains, language faces difficulties in communicating pain, and so both Daudet and Hitchens resort to metaphor, notably the imagery of battle, in an attempt to convey their experiences to their readers. Daudet's and Hitchens's respective works are but two examples of medical narratives, which tether together the health care professional and patient and also the writer and reader. Ultimately, Zinner draws some important implications for medical providers; they should recognize that "each illness is a solo journey in need of a community," realize that understanding the personal perspectives of their patients can in turn lead to a better medical outcome, and know that reading medical narratives can help one "understand[] the loss of the invaluable" and foster compassion.

In her contribution, "Suffering, Death, and the Significance of Presence," Autumn Alcott Ridenour similarly appeals for compassion for the suffering and dying but also explores the practice of grief after death and the hope of resurrection. Drawing especially from Augustine, she begins by portraying the human body as susceptible to suffering and death as a consequence of sin, as well as to change even prior to the fall of humankind. As she goes on to show, the notion that bodies are fundamentally prone to suffering and transience is echoed by physicians such as Bishop and Sherwin Nuland. However, Christians also look forward to the resurrection of our bodies after death; in Bishop's memorable words, the cadaver is an "anticipatory corpse." But as we await the fulfillment of this hope, Ridenour suggests, we are justified in expressing grief in the face of suffering and death, and we are called to be empathetically present to those struggling with these realities. Here again she finds common ground between theology and medicine, looking first to the words and deeds of Christ and Augustine, then to the insights of Nuland, Bishop, and other medical ethicists.

Next, D. Gareth Jones focuses on some issues that arise after death in "The Dead Body as an Object of Investigation, Intrigue, and Reverence." As he indicates, the theological literature has paid a good deal of attention to the nature of the living body and the relationship between body and soul but less to the way we respond (and ought to respond) to dead bodies. Jones's essay seeks to address this deficiency, and it functions as a corrective of sorts to certain medical abuses of the past. Regarding bodily dissection, he suggests that this can help us better appreciate "the body as made in the image of God" and can be morally justifiable as long as the individual during his or her life provided informed consent, which is crucial within a Christian worldview that takes "a high view of the dead body." On the retention of bodies and body parts post-mortem, he again highlights the importance of consent but also of an ethical awareness on the part of health care professionals and particularly a concern for the poor and marginalized that is inspired by the Bible. On the topic of plastination, Jones provocatively proposes that the informed consent of participants is not sufficient to warrant a donation aimed purely at attaining one's "own post-mortal desires" or the entertainment of spectators.

The third part of the book concludes with an interreligious perspective on the end of bodily life, Noam Stadlan's "Defining Death in the Context of Jewish, Christian, and Muslim Perspectives." As Stadlan notes, there are two primary competing views on the definition of death: death involves either the cessation of integrated function or the cessation of neurological function. He holds that only the latter position can be considered internally valid (for it has often proposed a specific concept, criteria, and tests), externally valid (for instance, it corresponds with our intuition that a dicephalous body actually should be considered two persons), and easily compatible with a reasonable basis for personal identity. Stadlan then uses this basic framework to critique various understandings of death in Jewish, Christian, and Islamic sources, and he finds himself most sympathetic to the "respiratory-brain" definition of death of the Chief Rabbinate of Israel. Stadlan's piece serves as a fitting finale to this collection, given the fact that it is the only essay to devote significant attention to all three of the aforementioned monotheistic traditions and given the extensive implications of his closing remarks, which suggest a contextual and non-literal approach to religious sources both within and outside the field of medicine.

In all, as you have and will read, these essays labor creatively and constructively toward responding to the principal questions concerning the nature of the human body in medicine.[4] Although the area over which this collection traverses might be great, the contributors' scholarly contributions do advance a particular narrative, one that impels us all to listen again to religious voices to discover (again) the ways we might treat the human person. Ultimately, we trust that this volume, and the essays therein, will stimulate considerable discussion and challenge problematic conceptions of the human body in medicine. Although the editing process necessarily strives for a certain degree of objectivity, mechanization, and control over the body of a work, it is our hope that its original spirit fully remains.

## Notes

1 The editors thank Matthew Vest and Jacek Mostwin for their assistance with the wording in the summaries of their particular chapters.
2 Gerald P. McKenny, *To Relieve the Human Condition: Bioethics, Technology, and the Body* (Albany, NY: State University of New York Press, 1997), 31.
3 Jeffrey P. Bishop, *The Anticipatory Corpse: Medicine, Power, and the Care of the Dying* (Notre Dame, IN: The University of Notre Dame Press, 2011), 313.
4 While the intersection of these questions with race and gender also certainly merits attention, it is not a specific focus of this anthology. That said, some of our chapters make some pertinent remarks in passing: Dorff on how "physicians need to see their patients not simply as bodies but as people" of particular genders and ethnicities, Mattson on the ritual purity of Islamic women, and Jones on the historical problem of the medical use of deceased bodies of different races without consent.

# Prologue
## Which medicine? Whose religion?

*H. Tristram Engelhardt, Jr.*[1]

### Always distinguish

What purposes should interreligious dialogues serve? What goals could they support? Are such dialogues meant to decrease the likelihood of religiously motivated violence?[2] Are they meant to disclose some overlooked unity or communality among religions and/or faiths? Do they point to a religious truth or set of goals that all should embrace? The answers to such questions are made more difficult if such interreligious dialogues are tied to a second issue such as medicine. Imagine, for example, an interreligious dialogue between Roman Catholics and Southern Baptists regarding the proper role of the free market. To give substance to this illustration, I will presume that Roman Catholics, unlike Southern Baptists, have a greater suspicion of the market and a greater inclination toward socialist, pro-labor union interventions,[3] although there are important exceptions such as Michael Novak and Samuel Gregg.[4] Imagine that the special issue of youth unemployment is chosen as a further focus of the dialogue. A preliminary issue is who in a dialogue should be invited to represent the Roman Catholics and the Southern Baptists. In the case of the Roman Catholics, there are persons in authority to answer this question, namely, a pope and bishops, so that the Roman Catholics can determine the legitimacy of those who claim to represent Roman Catholicism. For Southern Baptists who not only repudiate any papal claims but have no bishops, the issue of who is in authority to speak will be much less clear.

Let us suppose that these hurdles can be met and an interfaith dialogue does take place and that Cardinal Maradiaga attends, who with his colleagues follows sentiments expressed in *Evangelii Gaudium* and attributes the problem of youth unemployment primarily to free market greed, holding that Christianity on the basis of social justice should support a more robust welfare state.[5] Let us further suppose that the Southern Baptists who attend argue that youth unemployment is due to politicians' and labor unions' greed for power that shackles the market, leading to lower productivity, thus diminishing the number of new jobs and producing the high youth unemployment seen in Italy and Spain as compared with youth unemployment in Texas (which has a higher immigration rate than Italy or Spain), not to mention Germany before the immense migration of over one million Mohammedans in 2015–2016.[6] The Southern

Baptists also generally reject the Roman Catholic commitment to social justice, arguing among other things that it empowers a secular post-Christian state. Instead, I will presume for the purposes of this paper that the Southern Baptists ask Christians to give at least 10% of their income to the church and to the poor, while asking local churches to encourage their members to start for-profit businesses, which can employ the youth. What results will dialogue produce, given that the two parties are separated by different basic premises and rules of evidence about how to establish what Christianity is, as well as regarding what the market should be left to do? Perhaps some Roman Catholics will convert to the view that, to lower youth unemployment, the minimum wage for persons under twenty-five should be lowered, as well as laws changed so that employers with fewer costs can fire the youth once hired. Perhaps some Southern Baptists will convert to the view that Christians ought to have bishops and therefore become Roman Catholic, Orthodox Christian, or Methodist.

Any agreement among the dialoguing partners will require a conversion to a common paradigm through which to understand what should count as relevant information, such as regarding the significance of bishops and markets. The challenge is that the Roman Catholics and the Southern Baptists, as well as proponents of a socialist state versus those of a capitalist state, are separated by disparate paradigms of ecclesial, economic, and political reality. They live within different thought communities in different life worlds. On the one hand, everything religious looks different to each party. They do not mean the same thing by such words as "church" and "presbyter." For Roman Catholics and Southern Baptists, these and other theological terms have different intensions and extensions nested within quite different explanatory, metaphysical, and social frameworks. The same is the case regarding terms such as "just profits" and "appropriate labor markets." Differences are compounded by the circumstance that the crucial terms are framed by different epistemic and non-epistemic values in being aimed not just at explaining the world truly but at changing the world effectively. There is no common understanding as to what is effective because there is no common agreement regarding goals such as liberty, equality, and prosperity. The disagreements are not just about what it is to know truly but also, regarding the goals in terms of which one should shape the world, about what it is to act rightly and to achieve the good. The disputes involve not just the clarification and ranking of epistemic values or goals but the clarification and ranking of non-epistemic values and/or goals as well.

Aside from conversions, such dialogues may largely re-enforce judgments about the otherness of the other. The Southern Baptists may leave strengthened in their opinion that Roman Catholicism is distant from the Church of the Apostles and that Pope Francis I is moved by a left-of-center Argentine-Italian populist approach to economics and politics. Indeed, the Southern Baptists may hold that they now understand better why Argentina and Italy are marginally economically and politically functional. On the other hand, the Roman Catholics may be affirmed in their conviction that the Southern Baptists are plagued by an excessive individualism and concern with property that is an impediment to understanding the force and meaning of church and solidarity. Moreover, Roman Catholics will have a better appreciation of how, from their point of view, the continued conversion of Roman Catholics to evangelical communities in Brazil will – from their perspective – adversely affect Brazil.[7] On the other hand, the Southern Baptists will be confirmed in their view that any increase in the number of Roman Catholics in the United States will economically and politically adversely affect America. Both sides may come away with the view that they have a better understanding of why they disagree with each other.

## Whose medicine?

How will matters differ if the focus is on medicine rather than the market? In great measure, this will depend on the extent to which those in dialogue agree regarding what should count as medicine. Imagine that a focus of the dialogue of religion and medicine is on homeopathy versus the current dominant account of medicine and that half the participants favor homeopathy. In this dialogue, one can also imagine the proponents of the current dominant medical model refusing to be described as allopaths by the homeopaths, insisting that allopathy identifies the traditional Western medicine that the current dominant medical paradigm replaced.[8] Imagine that in response the homeopaths assert that they have a more holistic approach to patient care. The proponents of the dominant paradigm may then in riposte accuse the homeopaths of failing to acknowledge the importance of controlled clinical trials, the role of observer bias, etc. What goals could such a dialogue about religion and medicine serve? The answer will turn on the extent to which Roman Catholics versus Southern Baptists have differing views of scientific evidence and the problem of observer bias in the acquisition of empirical evidence for establishing claims about the nature of disease, as well as regarding the treatment of disease.

Now let us imagine that there is an interfaith dialogue on religion and medicine with a focus on the meaning of the body, with all physicians affirming the now-dominant medical-scientific paradigm, with the religious interlocutors being half Orthodox monks and the other half Southern Baptist pastors. Let us imagine further that the first presentation is made by a monk from Mount Athos who begins by stating that the purpose of Christianity is to produce relics. By this, he means that the Church is to produce holy saints, as holy as St. Paul, so that when one touches their bodies (as mentioned in Acts 19:11–12),[9] one will receive grace and diseases will be healed, God willing, of course. During his presentation, he quotes from the Ecumenical Patriarch Bartholomew I, who, the monk explains, is currently the true successor to the primacy once possessed by old Rome. Regarding relics and the body, Patriarch Bartholomew states: "Grace is not only obtained through the transformed relics of the saints, which is totally inexplicable without acceptance of the divine. Grace also radiates from living Saints who are truly in the likeness of the Lord [Luke 8:46]. . . . Grace can also be obtained by the presence of the Saints who have influenced and sanctified, and to a degree transformed, natural objects and places."[10] The body is appreciated as open to sanctification, a category foreign to the dominant medical paradigm.

The Southern Baptist pastor chosen to give a commentary on the monk's presentation, let us suppose, rejects the status of bishops and the ecumenical patriarch claimed by the Orthodox and the practice of having monasteries, along with the Orthodox Christian use of relics, not to mention the Orthodox Christian understanding of grace. This is not to suggest that this interfaith dialogue will not be informative for many participants. The monks will leave the interfaith dialogue likely reinforced in their initial view regarding how distant Southern Baptists are from Orthodox Christianity, which understands itself as the Church of the Apostles and the Fathers. They will understand their differences in greater substance and detail. The Southern Baptists for their part will likely be reinforced in their view that physicians should not take relics embedded in an icon with them for their patients to kiss. A Southern Baptist pastor, like others before him, may be brought to convert after being slipped a copy of the martyrdom of St. Polycarp with its portrayal of the early Christian veneration of relics.

Why do I make these remarks? Surely, they are not made to discourage dialogues on religion and medicine, at least insofar as such dialogue does not take the character of reductive reflections on spirituality that wish to understand the worth of religion in terms of how religion makes people happier and healthier. Non-reductive public reflections on religion can serve the important purpose of protecting and restoring a public space for taking religious questions seriously. In a culture that is now articulated as if God did not exist, this will involve entering the culture wars.[11] Such cultural conflicts are likely to be beneficial for whatever religion one holds to be true. Of course, reductive dialogues about religion or dialogues that treat religion as merely a cultural inheritance or tradition do the very opposite. One can imagine the first dialogue on Christianity and the market becoming reductive if it directed its focus to evaluate religion in terms of which beliefs support practices and attitudes most likely to reduce youth unemployment.

The reason for my asking these questions is to underscore some of the insights one may garner from asking the question *cui bono* regarding dialogues on religion and medicine. Greater clarity can inform one, depending on one's understanding of religion, as to which dialogues of religion and medicine one should support and why. The position likely to be affirmed will depend on the participants' view as to how and in what respects concern regarding medicine and religion can be rightly or wrongly directed. My expectation is not that there will be agreement on such matters but that an honest geography of differences and goals should be of interest.

## Cautiously affirm: taking differences seriously

The journal *Christian Bioethics: Non-Ecumenical Studies in Medical Morality* is now (2017) in its twenty-third year. When founded, its subtitle was regarded as more controversial than it is currently. *Christian Bioethics* received letters protesting the subtitle. How could one want to be non-ecumenical? The response made by those launching *Christian Bioethics* and by those who in its infancy guided its development was that with so many people trying to obscure the differences separating the various Christianities, it was difficult to determine clearly where there were points of disagreement regarding issues of bioethics. This remains the case. It is hard to understand clearly what constitutes Christian bioethics because there is no agreement as to what counts as Christian. To appreciate the nature of Christian bioethics, one needs to recognize where disagreements in Christian bioethics exist and what their nature is. One needs better accounts of the relevant substantive matters in dispute dividing the Christianities to see with any precision what different views regarding the content of Christian bioethics are in dispute. This is not to deny that many of the Christianities are divided into traditional and post-traditional wings, so that traditionalist Lutherans and Presbyterians might have more agreement on matters bioethical than either would have with their post-traditional nominal co-religionists. However, *Christian Bioethics* seeks more clearly to lay out the broad character of differences separating Orthodox Christian, Roman Catholic, and Protestant bioethics (as well as the various forms of Protestant bioethics). *Christian Bioethics* is committed to examining the full spectrum of agreements and disagreements in service of the goal of gaining a clearer view of how and why different views of Christianity ground different views of bioethics so as better to understand the field of Christian bioethics.

It turns out that frank interchanges can take place in which the dialoguing partners recognize each other respectively to be misguided (i.e., being in heresy) about that which is most important, namely, how properly to deport oneself regarding health care and the biomedical sciences in order to pursue salvation. The result has been a clearer appreciation of differences, including what the different positions entail. In addition, contributors have recognized that they are at liberty to develop scholarly articles from frankly confessional perspectives. The result is not a polite papering over of differences but an open acknowledgment of important differences to enable the development of a body of scholarship. The participants can recognize each other to be theological strangers while remaining scholarly friends. A dialogue that nurtures a better appreciation of differences can be quite useful for the development of a scholarly field.

## Notes

1 The editors gratefully acknowledge the assistance of the author's wife, Susan Engelhardt, in proofreading his chapter one final time after his passing in June 2018.
2 After decades of interreligious dialogues, there is no good evidence to support the view that such dialogue has diminished worldwide interreligious violence.
3 Since Pope Leo XIII, the popes of Rome have endorsed social-democratic approaches to resolving economic problems. See, for example, Francis, *Evangelii Gaudium* ["The Joy of the Gospel"] (Vatican City: Libreria Editrice Vaticana, 2013), especially §§ 50–60.

4  Samuel Gregg, *Tea Party Catholic: The Catholic Case for Limited Government, a Free Economy, and Human Flourishing* (New York, NY: The Crossroad Publishing Co., 2013); Michael Novak, *The Catholic Ethic and the Spirit of Capitalism* (New York, NY: Free Press, 1993).

5  Cardinal Maradiaga, who functions as the most prominent of Francis I's advisers, appears to have a marked sympathy for left-of-center approaches to economic problems. Óscar Andrés Rodríguez Maradiaga, "The Importance of the New Evangelization," *Whispers in the Loggia Blog*, October 25, 2013, https://whispersintheloggia. blogspot.com/2013/10/the-councils-unfinished-business.html.

6  Youth unemployment in Texas is 13.5%. "Youth Unemployment Rate, Figures by State," n.d., http://web.archive.org/web/20130915074103/http://www.govern ing.com/gov-data/youth-employment-unemployment-rate-data-by-state.html. In November 2014 in Western Europe, the lowest rates of youth unemployment were found in Germany (7.4%), Austria (8.9%), the Netherlands (9.7%), and Denmark (11.4%). These are all countries with a substantial Protestant population or with a connection to such a country (Austria, for example, has special ties to Germany and was subjected to the secularizing force of Josephism). In southern Europe, youth unemployment was much higher: Spain (53.5%), Italy (43.9%), and Portugal (34.5%). "Youth Unemployment Rate in EU Member States as of November 2014 (Seasonally Adjusted)," n.d., http://web.archive.org/web/20150606154106/https:// www.statista.com/statistics/266228/youth-unemployment-rate-in-eu-countries. There is no evidence that approaches to social justice inspired by Roman Catholicism have had a positive impact on youth unemployment in Western Europe. (Editors' note: Engelhardt relied on earlier versions of these two websites. To best preserve his thinking and writing here, archived webpages are provided.)

7  Approximately one out of every four Brazilians is now evangelical, and some hold that by 2020 half of the population will be evangelical. Andrea Marcela Madambashi, "Half of Brazil's Population to be Evangelical by 2020," *Christian Post U.S.*, February 20, 2011, www.christianpost.com/news/ half-of-brazils-population-to-be-evangelical-christian-by-2020-49071.

8  Homeopathy, founded by Samuel Hahnemann (1755–1843), rejected the old, traditional, Western medical axiom that diseases were cured by their contraries (*contraria contraribus curantur*) and instead held that likes were cured by likes (*similia similibus curantur*). Within this framework, those who were not homeopaths were allopaths. However, practitioners of the current dominant medical paradigm are not allopaths in the original sense of the term.

9  "God did extraordinary miracles through Paul, so that when the handkerchiefs or aprons that had touched his skin were brought to the sick, their diseases left them, and the evil spirits came out of them" (Acts 19:11–12 [New Revised Standard Version]).

10  Bartholomew I, "Joyful Light (Address at Georgetown University)," October 21, 1997, www.patriarchate.org/de/homily/-/asset_publisher/NrbYUGIG0n1r/content/ address-of-his-all-holiness-ecumenical-patriarch-b-a-r-t-h-o-l-o-m-e-w-phos-hilaron-joyful-light-georgetown-university-washington-dc-october-21-1997.

11  The deep secular character of our contemporary culture is examined in H. Tristram Engelhardt, Jr., *After God: Morality and Bioethics in a Secular Age* (Yonkers, NY: St. Vladimir's Seminary Press, 2017).

# Part I
# Understanding the body

# 1 Responsibility for the broken body

## Exploring the invitation to respond to the presence of the Other

*Ashley John Moyse*[1]

> I feel some hesitation to invite you to come with me into the body. It seems a reckless, defiant act. . . [as] the doctor to man stumbles, must often wound; his patient must die, as must he. . . . [But] . . . Soon you shall know surgery as a Mass served with Body and Blood, wherein disease is assailed as though it were sin. . . . So shall I make of my fingers, words; of my scalpel, a sentence; of the body of my patient, a story. . . . Here then is the doctor listening to the sounds of the body to which the rest of us are deaf. He is more than doctor. He is priest.
>
> – Richard Selzer, *The Surgeon as Priest*[2]

Richard Selzer's *The Surgeon as Priest* (1976) directed my attention toward the bodies of his patients, among others, as the physician takes the body of the Other into her hands as though it were her own. Yet the body is not to be possessed. Rather, the body, who is a person encountered, is to be loved. Put differently, the surgical sacrilege is to be redeemed by the agency of love and by the art of ritual. Consequently, through his essay, I think that I've been introduced once again to medicine, which is principally the practice of invading the body that is necessarily in communion with the world, with other human bodies pursuing wholeness.

Nevertheless, Selzer's narrative is not my focus. Rather, I merely want to use it as a springboard, highlighting the fact that medicine, in and of itself, offers particular stories worth exploring. And, I think it is worth doing so to correct the tendency to reduce the practice of medicine to the singular exercise of invading a mere body, for the body which the physician invades is much more than dead matter to be animated by the modern triumphs of will, reason, and technique.

Yet before thinking about these stories of medicine, I will consider how theology might respond with and for the modern institution of medicine and its commitment to scientific precision, one that is determined to reduce the body to an object for the gain of epistemic power over it.[3] Put differently, I would like to think about the implications of theology for medicine, bioethics, and the biomedical disposition toward the human body. In doing so, I will speculate about how theology might interrupt the practice of medicine and challenge it to recall its principal responsibility. I will labor to show the significance of the human body in Christian theology and also in medicine while arguing that we must stand with and for persons struggling for life at the crises confronted in the body itself. Finally, the implications of theology for medicine's understanding of the body will be set out, demonstrating the vital importance of the seen, albeit broken, body that invites responsibility.

## On being human[4]

E. L. Mascall has commented, "Christianity has consistently claimed to be concerned with body and soul at once. And, at a time when most people seem to have the idea that religion is a purely spiritual matter, it is essential to insist on the concern that it has *with* the body."[5] However, such consistency is marred by particular failings to attend to the body and soul at once, as in Gnostic writings and certain Neo-Platonic deviations of philosophical and theological anthropology, which consider the body, in and of itself, as evil or as a prison for the spirit/soul. The derision for the physical body, as for all of nature, follows after such perspectives while informing a particular belief that we should seek technological solutions to the problems of finitude and fate (the problems associated with *having* a body).[6]

Nevertheless, theological anthropology does tend toward an ontology that understands the human person not only as "a composite being, a soul-and-body unity"[7] but also as being a body who shares in the same condition as others.[8] Introducing the ontological composition of the human person as an integrated duality of body and soul, Karl Barth has argued that human existence is soulish, yet the soul exists in a particular bodily form.[9] That is to say, the human person is irreducibly the soul of her body; or in Saint Basil the Great's poetic expression, "As the flesh was molded, the soul was made."[10] Thus, when we address the nature of human persons, we must attend to the whole person, body and soul.[11] So, unlike certain dualisms, where the body and soul are "self-contained and qualitatively different in relation to the other,"[12] the co-inherence of body and soul is vital for understanding the properly ordered human being.

It ought to be accepted, therefore, that Christian anthropology holds the body and soul in unity.[13] As I continue to speak of the body, it is important not to forget but to hold that such conversation is also to be about the soul. So that we might not forget at the outset, let us turn to look at the face of Christ for further understanding. We must understand the body of Christ to be material, yet not merely material.[14] As material, it is "visible, outward, [and] earthly."[15] It is, therefore, aesthetic and empirical. It is ready for observation, yet not merely observation. Rather, it is ready for encounter. Accordingly, the body of Christ is a living body, which means it is a historical body.[16] It is the visible spectacle of God's being and is, therefore, substantially the whole person of Christ made available for encounter. Christ is quite literally the whole of God expressed in material performance – in the actuality of Christ's historicity.[17]

Let me explain this (all too) briefly: Barth has argued that the formula for defining human being may be regarded as: "*Ich bin indem Du bist* [I am as Thou art; I am by the fact that you are]."[18] This serves as the definition of the fully mature human. It is known principally in relation to the primal humanity (history) of Christ – a primal humanity in which the body is not something that *belongs* to but is actually *inherent* of being human – and being human in community. A human being, therefore, and principally Christ, is not complete without the body.[19] Yet in addition to our own body, as we learn from the body of Christ, we are introduced to the bodies of those Others who stand alongside us. In this, we learn that humanity is not made for a solitary and isolated existence. Rather, we are social beings – once again, this is conveyed by the relational definition of humanity offered by Barth: I am as Thou art. Accordingly, with this formula, we do not describe the relationship between two static and self-determining atoms. Instead, the formula describes two dynamic beings who move out from themselves for existence, encountering each other for their co-existence. This is to suggest that the "I am" and the "Thou art" encounter each other as two histories interrupting a particular solitude and inculcating a new experience, the real experience, of being. In such an encounter, theologically considered, our history is interrupted and transformed by the history of Christ, and we come to learn that we are as He is. We also come to learn to, with, and for whom we are responsible: moving out from ourselves, we discover our near and distant neighbor.

In other words, in the Christian tradition, we understand what it means to be and to act as humans by first looking and listening to Christ.[20] We are not to learn about being human by phenomena incumbent to general human existence. Rather we are to learn about being human through "the concrete human person to whom, according to Christian faith, God bound himself and entered into human history."[21] This is the "ontological undertone" of Christian theological anthropology that must be observed.[22] It is in the encounter with Christ that humanity is introduced to her indelible Counterpart – present among us all as both the divine and human Other.[23]

Accordingly, Jesus interrupts human existence with that of his own humanity, transforming ours. The transformational event is accomplished when correlating subjects interrelate, which is what Barth describes as history: "The history of a being begins, continues, and is completed when something other than itself and transcending its own nature encounters it, approaches it and determines its being in the nature proper to it, so that it is compelled and enabled to transcend itself in response and in relation to this new factor."[24] The Other whom we encounter in such interrelation, however, if we are opened toward transformation, must be considered as the one who speaks to us, who has the freedom to address and to claim us for response. In this way, history becomes the ground for ethics, such that "I" am claimed for responsibility as "Thou" encounters, approaches, and determines. History as encounter, in this way, claims us and demands that we see, hear, and share speech and life with our embodied counterparts, correlating with persons rather than abstracted moral apparatus. As we are open for encounter, we are compelled to act for the embodied Other, for she is not an abstract redundant subject divorced from all that is real. She is not a disembodied illusion to be merely contemplated. Rather she is my neighbor, my counterpart, to whom and with whom and for whom I am enabled, rather summoned, to exercise my humanity and she hers.

This speaks of a dynamic exchange between embodied counterparts, which we have been trained to see by humanity's principal encounter with Christ. It begins, continues, and is completed as we come to know our counterpart, not as a moral stranger but rather as a neighbor, as co-humanity who may edify and direct our action(s). Appropriately then, the question, "What shall I do?" is not to be answered as the "self-assertion of one or many solitary individuals"[25] retreating to the exercise of an autonomous, private, and dismembered will against an object to master. It is answered as a material performance of one with and for the Other whom we are granted permission to know and to act toward responsibly.[26] By such performance, community may be forged between two (or more) correlating persons whose particularity is mutually interrupted and transformed.

The question remains, however: What does such an anthropology have to do with medicine? That is to ask, why might a relational ontology, such as that offered by Karl Barth's exploration of Christology and creation, be relevant for our discussions concerning the body in medicine? The answer rests in the correlating relationships forged in medical clinics, surgical theaters, and other medical care facilities – the relationships forged between all those persons discovered in health care milieu, both sick and well, patient and professional. As I will continue to discuss below, the relationships are necessitated by the inabilities and incapacities brought on by injury and illness – limits that require correlation between counterparts.

## Theology and the body: medical stories of creatures and counterparts

We learn in illness that we are "unable to care for that which is most '[our] own' . . . [and] all those issues of trust and power and honesty that are the hallmark of every human relationship take on suddenly a dramatic importance." As David Schenck continues, "when gripped with illness, we find ourselves in new relationships with those who now care for our body."[27] Yet these people, these surgeons, doctors, specialists, and nurses, are most likely strangers – unfamiliar to us yet positioned precariously in control of our fate and finitude. We give to these others far-reaching and, at times, complete control over our embodied lives.

Here is the rub: The issues of trust, power, honesty, and dependency are complicated even further by the ways in which these medical professionals might speak over, around, and about the body. Those who care for the bodies of patients might speak of "it" as though the bodies were a cacophony of machines, with only names leading the chart to differentiate one from another.[28] Perhaps these same persons treat the body as such – a machine to be studied, surveilled, manipulated, and mastered.

Yet, following Schenck, the language we might use concerning the body when talking with others, be it relatives or friends for example, often includes discussions about the variety of roles of the body in private and public spheres and how it cannot be reduced to a mere object. In such spheres, the body is more than a mere object. Additionally, I find as a theologian that the language we might use concerning the body when gathered around the hallmarks of Christian pedagogy and praxis – the Eucharist, for example – precludes such instrumental reasoning and reductionist objectification. For the body *is* the expression of the soul.

So, one might ask as Schenck does: Might we retain confidence in such persons who continue to regard my body as mere object and not as the expression of my soul?[29] I think we can, and when ill we must. Yet the disposition of modern medicine, introduced by various scholars including Jeffrey Bishop, Gerald McKenny, Theodor Adorno, Gabriel Marcel, and Karl Barth, is one that does tend toward a view of the body as an object to control. It is a disposition that practitioners have adopted, whether wittingly or not. It is a disposition wrought from the modern preoccupation with power that comes by knowing and is exercised by doing.

We find ourselves laboring diligently to assert such power with the aim to bring about complete well-being and total control over the limits of human life – specifically the limits of biological existence that may be lamented and often grieved. In so doing, however, we have separated the body as object away from the soul as subject. It seems to me that we have shadowed a dualism, objectifying the body, effectively reducing human persons to a ghost in a machine. It is no wonder that we invite clinical spiritual care practitioners to provide counsel for the ghosts.

In so doing, I think we have lost a sense of the theological/spiritual significance of "physical" medicine. At a time when medicine is thought and discussed purely as a physical matter, many remain unaware that the physician, whose embodied agency through cutting and curative intervention, is providing spiritual care (or harm), too. To suggest that the physical care of the body at the hands of physicians is not also spiritual care is to inculcate a perspective that is, theologically speaking, false.

Therefore, I think that it is essential to insist that a theological intervention for medicine must be one that does not aim to colonize the field of practice but aims to remind the physician, for example, that all bodies are persons and the practice of medicine must be(come) grounded by love for such persons. For in the embodied exercise of a physician providing care for another who is ill and cannot care for her own body, it is essential to insist on the concern that medicine has with the whole person – united, indivisible body and soul. Likewise, to suggest that spiritual care attends to something other than physical illness is also misleading and perpetuates the division of care – spiritual and material – while maintaining relative silos from which physicians and clergy exercise their respective duties under the auspice of teams of professionals engaged in the exercise of (woefully modern) clinical competencies.

What is needed to reconcile the binary of spiritual and physical care? How might the narrative change? These are important questions to ask. The answer is not within range, given the limits of this essay. Yet, if you will, let me point toward an answer and encourage further exploration, dialogue, and discussion concerning such questions. The focus of such direction will be to see where and how theology might nurture the space for medicine to tell its stories again and again – stories of being redeemed by the agency of love and by the art of ritual, as Selzer directed us and where I, too, will point.

## On the body waiting to be seen, inviting responsibility

As discussed earlier, we learn as we encounter the visible spectacle of God's own self-revelation in Jesus Christ. We learn, in part, that the body of Christ is waiting to be seen (and heard). As we are as Christ is, so too must we attend to our own bodies as well as those of each other. The form of the soul, which is our body, is waiting to be seen: our own body, as that of our fellows, is waiting for and inviting response – it compels responsibility. This is true of all bodies that stand before us, including those with very little life left in them.[30] It is true even of bodies without life.[31] In each of these cases, there remains a call, which claims us for human action – claiming us for help, relation, and responsibility. The spectacle of our entire being speaks as the physical word of the soul. It speaks as the physical word of the command of God who speaks to us as well through his own body, both materially in his own self-revelation and mystically in his body, the Church.[32]

The principal word that we encounter, by no choice of our own, is that we exist – and our existence is coupled with and responsible to the existence of our fellows. That word to each of us is that we are alive – that we have been made, following the expression of our wholeness as soul and body, and set free upon our own feet to be with and for our fellows. The principal command of God for life, which is given as a permission, as a freedom, is made known by the concrete embodiment of our own being as with that of our neighbors. This command invites obedience; as God speaks to us as creatures, he not only recognizes our creatureliness but also wills something from us.[33] Therefore, in our here and now, in our existence as creatures, and in correlation with the creatureliness of our fellows, we can understand what is commanded to us – live!

In this way, the body *is* the spoken word. It commands attention and demands respect.[34] The physical word of the human body, which exists in unity with the soul, is made ready to be heard in its very existence. Yet the body as a "physical word" is often ignored. Perhaps Ludwig Wittgenstein's aphorism could be instructive for us here: "God grant the philosopher insight into what lies in front of everyone's eyes.' "[35] But, *what* lies in front of our eyes?

For the Christian trained to see the heart of salvation, to see the world rightly, what lies before our eyes is the face of Christ. Moreover, this face, this body of Christ, trains our gaze upon our own body and the body of our fellows. The body of Christ is that which we encounter as the reference point around which our world as whole creatures is arranged. Yet the body, whether our own or that of our fellows, often goes unnoticed until (in sickness, the forerunner of death) it becomes "terribly energetic and often so noticeable."[36] Schenck confirms this tendency:

> Only at moments of resistance, disruption or disintegration do we turn our attention directly to the body. [A person will sit down to read, or to listen to music, or to fall asleep] relatively unaware of [her] body. . . . That is, until she is jostled, has her foot stepped on, spills hot coffee on herself. Then, suddenly, the body demands attention – and she turns to it immediately, as we all would. For no demands are so urgent, so undeniable as those of the body.[37]

The institution of medicine steps in during these times of hyperawareness and – with vigilance, acuity, and assertive will – labors to control the experience and expression of such disturbance. But why? Certainly, there may be an assortment of reasons we might consider – some positive, some negative.

For example, it may be that under the pursuit of complete health and radicalized notions of technology-driven well-being reposes a discontentment. Those engaged in various forms of biomedical science and practice will become controllers of nature, including human nature. And some forecast overcoming the existential anxiety that accompanies finitude.[38] Such anxiety, however, may be legitimate, for human bodies are frail, limited, and often broken, limited by both decay and death. For many, such pending and final threats are grievous, stirring agency to attenuate such limits – to achieve control over the limits of objective flesh, over death and therefore life.[39]

In his book *The Anticipatory Corpse*, Bishop diagnoses how in the science and practice of modern medicine the dead body becomes epistemologically normative (and reviled). The continued movement of the body becomes the principal concentration for those positioned in fields of science and practice aimed against the sustained threat of death. Thus, in biomedical science and practice, that which is understood as good or right might correspond to the continued implementation of various techniques that affect the function of the moving parts of the human body, now reduced to pure material mechanics – to an otherwise dead (and meaningless) body that is a mere shell for one's being.

For the Christian rightly formed by the encounter with Christ, it is not as though we stand over our bodies, disincarnated from their corporeality. We are not, as the Christian tradition instructs, an abstract mind enslaved by a body – a true self trapped by a fleshly façade, whereby our real selves are active against an illusory external flesh to be domesticated for the dignity of our souls. Such a perspective is contrary to the Christian proclamation, which professes "that Christ shows us *what* it is to be God, in the *way* that he lives and dies as a human being."[40] That is, "[i]n the incarnation, Jesus took up this fleshly existence and transformed it into something that is 'quickening and living and meaningful.'"[41]

Accordingly, God became our counterpart, rather than a conceptual tool, general principle, or belief. He became human, rather than an abstracted ideal or prescriptive law. Accordingly, in God's condescension, in his coming to be human alongside fellow humanity, Dietrich Bonhoeffer has commented, "Christ does not abolish human reality in favor of an idea that demands to be realized against all that is real. Christ empowers reality, affirming it as the real human being and thus the ground of all human reality, in birth, in life, in death, and of course, in resurrection."[42] Such Christology opposes a vision of an unrealized, fragile, and unsatisfactory human existence, revealing rather, in Christ's own suffering, frailty, and limitedness, an authentic humanity.[43] Christ is *really* human – and in our encounter with Christ, we come to understand our own humanity.

This means that in Christian theology, Christ is not a projected ideal, disembodied spirit, or techno-evolved material reinterpretation of Nietzsche's *Übermensch*.[44] The Incarnation of Christ delimits and defines God's relation to the world, while also inviting all of humanity to take part.[45] Put differently, in an act of solidarity, if you will, God elects himself to occupy both time and space, while vindicating human embodiment as authentic, real, and good – "The message of God's becoming human attacks the heart of an era when contempt for humanity or idolization of humanity (sometimes these are held together) is the height of all wisdom."[46]

Such a theologically ordered human reality, however, requires our awareness and responsibility for it to be realized in our lives and in the lives of our fellows.[47] Such awareness might be realized by asking a principal question of theology, which is made acute as we are interrupted and transformed by the presence of God in Jesus Christ: "*Who* is my neighbor? Who is *my* neighbor?"[48] It is the question we are to ask again and again in the practice of theology and theological ethics that is unencumbered by the weight of real human, and therefore bodily, existence. It is also the question we are to repeatedly ask in the practice of ethics that attends to the particularity of persons gathered and encountered at the crises of embodied human life abutted by death.[49]

## Responsibility for the *broken* body

And so, perhaps the question, "Who is my neighbor?" is what we need to ask in the practice of medicine where the body does speak. It could very well be that such an interrupting question, and the relational ontology that grounds it, might make us aware of the "quickening and living and meaningful" body before us. It could be that such a question might *save* modern medical professionals from a diminished capacity to see, hear, and exchange moral speech with the meaningful, albeit ill and imperfect, body gathered in the medical clinic, surgical theater, or research laboratory.

That question challenges us to attend to the Other who claims our responsibility. It stirs us to attend to that ethical demand that is made known in the actuality and historicity of creaturely life. It is the command that comes to us as the physical word spoken by the body of Christ and, by permission, by our own bodies, whether sick or well, whether alive or dead. We learn this theologically as we become aware of the actuality and historicity of Christ who is known by the witness of Scriptures and by way of the practice (that is, embodied event) of the Eucharist, which also provokes us to ask the question, "Who is my neighbor?" But more acutely, the Eucharist summons us to ask, with gratitude, "*Who* is this broken body before me, who claims *my* responsibility?"

It might just be that medicine needs such an analogical practice that reminds those embodied medical professionals gripped and claimed by modern technology and the objectifying gaze of scientific rigor to look up and to see the wholly embodied *person* before them – to see the embodied soul and besouled body who demands, by her very existence, responsibility and care who demands to be seen, heard, and loved.

It is here that I am thankful for Selzer's essay, which was onto something important: "I make of my fingers, words; of my scalpel, a sentence; of the body of my patient, a story." We must once again not only tell but also listen to the stories of our fellows. I say this for in Christian theology, as presented above, the stories we tell and those we hear from others compel us to understand the spiritual significance of the body – our own and that of the Other. Yet we are not compelled merely to listen to stories; rather, the stories invite performance – performance that is, at once, both physical and spiritual in unity. Consider the ways in which the sacraments teach us to see the world rightly, while inviting both gratitude and responsibility. They train us, like habits of virtue, to *become* human. They nurture both body and soul in unity.

The principal measure of good medicine, and the principal responsibility of the good physician, therefore, must be for such practices and persons to give due care for those who cannot provide care for themselves.[50] If our bodies are always in communion with each other, such that we ought to attend to this communion, then medicine ought to be ever-vigilant to concentrate upon this *demanding* body that the physician invades in the most intimate of ways.[51] While disorder and impairment, disease, and disturbance are the "why" of medicine, the radical *responsibility* of medical professionals is to attend to the physical word of the soul as fellow or as friend.

And so, while the broken body *invites* response by the *physical word* of the soul, which is opposed by "the growth of death in us by physical decay and illness,"[52] medicine must learn again and again to attend to the broken body not as an object to possess, mutilate, and master. It must attend to the broken body not with an answer against death, as though death is defeated by biomedical understanding and assurance whether by sustaining life artificially or by mediating death.[53] Rather, it must attend to the broken body as a gift that contains permission or a summons, or quite possibly a demand, to act – it must attend to the broken body as our neighbor claiming us for love. Therefore, with gratitude and responsibility, we must again take seriously the historicity and particularity of embodied human beings struggling *together* amidst the ambiguities of present crises and toward the flourishing of human life even unto death.

## Notes

1 The following essay was made possible through the support of a grant from the John Templeton Foundation. The opinions expressed in this publication are those of the author and do not necessarily reflect the views of the John Templeton Foundation.

2 The epigraph offers a rearranged selection of prose from Richard Selzer, "The Surgeon as Priest," in *Mortal Lessons: Notes on the Art of Surgery* (New York, NY: Simon & Schuster, 1976), 24–36.

3 The argument that the body has been objectified in the medical milieu is one made by, among others, Jeffrey P. Bishop, *The Anticipatory Corpse: Medicine, Power, and the Care of the Dying* (Notre Dame, IN: The University of Notre Dame Press, 2011); Gerald P. McKenny, *To Relieve the Human Condition: Bioethics, Technology, and the Body* (Albany, NY: State University of New York Press, 1997).

4 This essay, and section in particular, is based on the second chapter of my book: "The Technique of Bioethics and the Freedom for Encounter," in *Reading Karl Barth, Interrupting Moral Technique, Transforming Biomedical Ethics* (New York, NY: Palgrave Macmillan, 2015), 59–94. Revised and reproduced with permission of Palgrave Macmillan.

5 E. L. Mascall, *Man: His Origin and Destiny* (Westminster, UK: Dacre Press, 1940), 44.

6 Charles Taylor, *The Ethics of Authenticity* (Cambridge, MA: Harvard University Press, 2003), 6.

7 Mascall, *Man*, 46.

8 John Dunhill, "Being a Body," *Theology* 105 no. 824 (2002): 110.

9 Karl Barth, *Church Dogmatics* [CD], trans. Geoffrey W. Bromiley, 4 vols. (Edinburgh, Scotland: T&T Clark, 2004), III/2, 325.

10 St. Basil the Great, *On the Human Condition*, trans. Nonna Verna Harrison (Crestwood, NY: St. Vladimir's Seminary Press, 2005), 50.

11 Barth, CD, III/2, 350, 367. In addition, while reflecting on the unity of the body and soul in regard to our health, Barth comments: "[We do] not have a specific physical life in the sound or disordered functions of [our] somatic organs, nervous system, blood circulation, digestion, urination, and so on, and then in an upper storey a separate life of the soul. [We] live the healthy and sick life of [our] body with that of [our] soul, and again in both cases, and in their mutual relationship, it is a matter of [our] life's history, [our] own history, and therefore [ourselves]." Ibid., III/4, 359. Wholeness, therefore, is central to Barth's anthropology.

12 Ibid., III/2, 380. Such dualism does tend to lead toward one of two conclusions, either (1) I am only a body, as in materialist philosophies, or (2) I am really a spirit, a thinking subject, as Descartes would have us give assent. In either case, Christian anthropology is not represented, for it is able to speak at once of both soul and body. For a more complete treatment on Barth's anthropology, and for particular treatments of different modes of dualism and holism, see Marc Cortez, *Embodied Souls, Ensouled Bodies: An Exercise in Christological Anthropology and Its Significance for the Mind/Body Debate* (London, UK: T&T Clark, 2011).

13 For additional reading on the unity of body and soul, see the following: Barth, CD, III/2, 344–436; Emil Brunner, *Man in Revolt: A Christian Anthropology* (Cambridge, UK: James Clarke & Co., 2002), 362–389; G. K. Berkouwer, *Man: The Image of God* (Grand Rapids, MI: Wm. B. Eerdmans, 1962), 194–233.

14 Barth, CD, III/2, 350.

15 Ibid., III/2, 367. See also Marc Cortez, "Body, Soul, and (Holy) Spirit: Karl Barth's Theological Framework for Understanding Human Ontology," *International Journal of Systematic Theology* 10 no. 3 (2008): 332–334.

16 Barth, CD, III/2, 377.

17 John B. Webster, *Barth's Ethics of Reconciliation* (New York, NY: Cambridge University Press, 1995), 86.

18 Barth, CD, III/2, 248.

19 Mascall, *Man*, 42–58.

20 Barth, CD, III/2, 132.

21 Wolf Krötke, "The Humanity of the Human Person in Karl Barth's Anthropology," in *The Cambridge Companion to Karl Barth*, ed. John Webster (New York, NY: Cambridge University Press, 2000), 159.

22 Barth, CD, III/2, 134.

23 Ibid., III/2, 135.

24 Ibid., III/2, 158.

25 Karl Barth, *Humanity of God* (Louisville, KY: Westminster John Knox Press, 1960), 71.

26 Paul D. Matheney, *Dogmatics and Ethics: The Theological Realism and Ethics of Karl Barth's Church Dogmatics* (Frankfurt am Main, Germany: Verlag Peter Lang, 1990), 139.

27 David Schenck, "The Texture of Embodiment," *Human Studies* 9 no. 1 (1986): 51–52.

28 After all, aren't we trained to speak as such? Unfortunately, I am guilty of such rhetoric when I have instructed both undergraduate and graduate students about the structure and function of the human body.

29 Schenck, "The Texture of Embodiment," 52.

30 Ibid., 46.

31  Cf. D. Gareth Jones, "The Human Body: An Anatomist's Journey from Death to Life," in *A Tangled Web: Medicine and Theology in Dialogue*, eds. R. John Elford and D. Gareth Jones (Bern, Switzerland: Peter Lang, 2009), 105–121.

32  Cf. Donald MacKinnon's two Signposts contributions: "God the Living and the True," and "The Church of God," in *Kenotic Ecclesiology: Select Writings of Donald M. MacKinnon*, eds. John C. McDowell, Scott A. Kirkland, and Ashley John Moyse (Minneapolis, MN: Fortress Press, 2016).

33  Karl Barth, *Ethics*, trans. Dietrich Braun (New York, NY: Seabury Press, 1981), 117.

34  Respect is the chief concern of the freedom for human life. Therefore, as Barth indicates, "respect is due to it, and, with respect, protection against each and every callous negation and destruction." Barth, CD, III/4, 397.

35  Ludwig Wittgenstein, *Culture and Value: A Selection from Posthumous Remains* (Oxford, UK: Wiley-Blackwell, 1998), 72. The aphorism is also quoted in Schenck, "The Texture of Embodiment," 44.

36  Barth, CD, III/4, 345.

37  Schenck, "The Texture of Embodiment," 43.

38  Beyond forecasting, some argue such pursuits are morally obligatory. The potential for improving the human condition has been discussed by several scholars from the humanities through the hard sciences. Both physical health and cognition are presented as the foci for both scientific and funding attention. For further interest, see John Harris, *Enhancing Evolution: The Ethical Case for Making Better People* (Princeton, NJ: Princeton University Press, 2007); Aubrey de Grey and Michael Rae, *Ending Aging: The Rejuvenation Breakthroughs That Could Reverse Human Aging in Our Lifetime* (New York, NY: St. Martin's Press, 2007).

39  Ernest Becker, *The Denial of Death* (New York, NY: Free Press, 1973), 33.

40  John Behr, "The Christian Art of Dying," *Sobornost* 35 nos. 1–2 (2013): 137.

41  Cortez, "Body, Soul, and (Holy) Spirit," 337.

42  Dietrich Bonhoeffer, *Ethics*, in *Dietrich Bonhoeffer Works*, ed. Clifford J. Green and trans. Reinhard Krauss, Charles C. West, and Douglas W. Stott (Minneapolis, MN: Fortress Press, 2005), 99.

43  Jens Zimmerman, "Being Human, Becoming Human: Dietrich Bonhoeffer's Christological Humanism," in *Being Human, Becoming Human: Dietrich Bonhoeffer and Social Thought*, eds. Jens Zimmerman and Brian Gregor (Eugene, OR: Pickwick, 2010), 27.

44  Ashley John Moyse, "A Theological Response for Ray Kurzweil's Future Perfect," *Religions: A Scholarly Journal* 5 (2013): 98–99.

45  Bonhoeffer, *Ethics*, 85, 159.

46  Ibid., 85.

47  Cortez, "Body, Soul, and (Holy) Spirit," 337.

48  Barth, *Ethics*, 351.

49  This question, "Who is my neighbor?" is a principal question that is considered throughout my book *Reading Karl Barth, Interrupting Moral Technique, Transforming Biomedical Ethics* noted above. At the very least, it is a vital question for biomedical ethics to consider, interrupting forms of moral discourse that compel solidarity toward principles rather than persons.

50  Schenck, "The Texture of Embodiment," 49.

51  Ibid., 45.

52  Alexander Schmemann, *For the Life of the World: Sacraments and Orthodoxy* (Crestwood, NY: St. Vladimir's Seminary Press, 1973), 100–101.

53  Ibid., 95–100.

# 2 Embodied soul and ensouled body
## Reflections on Ravaisson and theological methodology

*Matthew S. Vest*

This essay explores the thought of French philosopher Félix Ravaisson (1813–1900) on the topic of habit. Habit, for Ravaisson, presents an illuminating lens allowing us to peer deeply into human and material nature. Ravaisson's compact essay, *Of Habit*,[1] primarily addresses questions of natural science and philosophical anthropology, yet throughout this work – and especially at the conclusion – he challenges traditional boundaries of these two disciplines as he asks questions regarding the "freedom" and "will" inherent within the material, natural sphere (75), as well as the role of man as the freest and willing agent who is head of creation. While shunning materialism and idealism, Ravaisson sees in habit a middle way to grasp the ontological nature of all things – from base organic matter to human intelligence, morality, and God's indwelling of this entire order.

Ravaisson is not well-known outside French philosophy, yet his phenomenology of habit has much to offer to the dialogue surrounding the foundations of medicine, the field of bioethics, or any other endeavor that engages the relationship between body and mind/soul.[2] This is evidenced in at least three aspects from *Of Habit*: first, Ravaisson's thought explicitly challenges mind-body dualism and Kantian autonomous rationality, contesting by implication philosophy's post-Enlightenment hierarchy of discursive rationality over bodily knowledge. In this vein we might recall Wittgenstein's quote: "Nothing is more wrong-headed than calling meaning a mental activity."[3] Second, Ravaisson seeks to reunite the body and mind/soul and to demonstrate the relationship between this whole man and the natural world. Third, Ravaisson gives particular attention to a philosophical methodology that requires the body to play a meaningful role in epistemology. These three points are interrelated aspects of embodiment, which I reference in this essay to mean balancing the poles of the tangible and intangible, or the visible and invisible aspects of a person's body and soul. Embodiment can entail personification, realization, or incarnation as ways of expressing the invisible in concrete forms.

The first task of this essay is to summarize *Of Habit*, and at the end of this summary I will emphasize Ravaisson's exposition of human morality rooted in habit (67–71). This section on morality is notably relevant to the foundations and epistemology of a field such as bioethics, and it raises important questions regarding the philosophical and theological context of Ravaisson's thesis. Indeed, the way in which Ravaisson mysteriously speaks of desire, grace, or love as the hidden "impulse" within all nature (55, 75), and the way that he grounds this impulse in analogical reasoning – from man as microcosm to the cosmos on the whole (39, 65) – opens the door for Ravaisson's methodology and conclusion to be understood as a *theological* anthropology. At the same time, these claims raise the question, what *sort* of theological or philosophical knowledge is Ravaisson offering? What ontological grounding frames his theological claims? Ravaisson offers a few hints and yet remains predominantly silent toward such questions, leading some to deny any sincere theological meaning in *Of Habit*.[4] In response to these questions, I propose that Ravaisson's challenge to Kantian rationalism aligns with a pre-modern understanding of philosophy that is not rigidly distinct from theology. As such, Ravaisson's phenomenology of habit must be understood within a theological context where "theory" remains deeply rooted in the ancient Greek term *theoria* (θεωρία). I suggest that Ravaisson's habituated, embodied understanding of life is ripe for comparison with ascetic modes of virtue and knowledge – and that this may offer a specific Christian context and tradition for understanding Ravaisson's otherwise ambiguous theological claims.

## *Of Habit*

The opening and closing lines of Ravaisson's essay give testimony to its Aristotelian roots, and they indicate the metaphysical turn of the essay. *Of Habit* opens: "Habit, in the widest sense, is a general and permanent way of being, the state of an existence considered either as the unity of its elements or as the succession of its different phases" (25). Likewise, Ravaisson concludes by stating that habit functions as "the tendency to persevere in the very actuality that constitutes being" (77). Against the predominant Enlightenment view of habit as a "stultifying mechanism,"[5] habit for Ravaisson carries the ontological and ethical import that Aristotle envisioned in virtue or excellence (*arête*).

   In this way habit is more than "a state"; it is something "contracted" (25), a movement that synthesizes, draws together, and harmonizes. It is a "disposition, a virtue [that is] relative to change," and all "things" change through time and space toward "permanence" (27). Habit is not a state, or even changing states, but rather is a spontaneous disposition or tendency that emerges amidst change.[6] The key to tracing this disposition or tendency is the phenomenon of double movement in passivity and activity evidenced within change. "Life continually suffers external influences; and yet it nevertheless surmounts them and endlessly triumphs over them. . . . Life implies the opposition of receptivity and spontaneity" (31). In one sense, *Of Habit* revolves around this phenomenological distinction between receptivity and spontaneity. At the lowest end of the hierarchy of nature – organic matter – spontaneous activity is low, hence habit has "marginal access to vegetative life" (33). As the complexity of life increases, however, the principle of habit becomes more visible; passive receptivity is always present, yet in intricate, flourishing human life spontaneous activity is more evident (31).

These formulations may seem abstract and dense, yet they play into the overall scheme of Ravaisson's work. Part I focuses on "primary nature" without reference to a particular being as Ravaisson theorizes on the function of habit in nature. The editors comment:

> This abstraction is a function of Ravaisson's ultimate aim to show that habit is a power that stretches all the way down, from human life to vegetal life, and that this power cannot be straightforwardly understood in terms of any of the faculties – sensibility, imagination, understanding, reason or the will – advanced in many traditional forms of psychological and philosophical thinking. Habit will, in fact, be shown to be a power that underlies the operation of these faculties.
>
> (78)

Additionally, at the end of Part I, Ravaisson admits that looking to nature alone means seeing "only from the outside" and to see the "dispositions and powers" of the cosmos we must look to "ourselves" as the microcosm (39). Part II then focuses on the human experience, an experience revealing further the nature of habit that is manifest as a "spiral," spanning from the depths of basic, organic nature to the "flourishing consciousness" in humans (77). In effect, the organization of the essay presents a mirrored inversion of two key methodological steps. The first step is a phenomenology of habit that reveals continuity from human will to bodily instinct (Pt. II). In the second step, this continuity between will and instinct analogously corresponds to all nature (Pt. I).[7]

What does it mean, however, for habit to reveal continuity from the human will to bodily instinct? Within the framework of the double movement of passive receptivity and active spontaneity, Ravaisson articulates the heart of the matter in the "double law" of habit: *as habit works its way through life, the continuity or repetition of habit reduces receptivity and increases spontaneity*. In a lengthy but critical paragraph, Ravaisson summarizes this double law:

> The general effect of the continuity and repetition of change that the living being receives from something other than itself is that, if the change does not destroy it, it is always less and less altered by that change. Conversely, the more the living being has repeated or prolonged a change that it has originated, the more it produces the change and seems to tend to reproduce it. The change that has come to it from the outside becomes more and more foreign to it; the change that it has brought

upon itself becomes more and more proper to it. Receptivity diminishes and spontaneity increases. Such is the general law of the disposition, of the habit, that the continuity or the repetition of the change seems to engender in every living being. If, therefore, the characteristic of nature, which constitutes life, is the predominance of spontaneity over receptivity, then habit does not simply presuppose nature, but develops in the very direction of nature, and concurs with it.

(31)

As Michael Moore suggests, a long-distance runner would find it easy to agree with the above explanation of the double law of habit. As the runner's body and mind are habituated to "pain, effort, and endless repetitions," the running movements become easier to perform. The runner becomes smoother and more relaxed as his activity becomes routine and expected. The idea or mental process of running does not disappear but rather is dissipated into the body, and this leads to Ravaisson's claim that "the *idea* becomes *being*" (55).[8] Interestingly, as such "movement . . . becomes a habit, [it] leaves the sphere of will and reflection . . . [but] does not leave that of intelligence" (55). Thus, habit is not a mechanical, thoughtless action but rather becomes "the effect of an inclination that follows from the will," and every goal-focused inclination "implies intelligence" (55).

In this way, Ravaisson seeks nothing less than a definition of intelligence centered on the doubly moving passive and active body. As the goal or "end" of a movement is "fused" with the movement, "habit becomes more and more a substantial idea" (55); thus we may envision a virtuoso violinist who performs not in any "mechanical" manner but *as* the music itself. This ontological view of habit now clarifies the opening of Ravaisson's essay: "the universal law, the fundamental character of a being, is the tendency to persist in its way of being" (27). Moreover, as ideas become realized in bodies, the bodies – even to particular organs – are formed in this new "way of being." "The spontaneity of desire and intuition is dispersed, in some way, as it develops, within the indeterminate multiplicity of the organism" (57). Taking over from acts of will, habits are "inclinations" born, for example, from custom and then pass away when customs are interrupted or no longer practiced. At that point, the movements and acts may continue, but after some time they would "return" to the sphere of the will and consciousness. This process of passing beyond and returning to the sphere of the will is ongoing throughout all of life.

## Habituated morality and bioethics

More can be said of Ravaisson's overarching thesis, yet another way to summarize his essay is to attend to his discussion of morality grounded in habit. This discussion carries significance for a field such as bioethics that engages bodies, actions, and morality while also presenting Ravaisson's most explicit theological statements.

Morality, as with all of nature, is suspended between action and passion because morality is a continuation of the order evidenced in nature. The moral life is not completely other than organic, natural life but is, rather, an example of the relationship of all things. This relationship, however, spans great lengths as Ravaisson states moral life is a "superior life" and a "world" unto itself that "increasingly separates and detaches itself from the life of the body, and in which the soul has its own life, its own destiny and its own end to accomplish" (67).[9] The end of morality is the triumph of action over passion – which takes root in pleasure and pain, corresponding to good and evil (69). Just as physical feelings manifest the habituated process of coming into being, so, too, feelings – *sentiments*, such as pity or sorrow – in the moral spheres manifest the progression of the soul into being. Continuing with the analogy, just as the repetition or continuity of the physical body reduces receptivity and increases spontaneity, so, too, moral habits become easier as pleasurable action replaces passive sensibility. "In this way, as habit destroys the passive emotions of pity, the helpful activity and the inner joys of charity develop more and more in the heart of the one who does good" (69).

This formulation of moral activity, of course, aligns with Aristotelian virtue, which at first is "an effort and wearisome" but then becomes "something attractive and pleasurable" (69), and, as in the formative art of education, a second nature is mysteriously formed through virtuous practices. This pursuit of virtue, moreover, is no mechanical virtue; behind (or within) the habituating activity of nature, the persistence within a thing's way of being, lies a mysterious "force" that serves to unify and bring together the physical and mystical. We must remember that, for Ravaisson, "both physical and rationalistic theories" are insufficient to explain this "force that, without losing anything of its higher unity in personality, proliferates without being divided; that descends without going under; that dissolves itself in different ways, into its inclinations, acts and ideas; that is transformed in time, and that is disseminated in space" (55, 57). To explain this force in habit, Ravaisson points to grace: "[Habit] is, indeed, a law, a *law of the limbs*,[10] which follows on from the freedom of spirit. But this law is a *law of grace*. It is the final cause that increasingly predominates over efficient causality and which absorbs the latter into itself. And at that point, indeed, the end and the principle, the fact and the law, are fused together within necessity" (57). Likewise, speaking of habituated morality specifically, Ravaisson names love as that which "augments its own expressions":

[T]he unreflective freedom of Love constitutes all of its substance, and love can no longer be distinguished from the contemplation of what it loves, nor contemplation from its object; and it is this that forms the source, the basis and the necessary beginning: this is the state of nature, whose primordial spontaneity envelops and presupposes all will. Nature lies wholly in desire, and desire, in turn, lies in the good that attracts it. In this way the profound words of a theologian might be confirmed: "Nature is prevenient grace." It is God within us, God hidden solely by being so far within us in this intimate source of ourselves, to whose depths we do not descend.

(71)[11]

In light of these quotes, we may see how morality summarizes Ravaisson's whole view of habit, and we can note at least two immediate connections to bioethics. First, as stated above, any essential separation of mind, soul, and body has no place within this paradigm of habit. Therapy of the body is intimately related to therapy of the soul such that physicians and patients come together not merely around physical needs.[12] The boundaries of the physician-patient relationship in this framework certainly challenge many contemporary medical categories and specializations, and physicians approaching questions regarding patient desires, quality of life, and contextual circumstances would be obliged to take theology and spirituality seriously. Without functioning as priests – and certainly not ignoring the lack of moral consensus in today's post-modern, pluralistic society[13] – physicians would be obliged to engage in moral issues stemming from a patient's habits. The current cultural *Zeitgeist* favors physicians engaging patients morally on habits such as smoking,[14] yet countless other topics with clear health implications for embodied, spiritual persons are predominantly taboo for physicians and health care institutions to discuss on moral grounds that extend beyond medical techniques and possibilities. Here one thinks especially of the challenges for physicians to speak with their patients regarding sexual health, the psychological and spiritual effects of abortion, reproductive technologies, the post-modern redefinitions of marriage, family, and more.[15] If Ravaisson's "spiral" does indeed unite the physical to the moral within a progression or revealing of unified being, the clinical, scientific logic in today's physician-patient relationship would be radically challenged.[16]

Second, Ravaisson's progression of moral being may enter into the epistemological conversations of bioethics with particular relevance for a phenomenological approach to bioethics advocated by Drew Leder, Richard Zaner, George Agich, and others.[17] Drawing on Husserl's phenomenology to heal the sick and Merleau-Ponty's pre-rational language, these philosophers seek moral knowledge for bioethics through the experience and perception of the lived body, and amidst this dialogue Ravaisson offers an explicit path toward grasping morality in perceiving bodies.

### The theological roots of Ravaisson's taxonomy?

At the same time, while noting the advantages of Ravaisson's phenomenon of habit for contesting Enlightenment rationalism and physicalism, or for furthering dialogue within the field of bioethics, we should carefully attend to Ravaisson's claims that move boldly from spirited, organic nature to incarnational embodiment. What does Ravaisson intend by stating that the phenomenon of habit reveals "God within us"? Two contemporary academics, Catherine Malabou and Kam Shapiro, dismiss any substantive connection between *Of Habit* and Christian theology,[18] and in a way this is understandable. Ravaisson's essay opens in a most abstract way; even as he moves his focus from being to beings, at no juncture does he address or name a particular being.[19] Ravaisson focuses almost exclusively on the phenomenon of habit, and it is this abstract phenomenology that informs his anthropology. Toward the climax of his argument, however, he then appeals to the divine presence in nature.

The question that comes to mind at this juncture concerns the boundaries and proper relationship between Ravaisson's philosophy and theological inquiries. Some may find it simplest to say that Ravaisson reached the end of his philosophical pursuit and then handed off, so to speak, to theology. That ordering could be aligned with some practices within the Scholastic university in the West where philosophy and theology became sciences (*Wissenschaften*) with their own distinct objects, methodologies, and hierarchy. This ordering, however, is problematic in light of the technical history of the term "science" that was associated with holistic "knowledge" long before it garnered the logical, cognitive associations of the Galilean and Baconian revolution.[20] Ravaisson's inquiry does not seem to align well with the modern concept of scientificity born from such an Enlightenment emphasis upon a priori or experimental science. On the contrary, Ravaisson's methodology seems more to align with Husserl's later explicit goal of seeking a general theory of knowledge (*connaissance*) through phenomenology. "By suggesting that [phenomenology] founds *the* science par excellence, Husserl in fact takes leave of the modern concept of scientificity. The sciences in crisis that concern [Husserl's *The Crisis of European Sciences and Transcendental Phenomenology*] are only sciences. Phenomenology thus takes leave of the modern concept of science all together."[21]

This point by Jean-Yves Lacoste regarding phenomenology's seeking a general theory of knowledge is helpful as a way of grasping Ravaisson's habit. As Ravaisson's conclusions push the line toward theology, Malabou and Shapiro seem to read *Of Habit* non-theologically from a modern standpoint with discrete, disciplinary lines between philosophy, theology, and science. A general theory of knowledge that would align with Ravaisson's Aristotelian roots, however, freely transgresses the lines between the aims of a "philosopher" and a "theologian" first and foremost because the definition of philosophy in the Greco-Roman world was not overly specified. Recalling an image from the *Meno*, ancient philosophy stuns and mystifies like a torpedo fish, and, to express rightly perplexity in ancient philosophy, Lacoste reminds us of the need to move from one (modern) language to another "to wonder, not about what 'theory' and 'science' signify in our languages, but about what *theoria* and *episteme* mean in Greek."[22] *Theoria* and *episteme* invoke a whole other (ancient) tradition of knowledge that unites where the modern sciences and disciplines have fragmented. We could proceed further to catalog other categories or modes of knowledge such as *gnosis, phronesis, techne, aisthesis,* and *noesis,* and yet the point here is to make the distinction between *theoria* and theory and *episteme* and science. In the modern sense of the term theory, we gravitate toward discursive reason (*dianoia*) as emphasized in Scholastic *scientia* and Enlightenment rationality, and while *theoria* is never separated from such conceptual knowledge, *theoria* in Greek entails a mystical contemplation of "the real in its unfolding or budding forth" and not of "reality as completed, accomplished, and at our disposal."[23] To behold this unfolding of the real, *theoria* implies an active practice of contemplation, a *vita philosophica* or way of life and a manner of being in the world, and this methodological context seems most fitting to Ravaisson's analysis of habit. If Ravaisson's understanding of philosophy indeed falls primarily within the bounds of discursive rationality, Malabou's Nietzschean reading or Shapiro's secular interpretation of Ravaisson becomes more possibly viable,[24] for discursive reason and Scholastic *scientia* do emphasize a logic and rationality that may be employed as a tool within varying presuppositional groundings. *Theoria* and *episteme,* however, direct our attention to the *logos,* and, be it the pagan *logos* or the Christian *logos,* what is critical to note in *theoria* is the interwoven presence of theology and religion in ancient philosophy.[25] Moreover, within such a philosophical context, Ravaisson's transition from organic matter to incarnational embodiment may find root in a more coherent theological soil.

## *Theoria* or *theosis?*

More could be said of the blending of philosophy and theology in *theoria* amidst contexts such as the schools of the Cynics, Epicureans, or Neoplatonists.[26] My argument here, however, is that the ambiguity in the role of a "philosopher" and "theologian" in antiquity is helpful for understanding the "presence of the divine" that Ravaisson sees in habit. At the same time, while seeking a coherent theological context for Ravaisson, how far can we take his theological discourse within the Christian tradition? This question is important as thus far I have used the term "theology" in reference to Greek *theoria,* and it should be clear that Ravaisson's theological ways of habituated embodiment are distinct from Christian asceticism; at the same time, a parallel or analogous relationship can be discerned that is worth examining. Ravaisson's treatment of habit for persons emphasizes the progression and formation of body and spirit that are an embodied ontological unfolding of human nature, and this process notably aligns with asceticism as "self-mastery" that enables man to fulfill his purpose. Hence Eastern Orthodox Bishop Kallistos Ware quotes Nicolas Berdyaev – "asceticism means the liberation of the human person" – to make the point that ascetic self-denial is a necessary aspect for all of life, including athletics, politics, scholarly research, and particularly prayer.[27] Far from the gloomy connotations of severe austerity, Ware points to the ascetic practices of *anachoresis* (withdrawal) and *enkrateia* (self-control) as ways of "building the soul" and seeking the conversion of one's self. *Anachoresis* is for the sake of the world or even a "return" for greater service to one's neighbor; likewise, *enkrateia* functions for greater human freedom.[28] As indicated above, a virtuoso (*virtus*) musician and endurance athlete would be well suited to grasp Ravaisson's habit and the meaningfulness of asceticism as the transfiguration of man. Indeed, when asceticism is understood as transfiguration rather than undue mortification, asceticism is "universal in its scope" and can rightly be said to be a "vocation" for all and a gateway to flourish as authentic human beings.[29]

To be sure, the relationship between Ravaisson's habit and asceticism is not essential but rather analogous, and the goal here is to explore what I contend is a positive and helpful context for furthering a reading of Ravaisson within Christian theology. Turning to Saint Gregory the Theologian (330–390 A.D.) is helpful for he defines theology experientially in reference to an inner, noetic illumination, a knowledge and light kindled through holiness. Theology begins with the person and character of the one theologizing such that Saint Gregory speaks first of "theology to cleanse the theologian": hence true theology is kindled through ascetic formation, seeking the purity of holiness.[30] Theology practiced without restraint and purification of body and soul is dangerous just as it is dangerous to gaze at the sun with weak eyes, and only "when we are free from the mire and noise without" are we still enough to know God (Ps 45.11 LXX) and "to judge uprightly" (Ps 74.3 LXX) in theology.[31] Moreover, knowledge of God cannot be deduced from a logical process of discursive reasoning, but rather the theologian must be purified (*katharsis*) in soul and transformed within, discerning knowledge through *noesis* (intellection) and *theoria* (contemplation) as the knower is united to God. The intent of ascetic practices is to seek the highest possible knowledge in *theosis*, the mystical union with God through the person of Christ; in this way Saint Gregory particularizes *theoria* within the economy of Christian *theosis*. In the words of Saint Maximus: "God made us so that we might become 'partakers of the divine nature' (2 Pet. 1:4) and sharers in His eternity, and so that we might come to be like Him (cf. 1 John 3:2) through deification by grace. It is through deification that all things are reconstituted and achieve their permanence; and it is for its sake that what is not is brought into being and given existence."[32]

Here we do well to recall Ravaisson's language regarding the culmination of the *law of the limbs* into the *law of grace* (57) and the union of embodied "love" ascending into the "object of love" (71). Likewise, as Ravaisson speaks of education and forming the soul toward the good (69), "it is the good itself, at least the idea of the good, which descends into these depths, engendering love in them and raising that love up to itself." The "idea" of the good is perhaps slippery language to substitute for the good *itself*, yet shortly thereafter Ravaisson specifies how habit reveals "God within us, God hidden solely by being so far within us in this intimate source of ourselves, to whose depths we do not descend" (71). What seems clear is that Ravaisson sees habit as embodied knowledge and even *the* form of participation with God. Tying down such language within Christian theology may lie beyond the reach of Ravaisson's analysis of habit, yet his significant hints toward theological – though not Christological – macrocosm and microcosm all but beg for a furthering of his thought within the Christian tradition. Ravaisson posits a grace-filled journey in and through the cosmos aimed at nothing less than an experiential union with God as the active, habitual lover is conformed to the object of love. For many reasons, this vision of union in Love is compelling, yet some may question whether the experience of God through habit hangs suspended in ambiguity without some more particular grounding. Ravaisson has offered a methodological way beyond Kantian rational morality, but what will distinguish between the habitual experience and formation of daily meditation for a Buddhist and daily prayer for a Christian monk? Ravaisson gives practical advice regarding the initial "effort" and weariness of seeking the virtues that later "becomes something attractive and a pleasure only through practice" – leading eventually to the "holiness of innocence" (69) – but how are we to discern this experience of an unnamed good?

One suggestion may be to read *Of Habit* within the nuanced paradigm of natural theology as articulated by Anglican bishop Rowan Williams.[33] Williams notes with concern the type of natural theology that seeks knowledge of God apart from revelation *as* an intentionally democratizing and demystifying maneuver, and he distances his point from this anti-revelationist framework by allowing for the possibility of contemplating God through and in light of revelation. Following Cornelius Ernst, Williams turns especially to the habits of language that uncover layers of complexity in biblical speech.

> There is an underlay of language [in the Scriptures] taken for granted, a world in which people talk about "God," but precisely this language is being disrupted and transformed because of certain events that give the word a new and difficult context. Here "God" comes to work like a metaphor, in fact: a word whose territory we think we know is invited to play away from home in order to capture something that more familiar usage can't cope with. When Hebrew Scripture says that YHWH (the enigmatic and unpronounceable designation of Israel's Lord and Saviour) is God, *elohim*, or that YHWH *elohim* does or says this or that, there is a presupposition that we already know something of what *elohim* means. We are saying that the one we identify as the YHWH who does or says this or that is appropriately called *elohim*. An implicit grammar is at work . . . .[34]

Williams's point is that our language presents puzzles that simultaneously (a) challenge our presumptions of the static, universal, or normalizing nature of language while (b) directing us to see ourselves experientially within the middle of these puzzles. "What we live out in our 'ordinary' experience of the world appears under a certain kind of light as profoundly puzzling," and the contemplation of God and His creation amidst this puzzling intellectual climate can lead to the activity of pondering habits of nature such as we see in Ravaisson's work. In this way, Williams sees a "defensible natural theology" as a "discourse that attempted to spot where routine description failed to exhaust what 'needed to be said' (however exactly we spell out the content of this phrase)." Such a discourse is "emphatically" not about providing "explanatory gaps" in the normal sense but is rather about seeking a "faithful description of the world we inhabit" and "respond[ing] to our environment by gesturing towards a context for the description we have engaged in."[35]

While it does not seem that Williams had Ravaisson in mind while addressing such a defensible natural theology, the habits of language Williams ponders align reasonably. The habits of language do not reveal clearcut philosophical protocols as much as they reveal a "bundle of activities, linguistic and symbolic practices"[36] including rituals, prayer, and all other repetitive activities that characterize the phenomenon of language. Within such a context described by Williams, Ravaisson's theological phenomenology and anthropology may rightly be read as an exploration and contemplation of how life – as grace-filled, energized (ενέργεια), intelligent materiality – exists within a hierarchical spiral of love (71).

To be clear, my suggestion for reading Ravaisson within the framework of Williams's defensible natural theology or as a parallel to Christian asceticism does not mean that *Of Habit* is unquestionably free of drastically different approaches such as Shapiro's or Malabou's atheistic or Nietzschean readings referenced above. Moreover, even if the framework of "natural theology" suggested here is deemed reasonable, I agree with Goss and Vitz's discussion of natural law in bioethics that maintains that natural law thinking itself requires the context of the "noetic, liturgical-ascetic moral epistemology" that stems from the way of life in traditional Christianity.[37]

Such clarifications aside, *Of Habit* stands as an illumining exercise in thinking along the lines of Saint Gregory's definition of embodied theology. Perhaps an even more helpful context for Ravaisson's project can be envisioned in Saint Maximus's threefold account of deification or *theosis*. Deification for Saint Maximus starts with the practiced virtues (πρακτική), moves to contemplation of the natural world (θεωρία), and ends properly in theology (θεολογία). This threefold path clarifies both the paradigm and language of what is theology and philosophy simply through the names for these three categories: the first may be termed ascetic or practical philosophy (πρακτική φιλοσοφία), the second is natural philosophy (φυσική φιλοσοφία), and the third is theological philosophy (θεολογική φιλοσοφία).[38] The first stage of acquiring the virtues redirects the passions, forming a desire for God that fuels contemplation.[39] In the second stage, this desire to contemplate God opens deeper dimensions to the study of nature where the inner principles and laws of nature allow the purified man to discern the wisdom and harmony in created nature.[40] With the first two completed, the third stage moves to *theosis* proper and the direct knowledge of God in the fullness of participating in the divine energies.[41] In essence, what Saint Maximus articulates is an ordering of modes of knowledge whereby one seeks with the *nous* after the *logos*, or "essence which lies within every creature" and so finds God, "for from the manifest magnificence of created beings he learns what is the Cause of their being."[42]

Drawing these strands together, the point in suggesting the context of ascetic theology according to Saint Gregory and Saint Maximus for Ravaisson's habit is not an attempt to move outside the terms of his project but to expand it; perhaps it is most fitting to align Ravaisson with Husserl's phenomenology as a framework of general knowledge. If it is left primarily within phenomenology, I remain sympathetic to Ravaisson's Enlightenment critique and analysis of habit, yet as he concludes with a mysterious appeal to "God within us," the question should be asked: how might we read Ravaisson's phenomenology, anthropology, or theological intimations in a way that fittingly addresses that mystery? *Pace* Malabou and Shapiro, this question seems significant toward framing our expectations of what Ravaisson may offer, especially for fields such as bioethics that interact significantly with questions of life – both biological *(bios)* and spiritual *(zoe)* – medicine, religion, and morality. If we abandon or ignore the concluding mystery of Ravaisson's grace-led nature, how are we to think of all that came before? If habit does not reveal "God within us," all Ravaisson's detailed analysis of habit is called into question for the profound reason that, for Ravaisson, the principle revealing morality and nature is one and the same.

## Notes

1  Félix Ravaisson, *Of Habit*, trans. and commentary by Clare Carlisle and Mark Sinclair (London, UK: Continuum, 2009). References to *Of Habit* will be noted in the text and endnotes of this paper in parentheses.

2  Strictly speaking, Ravaisson of course does not speak of his work as "phenomenology" even though his method is to trace the experience and phenomena of intelligence throughout nature. Further, given the implications in Ravaisson's thought for seeking ultimate meaning in nature and humankind, we should equally think of his work in terms of ontology.

3  Ludwig Wittgenstein, *Philosophical Investigations*, trans. G. E. M. Anscombe, P. M. S. Hacker and Joachim Schulte (Oxford, UK: Wiley-Blackwell, 2009), 181 (PI 693). "Wittgenstein was placing his explorations of the epistemological predicament of the self in the context of a narrative which, as it interweaves biblical language with metaphysical dualism, autobiography with doxology, establishes the sense of the 'I' in the sight of God which remains the paradigm for the self even where the theology has been abandoned . . . to probe the epistemological predicament of the soul in the *Confessions* was [for Wittgenstein] to open up a seam in the theological anthropology that has shaped Christian self-understanding since the fifth century." Fergus Kerr, *Theology After Wittgenstein*, 2nd ed. (Oxford, UK: Wiley-Blackwell, 1997), 42; see also 42–45.

4  I discuss such a non-theological reading of Ravaisson in more detail below. See also endnote 18.
5  "Ravaisson redeems habit from Enlightenment detractors who saw it as a stultifying mechanism, recovering the ontological and ethical centrality it had for Aristotle while merging it with a pantheistic Christian metaphysics. His work occupies a key place in post-Kantian philosophy, its influence passing through Hegel to the phenomenology of Heidegger and the vital materialism of Bergson and Deleuze. It therefore provides us with an occasion to reflect on the importance of habit in the philosophy of these later thinkers and in the political thought their work inspires." Kam Shapiro, "Reviving Habit: Félix Ravaisson's Practical Metaphysics," *Theory & Event* 12 no. 4 (2009).
6  Ravaisson clarifies that not all change is the same:

> With the exception of change that brings something from nothing into existence or from existence to nothingness, all change is realized in time; and what brings a habit into being is not simply change understood as modifying the thing, but change understood as occurring in time. . . . Nothing, then, is capable of habit that is not capable of change; but everything capable of change is not by that fact alone capable of habit. A body changes place; but if we throw a body 100 times in the same direction, with the same speed, it still does not contract a habit; it still remains the same as it was with regard to the movement that has been imparted to it 100 times.
>
> (25)

Gaitán and Castresana hence summarize: "The habit, according to Ravaisson, is not possible at the inorganic level (physical, chemical, and mechanical), but it is organically possible. This is because the physical bodies are subject to external influences, i.e., to the general laws of matter, while living things have a nature that remains constant in the midst of change. For this reason, there is individuality only where there is life." Leandro M. Gaitán and Javier S. Castresana, "On Habit and the Mind-Body Problem: The View of Felix Ravaisson," *Frontiers in Human Neuroscience* 8 no. 684 (2014), www.frontiersin.org/articles/10.3389/fnhum.2014.00684/full. See also Aristotle, *Eudemian Ethics*, II.2.
7  For Ravaisson, [these two methodological steps present], "properly speaking, the method of high philosophy, of metaphysics. . . . This intimate constitution of our being which consciousness allows us to know, is found, by analogy, to reside elsewhere, and then everywhere." Continuity cannot be observed directly in the hierarchy of beings – presented in Pt. I of the text – because we do not see the "dispositions or powers" of other beings, and thus the continuity of nature "is only a possibility, an ideality that cannot be demonstrated in nature itself." However, this ideality can be known "by the most powerful of analogies," for it "is presented in the reality of the progression of habit" (p. 65).

(Editor's Introduction, 16)

8  Michael Edward Moore, "Félix Ravaisson, *Of Habit*," *The European Legacy: Toward New Paradigms* 15 no. 6 (2010): 820.
9  The way Ravaisson speaks of moral life as "superior" and a world unto its own may strike some as problematically gnostic, yet Ravaisson's point is not to speak of morality and spiritual realities apart from the body. For Ravaisson, a moral life apart from the body is inconceivable as the "lower limits" of life are necessary for the horizons of the higher. Habit descends and ascends along the whole series of life beings, and "in doing so reveals [an] intimate essence and . . . necessary connection" amongst all things inanimate and animate, bodily and spiritual (67).

10  The editors point out that Ravaisson may be alluding to Saint Paul in Rom. 7.23: "But then I find quite another law in my members which conflicts with the law of my mind" (121 n. 35).

11  A footnote to the text points to Fénelon as the "theologian" in reference (127 n. 61; Fénelon, *De l'exist. de Dieu*, XCII).

12  The analogy between therapy of the soul and body of course stems from a rich classical history in ancient medicine. Ludwig Edelstein, *Ancient Medicine: Selected Papers of Ludwig Edelstein* (Baltimore, MD: Johns Hopkins University Press, 1987); Martha Nussbaum, *The Therapy of Desire: Theory and Practice in Hellenistic Ethics* (Princeton, NJ: Princeton University Press, 1994).

13  H. Tristram Engelhardt, Jr., *The Foundations of Bioethics*, 2nd ed. (New York, NY: Oxford University Press, 1996).

14  Huddle, Kertesz, and Nash argue convincingly that the rationale behind health care institutions excluding (or not) smokers from employment is a distinctively moral issue – hence the lines between a "public health" argument and a "moral" argument are shown to be not as discrete as some might envision. Thomas Huddle, Stefan Kertesz, and Ryan Nash, "Health Care Institutions Should Not Exclude Smokers from Employment," *Academic Medicine* 89 no. 6 (2014): 843–847.

15  Ana Iltis and Mark Cherry, "Bioethics and the Family: Family Building in the Twenty-First Century," *Christian Bioethics* 21 no. 2 (2015): 135–143.

16  Admittedly, envisioning such a theological turn in modern, Western medicine is difficult. To step outside the modern, secular life-world of Western medicine is nothing short of a worldview paradigm shift akin to Michael Hanby's *No God, No Science? Theology, Cosmology, Biology* (Oxford, UK: Wiley-Blackwell, 2013). Hanby's radical work seeks to recover a pre-Baconian, pre-Galilean, and theologically grounded metaphysics of science.

17  Drew Leder, ed., *The Body in Medical Thought and Practice* (Dordrecht, The Netherlands: Kluwer Academic Publishers, 1992); Richard M. Zaner, *Ethics and the Clinical Encounter* (Englewood Cliffs, NJ: Prentice Hall, 1988); George Agich, "A Phenomenological Approach to Bioethics," in *Case Analysis in Clinical Ethics*, eds. Richard Ashcroft, Anneke Lucassen, Michael Parker, Marian Verkerk, and Guy Widdershoven (New York, NY: Cambridge University Press, 2005), 187–200.

18  See Malabou's preface to Carlisle and Sinclair's English translation of Ravaisson's work. Malabou acknowledges Ravaisson's spiritualism while seeing habit as a nearly autonomous force of mutation. She picks up particularly on Ravaisson's inclusion of tics and illness within habit to highlight the open-ended self-determination in habit (vii–xx). Shapiro, also, does not hesitate to imagine Ravaisson without Christian grace, suggesting instead an "Epicurean gratitude for the chance arrangement of atoms that give life and pleasure." Shapiro, "Reviving Habit."

19  "Ravaisson will admit, at the end of Part I, that it is only in reflecting on our own experience that we can gain a full and adequate grasp of habit, but here habit is discussed without any deliberate reference to the human being – nor, for that matter, to any particular being at all" (Editor's Commentary, 78).

20  Jean-Yves Lacoste, *From Theology to Theological Thinking*, trans. W. Chris Hackett (Charlottesville: University of Virginia Press, 2014).

21  Ibid., 67.

22  Ibid., 1.

23  Ibid., 2.

24  For these interpretations, see Malabou's preface (xvi–xx) and Shapiro, "Reviving Habit." Malabou's "plasticity" reading may gain some ground, and yet we do well to remember that everything in Ravaisson pivots on the distinction

between good and bad habits, one that is not merely a human, subjective distinction. Nature for Ravaisson must be understood teleologically, and as "laws" are secondary to habits, the understanding of what is a good habit for us is not merely mechanical. Malabou's reading seems a stretch within the internal logic of Ravaisson's system.

25 See also Pierre Hadot, *Philosophy as a Way of Life*, ed. Arnold I. Davidson and trans. Michael Chase (Oxford, UK: Wiley-Blackwell, 1995); John Milbank, *Theology and Social Theory*, 2nd ed. (Oxford, UK: Wiley-Blackwell, 2006).
26 Likewise, it would be informative to pursue in detail the genealogy of when the term "theologian" came into more common use following the first centuries of Christianity.
27 Kallistos Ware, "The Way of the Ascetics: Negative or Affirmative?," in *Asceticism*, eds. Vincent Wimbush and Richard Valantasis (Oxford, UK: Oxford University Press, 1995), 3.
28 Ibid., 8.
29 Ibid., 13.
30 Saint Gregory of Nazianzus, *On God and Christ*, trans. Lionel R. Wickham and Frederick Williams (Crestwood, NY: St. Vladimir's Seminary Press, 2002), Oration 28.1.
31 Ibid., Oration 27.3.
32 Maximus the Confessor, *Capita theologica et oeconomica* I.42 in *Philokalia*, vol. 2, ed. Saint Nikokimos of the Holy Mountain and Saint Makarios of Corinth and trans. G. E. H. Palmer, Philip Sherrard, and Kallistos Ware (London, UK: Faber & Faber, 1977), 173.
33 Rowan Williams, *The Edge of Words: God and the Habits of Language* (London, UK: Bloomsbury Publishing, 2014).
34 Ibid., 6.
35 Ibid., 8.
36 Ibid., 9.
37 Boaz Goss and Rico Vitz, "Natural Law among Moral Strangers," *Christian Bioethics* 20 no. 2 (2014): 283–300. Furthermore, *pace* Rowan Williams's nuanced exploration of a defensible natural theology, the history of natural theology's paralleling natural science remains an issue when adopting the term natural theology. Such an enterprise seems inevitably bound at some level to presuppose a univocity of being and some form of shared rationality between God and man. In however subtle a way, the inherent danger remains that one turns to methods of science and theoretical philosophy to substantiate theological thinking.
38 Maximus the Confessor, *Capita theologica et oeconomica*, 2.94, 96; cf. Frederick Aquino, "The *Philokalia* and Regulative Virtue Epistemology: A Look at Maximus the Confessor," in *The Philokalia: Exploring the Classic Text of Orthodox Spirituality*, eds. Brock Bingaman and Bradley Nassif (New York, NY: Oxford University Press, 2012), 240–251.
39 Maximus the Confessor, *Capita theologica et oeconomica* 1.37, in *Philokalia*, vol. 2, 122. See also Aquino, "The *Philokalia* and Regulative Virtue Epistemology," 243.
40 Maximus the Confessor, *Capita de caritate* 3.24, in *Philokalia*, vol. 2, 86.
41 Maximus the Confessor, *Capita de caritate* 2.26, in *Philokalia*, vol. 2, 69.
42 Maximus the Confessor, in *Philokalia*, vol. 2, 189.

# 3 Judaism on the body and the practice of medicine

*Elliot N. Dorff*

## Why visions matter

American Jews inherit two perspectives on life – that of Judaism (the Jewish side of their identity) and that of Western liberalism (the American side of their identity). In American liberalism, medicine is a pragmatic way to respond to physical and mental illness. In Judaism, physicians are nothing less than the agents and partners of God in preventing and curing diseases. Americans generally appreciate and trust their physicians, but in Judaism doctors are held in even higher esteem, and both clinical care and medical research are strongly encouraged. This perception of medicine affects the way Jews understand the respective roles of patients and physicians as well as the extent to which they think that society as a whole has a vested interest in, and a responsibility for, providing health care.

In my book *Matters of Life and Death: A Jewish Approach to Modern Medical Ethics*,[1] I have described this Jewish view of medicine in some detail and applied it to a range of issues in modern medical practice. In this essay, I will borrow from that discussion as I describe the picture that emerges from Jewish reflection on the body. While in the book I focus on the moral issues that arise at the beginning and end of life and on the distribution of health care, in this essay I will elaborate on how Judaism perceives the profession of the physician and examine some of its tensions and moral conundrums from a Jewish point of view.

## The body in Jewish sources

### The body belongs to God

Jewish sources maintain that God owns everything, including our bodies.[2] God loans our bodies to us for the duration of our lives, and we return them to God when we die. Medieval Jewish thinkers disagree as to whether after death we are resurrected in bodily form, as Saadia Gaon (882–942, Babylonia [modern-day Iraq]) maintains, or whether we are resurrected only in a spiritual body, as Maimonides (1135–1204, Spain and Egypt) sometimes appears to claim.[3] Modern Jews and Jewish thinkers disagree as to whether the classical doctrine of resurrection after death is to be believed literally, metaphorically, or not at all.[4] In any case, in this life neither men nor women have the right to govern their bodies as they will; because God created our bodies and owns them, God can and does assert the right to restrict how we use our bodies according to the rules articulated in Jewish law.

One set of these rules requires us to take reasonable care of our bodies. Just as we would be obliged to take reasonable care of an apartment on loan to us, so too we have the duty to take care of our own bodies. Rules of good hygiene, sleep, exercise, and diet are not just words to the wise designed for our comfort and longevity but rather commanded acts that we owe God. For example, Hillel regards bathing as a commandment (*mitzvah*), and Maimonides includes his directives for good health in his code of law, considering them just as obligatory as other positive duties like caring for the poor.[5]

Just as we are commanded to maintain good health, so we are obligated to avoid danger and injury.[6] Indeed, Jewish law views endangering one's health as worse than violating a ritual prohibition.[7] So, for example, anyone who can survive only by taking charity but refuses to do so out of pride is, according to the tradition, shedding his or her own blood and is thus guilty of a mortal offense.[8] Similarly, Conservative, Reform, and some Orthodox authorities have prohibited smoking as an unacceptable risk to our God-owned bodies.[9]

Judaism also teaches that human beings do not have the right to dispose of their bodies at will (i.e., commit suicide), for to do so would totally obliterate something that belongs not to us but to God.[10] This extends to inanimate property as well: we may use what we need, but we may not destroy any more of God's world than we need to in order to accomplish our purposes in life.[11]

### *Being created in God's image imparts value to life, regardless of the individual's physical or mental level of capacity or incapacity*

The Torah declares that God created each of us in the divine image: "God created the human being in His image, in the image of God He created him; male and female God created them" (Gen. 1:27).[12] Exactly which feature of the human being reflects this divine image is a matter of debate within the tradition. The Torah itself seems to tie it to humanity's ability to make moral judgments – that is, to distinguish good from bad and right from wrong, to behave accordingly, and to judge one's own actions and those of others on the basis of this moral knowledge.[13] Another human faculty connected by the Torah and by the later tradition to divinity is the ability to speak.[14] Maimonides claims that the divine image resides in our capacity to think, especially discursively.[15] Locating the divine image within us may also be the Torah's way of acknowledging that we can love, just as God does,[16] or that we are at least partially spiritual and thus share God's spiritual nature.[17]

Not only does this doctrine describe aspects of our nature, it also pre-
scribes behavior founded on moral imperatives. Specifically, because human
beings are created in God's image, we affront God when we insult another
person.[18] More broadly, we must recognize each individual's uniqueness and
divine worth because all human beings embody the image of God:

> For this reason Adam was created as a single person, to teach you that
> anyone who destroys one soul is described in Scripture as if he destroyed
> an entire world, and anyone who sustains one soul is described in Scrip-
> ture as if he sustained an entire world. . . . And to declare the greatness
> of the Holy One, praised be He, for a person uses a mold to cast a num-
> ber of coins, and they are all similar to each other, while the Sovereign
> of all sovereigns, the Holy One, praised be He, cast each person in the
> mold of the first human being and none is similar to any other. There-
> fore each and every person must say: "For me the world was created."[19]

No amount of ability or disability is relevant to the divine value in each
of us. The tradition mandates that we recite a blessing when seeing someone
with a disability: "Praised are you, Lord our God, *meshaneh ha-briyyot*, who
makes different creatures," or "who created us different." Precisely when
we might recoil from a deformed or incapacitated person, or thank God for
not making us like that, the tradition instead bids us to embrace the divine
image in such people – indeed, to bless God for creating some of us so.[20]
Treating others as images of God thus has significant moral implications.

### The human being is an integrated whole, combining one's body, mind, emotions, and will, and must be viewed within his or her social and cultural context

Western philosophical thought and Christianity have been heavily influenced
by the Greek and Gnostic bifurcation of body and mind (or soul). In these
systems of thought, the body is seen as the inferior part of human beings,
either because it is what we share with animals in contrast to the mind which
is distinctively human (Aristotle) or because the body is the seat of our passions and hence our sins (Paul in Romans and Galatians[21]), whereas the
soul can be saved. The Greeks glorified the body in their art and sculpture,
but that was only because developing the body was a means to an end, a
necessary prerequisite to cultivating the mind (as, for example, in Plato's
pedagogic program in *The Republic*). Similarly, Paul regarded the body as
"the temple of the Holy Spirit" (1 Cor. 6:19) but only because it serves to
sustain the soul so that it can accept faith in Jesus; the body *per se* "makes
me a prisoner of that law of sin which lives inside my body" (Rom. 7:23).

These views articulated in Western and Christian classics have shaped
these traditions from ancient times to our own. In Christianity, Augustine,
Luther, and Calvin, following the lead of Paul, all maintain that the body's

needs are to be suppressed as much as possible; indeed, asceticism has been a recurring and honored practice in Christian history.[22] In secular philosophic thought, "the mind-body problem" continues to be a stock issue in philosophic literature – i.e., how is it that the two, presumed to be so obviously different and separate, are related in some ways to each other?

Because Jews in ancient and medieval times lived among and interacted with Greeks, Romans, Gnostics, and Christians, Judaism was inevitably influenced by these conceptions. Two of the most prominent Jewish thinkers to reflect these influences are Philo, a Jew writing in first-century Alexandria – a city avidly pursuing Greek thought – and Maimonides, a twelfth-century Jewish philosopher who effectively translated Aristotle into Jewish terms. Such Jewish thinkers echo the widespread Greek and Christian notions that the soul is divine and the body animal; Philo even calls the body the "prison house" of the soul, as do many of his Hellenistic contemporaries in Alexandria. Philo and Maimonides also draw some of the same moral conclusions as their non-Jewish counterparts, defining the ideal life as one that cultivates the soul and abstains from the pleasures of the body as much as possible.[23]

In contrast, the Bible and the classical Rabbis of the Mishnah, Talmud, and Midrash – commonly referred to as "the Rabbis," with a capital "R," in contrast to "rabbis" with a lower-case "r," which is used to refer to their medieval and modern successors – do not share in this understanding of the human being. The Bible speaks of a person's *nefesh*, which translators often render "soul" but which actually has many meanings (including bodily parts like the throat). Even when the word specifically refers to a person's inner being, it stands in contrast not to the body but to a person's identity in the outside world. In this sense, the relevant correlatives in the pair are *shem* – that is, a person's name, or public identity, within the community – and *nefesh* – his or her inner being, self-identity, and private thoughts. Another Hebrew term often translated "soul" is *neshamah*, which, in its narrowest meanings, denotes "breath" but, more broadly, means one's inner being, roughly equivalent to that meaning of *nefesh*.

In the Talmud and Midrash, our soul is, in some senses, separable from our body. For example, when the Torah says that God "blew the breath of life into his [Adam's] nostrils" (Gen. 2:7), Rabbinic sources understand that to mean not only physical life but consciousness. God repeats that process each day when taking our souls away during sleep and returning them to us again when we awake. Moreover, according to one strain of Jewish thought, at death the soul leaves the body only to be united with it again at the time of resurrection. So, for example:

> Our Rabbis taught: There are three partners in [the creation of] a person: the Holy One, blessed be He; his father; and his mother. His father supplies the source of the white substance [probably because semen is white] out of which are formed [white things like] the child's bones,

sinews, nails, the brain in his head, and the white in his eye. His mother supplies the source of the red substance [probably because menstrual blood is red] out of which are formed his skin, flesh, hair, blood, and the black of his eye. And the Holy One, blessed be He, gives him breath [*ru'ah*] and spirit [*neshamah*], beauty of features, eyesight, the power of hearing, the ability to speak and to walk, understanding, and discernment. When his time to depart from the world approaches, the Holy One, blessed be He, takes away His share and leaves the shares of his father and mother.[24]

Similarly, when the morning prayer "*Elohai Neshamah*" thanks God for returning us to life after death, it is analogizing sleep with death and the return to consciousness with the renewal of life within "dead corpses" (the Hebrew words are deliberately redundant): "My God, the life-breath [soul; Hebrew: *neshamah*] You have given me is pure. You created it, You fashioned it, You breathed it into me, You preserve it within me [that is, You keep my body and soul together], and one day You will take it from me and return it to me in the future that is to come [after death]. So long as this life-breath is in me I thank You, Lord, my God, and God of my ancestors, Ruler of all creation, and Sovereign of all life-breaths [souls]. Praised are You, Lord, who returns life-breaths to dead corpses."[25] Rabbinic sources conflict, however, as to whether the soul can exist apart from the body, and even those who say it can exist independently depict the soul in physical terms, capable of performing many of the functions of the body.[26] Even according to this latter group, the body and soul are one, thoroughly intertwined entity.

In any case, in sharp contrast to strains within the Greek and Christian traditions, classical Rabbinic sources maintain that the soul is not superior to the body. One Rabbinic source speaks of the soul as a guest in the body here on earth: one's host must accordingly be respected and well treated.[27] Moreover, since the Rabbis regarded the human being as an integrated whole, the body and the soul are to be judged as one: "The Holy Blessed One brings the soul and throws it into the body and judges them as one."[28] Furthermore, although the Rabbis emphasized the importance of studying and following the Torah, even placing it on a par with all of the rest of the commandments,[29] they nonetheless believed that the life of the soul or mind by itself is not good, that it can be the source of sin: "An excellent thing is the study of Torah combined with some worldly occupation, for the labor demanded by both of them causes sinful inclinations to be forgotten. All study of Torah without work must, in the end, be futile and become the cause of sin."[30] In nineteenth-century Germany, when the government paid full-time clergy, the rabbinate took on many new tasks and became a way that people earned a living; before then, both the classical Rabbis and medieval and early modern rabbis earned their livelihood doing other things. Some of the classical Rabbis, for example, worked as shepherds, blacksmiths, or shoemakers; in medieval France, many were involved in producing wine.

This Jewish view of the body and soul being integrated has a direct effect on how Judaism understands mental illness and the care of people who suffer from it. Largely because Jews needed to determine when a person could be held legally responsible, Rabbinic sources seek to determine a definition – or at least some clear examples – of who is considered "insane."[31] Despite a strong emphasis on intellectual activity within the Jewish tradition, it does not see insane people or those with limited intellectual capacity as any less human than sane and intelligent people. It also sees mental and emotional health – and efforts to help people who have difficulties in those areas – as just as important as physical health.[32] The heavy involvement of Jews in psychiatry, psychology, and social work is evidence of this Jewish tenet, one that graphically illustrates the Jewish concern with both the body and the inner parts of our being – our mind, our emotions, and our will.

Furthermore, in medical contexts, this integration of our body, mind, emotions, and will and the family and social context that shapes a given person and his or her health situation mean that physicians need to see their patients not simply as bodies but as people. This is the goal, for example, of the element of the curriculum at UCLA Medical School called "Doctoring," required of all medical students all four years of medical school and created in the early 1990s by a committee of four faculty members, all of whom happened to be Jewish. The program consists of a series of specific cases in which the patient's social and economic status and/or religious and moral convictions play a significant role in the etiology of the person's illness (or other medical issue) and its potential cures or resolutions. For example, one of the cases in the curriculum is a fifteen-year-old female who visits your office complaining of stomach problems. You, the doctor, examine her and find that she has no stomach problems whatsoever; she is just pregnant. From a purely physical point of view, it would be better if she were eighteen or older, but at fifteen, if she is otherwise in good health and if she is monitored adequately during her pregnancy, she and the fetus will probably be fine. But in the case, the woman is unmarried, Catholic, and Hispanic, and all her health outcomes and those of her fetus will depend on those factors. The fact that she is Catholic probably means that an abortion is not a possibility, but not all Catholics agree with their Church on this teaching. Assuming she is not going to abort, will she get kicked out of her house because she got pregnant out of wedlock? If so, where will she live while she is pregnant? Given that she is Hispanic, she probably will not be forced out of her home, but will she give up the child for adoption or raise it herself, perhaps with the help of her family? Will she be able to finish high school? Where is the father of the child in all of this?

### The body is morally neutral and potentially good

The body is neither bad nor good. Rather, its energies, like those of our other faculties, are morally neutral. But the body, like all our other faculties, can and should be used for divine purposes as defined by Jewish law and tradition. Within these constraints, the body's pleasures are God-given and are not to be shunned, for to do so would be an act of ingratitude toward our Creator. The body, in other words, can and should give us pleasure to the extent that such pleasure enables us to live a life of holiness. In fact, according to the Rabbis, it is a sin to deny ourselves the pleasures that God's law allows. Just as the Nazirite was to bring a sin offering after denying himself the permitted delight of wine, so we will be called to account in the World to Come (here meaning life after death) for the ingratitude and haughtiness involved in denying ourselves the pleasures that God has provided.[33]

The Jewish mode for attaining holiness is thus not to endure pain but rather to use all our faculties, including our bodily energies, to perform God's commandments. For example, though we eat as all animals do, our eating takes on a divine dimension when we observe Jewish dietary restrictions and surround our meals with the appropriate blessings. Some bodily pleasures are even commanded. With the exception of Yom Kippur, the Day of Atonement, we may not fast on the Sabbath, and we must eat three meals to celebrate it. We should also bathe and wear clean clothes in honor of the day.[34] Sexual intercourse in marriage is commanded not only for purposes of propagation but also to enhance the spouses' mutual enjoyment.[35] Marital union thus not only produces the next generation but also strengthens the couple's bond to each other, a benefit not only for the couple but also for the children, for the people involved in a strong marriage are more likely to have the emotional strength to nurture and educate their children, both emotionally and Jewishly.

According to Maimonides, bodily pleasures are most appropriately enjoyed when we have the specific intent to enhance our ability to do God's will:

> He who regulates his life in accordance with the laws of medicine with the sole motive of maintaining a sound and vigorous physique and begetting children to do his work and labor for his benefit is not following the right course. A man should aim to maintain physical health and vigor in order that his soul may be upright, in a condition to know God. . . . Whoever throughout his life follows this course will be continually serving God, even while engaged in business and even during cohabitation, because his purpose in all that he does will be to satisfy his needs so as to have a sound body with which to serve God. Even when he sleeps and seeks repose to calm his mind and rest his body so as not to fall sick and be incapacitated from serving God, his sleep is service of the Almighty.[36]

The medical implications of this teaching are clear. We have the obligation to maintain our health not only to care for God's property but also so that we can accomplish our purpose in life: to live a life of holiness. Moreover, because pain is not a way to attain holiness, it is our duty to relieve it.

*Jews are not only permitted but obliged to pursue medical
interventions to avoid or cure diseases, so physicians are
members of an honored profession*

Because God owns our bodies, we are obliged to do what we can to escape
sickness, injury, and death and to help other people do so as well.[37] We
are to help others do this not for some general (and vague) humanitarian
reason or for reasons of anticipated reciprocity. Nor are physicians obliged
to heal the sick to honor a special oath they take, to pay back the society that trained them, or to fulfill a contractual promise that they make in
return for remuneration. Rather, we have a duty to heal others because we
are all under the divine imperative to help God preserve and protect what
is God's.

This is neither the only possible conclusion to be derived from the Bible
nor the obvious one. On the one hand, the Torah says that illness is one of
the divine punishments for disobedience; on the other hand, God announces
Himself as our healer in many places in the Bible.[38] We might conclude that
medicine is an improper human intervention in God's decision to cause illness or cure it, indeed an act of human hubris. Although the Rabbis were
aware of this line of reasoning, they counteracted it by pointing out that
God Himself not only authorizes us to heal but commands that we do so,
basing their assertions on two biblical verses: Exod. 21:19–20 (according to
which an assailant must ensure that his victim is "thoroughly healed") and
Deut. 22:2 ("And you shall restore the lost property to him"). The Talmud
understands the Exodus verse as giving permission for the physician to cure.
(It further argues that the command to "Love your neighbor as yourself" in
Lev. 19:18 even permits curative measures that require inflicting a wound
in the process.) The Talmud interprets the Deuteronomy passage to include
the obligation to restore another person's body as well as his or her property, hence there is an obligation to come to the aid of someone else in a
life-threatening situation.[39]

The following midrash is a beautiful Rabbinic response to the theological problem of balancing God's role in healing with that of physicians. It
asserts, as does Jewish law, that engaging in medicine is not a violation
of God's prerogatives but rather exactly what God would have us do in a
divine-human partnership:

> It once happened that Rabbi Ishmael and Rabbi Akiva were strolling in
> the streets of Jerusalem accompanied by another person. They were met
> by a sick person. He said to them, "My masters, tell me by what means
> I may be cured." They told him, "Do thus and so until you are cured."
> The sick man asked them, "And who afflicted me?" They replied, "The
> Holy One, blessed be He." The sick man responded, "You have entered
> into a matter which does not pertain to you. God has afflicted, and you
> seek to cure! Are you not transgressing His will?"

Rabbi Akiva and Rabbi Ishmael asked him, "What is your occupation?" The sick man answered, "I am a tiller of the soil, and here is the sickle in my hand." They asked him, "Who created the vineyard?" "The Holy One, blessed be He," he answered. Rabbi Akiva and Rabbi Ishmael said to him, "You enter into a matter which does not pertain to you! God created the vineyard, and you cut fruits from it."

He said to them, "Do you not see the sickle in my hand? If I did not plow, sow, fertilize, and weed, nothing would sprout."

Rabbi Akiva and Rabbi Ishmael said to him, "Foolish man! . . . Just as if one does not weed, fertilize, and plow, the trees will not produce fruit, and if fruit is produced but is not watered or fertilized, it will not live but die, so with regard to the body. Drugs and medications are the fertilizer, and the physician is the tiller of the soil."[40]

Ultimately, Rabbi Joseph Caro (1488–1575), the author of one of the most important Jewish legal codes, the *Shulḥan Arukh*, teaches this: "The Torah gave permission to the physician to heal; moreover, this is a religious precept and is included in the category of saving life, and if the physician withholds his services, it is considered as shedding blood."[41] This positive – indeed, mandatory – view of medicine has led Jews to be downright aggressive in the use of medicine, and it has also led Jews to honor doctors – to the extent that historically many rabbis have also been physicians.[42]

### Our bodies are mortal

There are, however, clear limits to both the ability of physicians to heal and their license to try to do so. The ultimate limit to medical practice is the fact that our bodies are mortal, a fact recognized already in the Garden of Eden story (Gen. 3:22) and later in the biblical book of Ecclesiastes: "There is a time to give birth and a time to die" (Eccles. 3:2). Furthermore, although physicians were unable to cure most diseases or even help people manage them until recently in human history, preventive medicine was quite good, beginning with such measures as quarantine for communicable diseases (Lev. 13–14) and extending to Rabbinic recommendations about limiting the amount of meat one eats while eating plenty of fruits and vegetables.[43] Physicians' ability to cure diseases, however, was very limited, largely taking the form of blood-letting, which cures only polycythemia, and surgery, which often led to the death of the patient through losing too much blood or infections. With major advances in medicine over the last century, however, physicians, patients, and families now often face the question of how much, if at all, to intervene to extend life, particularly when it is painful and compromised.

### The roles of physicians and patients in determining therapy

In light of doctors' expertise, patients must follow the physician's instructions in taking care of their bodies; to do otherwise would be to be derelict in their duty to God to preserve and protect God's property. This might produce a very paternalistic view of the physician-patient relationship, for the doctor's instructions are no less than God's! (Many physicians, I am sure, would love their patients to follow their orders that way, just as rabbis sometimes wish that their congregants would accept their authority as the *mara d'atra*, the master of the community, without question.) In the Mishnaic period, though, when a positive attitude toward medicine was first being formed, it was clear that the doctor had to enlist the cooperation of the patient if the doctor had any realistic hope that his or her orders would be followed (and contemporary doctors and rabbis need to learn this as well). Moreover, Jewish sources recognize patient authority on some aspects of their care.

Thus, the Talmud tells the story of Rabbi Judah, President of the Sanhedrin and editor of the Mishnah, and his doctor, Samuel Yarḥina'a. The rabbi was afflicted with an eye disease, and the physician suggested an injection into the area, but the rabbi objected: "I cannot endure it." The doctor then proposed a salve, which the rabbi also refused. Finally, the doctor suggested a third treatment, and the rabbi agreed to the therapy.[44]

In another case probing the relative authority of the patient and physician, the Mishnah permits feeding a sick person on the fast of Yom Kippur (and, by extension, any of the other fast days of the Jewish liturgical calendar) "on the basis of [the opinion of] experts."[45] The Talmud makes explicit how the process of justifying eating on the fast must work:

> Rabbi Yannai asserts that if the patient says, "I need food," while the physician says, "He does not need it," we listen to the patient. What is the reason? "The heart knows its own bitterness" (Prov. 14:10). . . . If the physician says, "He needs it," while the patient says that he does not need it, we listen to the physician. Why? [We presume] that stupor seized him [so that he does not feel the lack of food].[46]

On the other hand, with regard to medication Rabbi David Ben Zimra (1479–1573) rules this: "If the patient says, 'I need a certain medication,' and the physician says, 'He does not need it,' one listens to the patient. But if the physician says that the medication will harm him, one listens to the physician."[47] In modern times, this would mean, for example, that despite a patient's request for an antibiotic, physicians should not prescribe one for viral infections because every medication comes with side effects; the antibiotic may actually harm the patient, who may, for example, be allergic to it. Moreover, the physician has a duty to public health, and overuse of antibiotics has already meant that some drugs no longer work on patients who formerly could have benefited from them. With regard to food, however, Rabbi Ben Zimra rules that one listens to the patient even if the physician says that it will harm him,[48] presumably because patients know something about food but must bow to the medical expertise of physicians with regard to medications.

This is a far cry from modern American medicine, in which patients own their bodies and thus patient autonomy is the gold standard of medical care – to the extent that doctors have trouble asserting their opinion that a given intervention makes no medical sense, and efforts to define "futile care" to enable them to do that have encountered many difficulties. In Jewish tradition, the doctor is still in charge. Physicians, though, must recognize that their authority is persuasive, not coercive, so they must enlist the cooperation of the people they would serve if they have any reasonable hope of serving them effectively. (The same is true for rabbis.)

## The roles of the family and community in aiding physicians and their patients

Recognizing the patient as a person, though, is not limited to the person whom the physician sees in his or her practice. American ideology emphasizes our individual rights and freedoms; Judaism speaks of the divine worth of each individual as created in the image of God, but it puts great emphasis on the familial and communal context in which we live.[49] People, after all, usually live in families and communities, and those contexts can aid or hinder physicians in their work. We have good evidence, for example, that married men are more likely to see a physician when sick than bachelors are and as a result live longer then their unmarried counterparts do.[50] Hospice care was developed in the last several decades precisely to enlist the aid of family members, social workers, clergy, and friends as well as doctors and nurses in the care of the dying.

It is primarily in the commandment to visit the sick (*biqqur holim*), though, that Judaism manifests its recognition that neither doctors nor patients exist in isolation and that overcoming a patient's illness depends on cooperation not only between physicians and patients but also by the people who make up the context of the patient. Because visiting the sick, especially in hospitals, is seldom experienced as a pleasant task, the tradition mandates that we do this by making it a commandment. Maimonides codifies the law this way: "Visiting the sick is an obligation incumbent on everyone. Even the great [those of high social status] visit the small [those of low social status]. And we should visit many times each day, and all who add visits are to be praised as long as they do not burden [the sick person]. And anyone who visits the sick is as if he took away a part of his illness and made things easier for him; anyone who fails to visit the sick is as if he sheds blood."[51] To fulfill this law, many synagogues establish "*Biqqur Holim* Groups," consisting of volunteers who make sure that even those lacking family and friends who regularly visit them will have someone to pay attention to them, and not just medically.

The commandment to visit the sick is based in Jewish sources on the model of God Himself, who visited Abraham after his circumcision.[52] A Jew is supposed to visit the sick not only to support the patient psychologically and to fulfill the commandment but to imitate God's own example.

The commandment is a recognition of the fact that illness is *isolating*. A person's family and friends will not see the patient in the usual settings; they will need to make a special effort to see the person, and not everyone can or will do that. The Jewish tradition, however, knew that people need company, that, in the words of Genesis explaining why God created Eve, "It is not good for man to be alone" (Gen. 2:18). Short of execution or torture, solitary confinement is the harshest penalty in prison, and patients do not deserve punishment. Seeing them as persons and not just as malfunctioning bodies requires that family and friends visit them to overcome this sense of isolation.

Illness is also, of course, *debilitating*. Recognizing this, Maimonides, himself a physician as well as a rabbi and a philosopher, wrote this in his law code about how one should visit a patient – even when serving as the person's doctor: "One who enters a room to visit a sick person [who is lying on the ground with his or her head on a pillow] should not sit on the bed or on a chair or a bench or in an elevated place or above the sick person's head but rather should wrap himself in humility [for, according to the Talmud (*Shabbat* 12b), 'the Presence of God rests above the head of a sick person'] and sit lower than the sick person's head [in this case, by lying on the ground without a pillow] and ask God's mercy for him before leaving."[53] After quoting this, Rabbi Joseph Caro, in his later code, adds: "This, though, applies only when the ill person is lying on the ground such that a visitor who sits will be higher than him or her; but if the patient is lying on a bed, it is permissible to sit on a chair."[54] Notice, though, that all visitors, including physicians, were not allowed to stand in the patient's presence because that body language communicates that the person standing is powerful and the patient is not, and the last thing that a person should do when visiting the sick is to reinforce their sense of disability any more than their illness already has.

Illness is also *infantilizing*. In robbing someone of what he or she was able to do before, sickness makes one feel like a child or even, as in the case of incontinence, an infant. Moreover, illness is *boring*; one cannot do what normally occupies one's day and week, so one seeks anything that will pass the time in an interesting way. Both patients and their visitors tire of talking about the food and the weather very quickly.

To counteract both the sense of diminishment that illness conveys and its boredom, *visitors should talk about the same adult topics that they would discuss with the ill person if he or she were not sick*, whether that is the family, business, politics, sports, movies, novels, synagogue affairs, or anything else that would normally be discussed. One can even do things that will stretch the minds of the ill to consider things they had never studied before, for unless a person suffers from a mental illness like Alzheimer's or another form of dementia, the mind continues to like to be stimulated. I once taught four sessions on Jewish theology to a group at the Jewish Home for the Aged, and when I asked the social worker why the residents wanted this topic, she said, "Because they are sick of Bingo!" None of the residents had studied Jewish theology previously, but they all read the assignment for each lesson, and they energetically and enthusiastically interacted with me during those sessions. Adult conversation, even on subjects unfamiliar to patients, can capture their interest and reinforce a sense of dignity and adulthood in them.

The Jewish tradition also provides visitors with another suggestion, especially for visiting patients with chronic illnesses who can benefit from a long-term agenda for conversations – namely, help the patient create an ethical will. A product of Jews of the Middle Ages, ethical wills were originally letters that a parent wrote to his or her children, and it can still take that form. Nowadays, though, many instead use an audiotape or a videotape. An ethical will includes the family story; this involves helping the patient recall early memories of childhood, including descriptions and stories of all the relatives, as well as the patient's account of his or her later life. Ethical wills commonly include mention of the person's convictions and moral values (hence the name "ethical will") as well as his or her suggestions and hopes for the future of the family and expressions of love. Even if the person's adult children may be tired of hearing the stories, the patient's grandchildren will eagerly want such a record. Patients who know that someone is coming to help them with this project have a real reason to get up in the morning and look forward to the day, for they are clearly doing something meaningful. This will help combat the depression and boredom that typically accompany long-term illness. Conversely, because creating such a document or tape can take days or weeks, it helps visitors pass the time and even look forward to the visits. Physicians can suggest this to their Jewish patients – and to their non-Jewish patients as well.[55]

## The limits of medicine

The very first time I heard a doctor say that he needed not only to seek to cure but to care occurred when I was serving on the first Jewish Hospice Commission in the nation, created in Los Angeles in 1983. The physician, Lawrence Heifetz, is an oncologist who specializes in brain surgery. He told me that at the time some three-quarters of the cases he saw he could not cure, but he realized that even when he could not cure, he could care. That is what motivated him to be involved in creating a hospice option at Cedars-Sinai Medical Center, on whose staff he served at the time.

Hospice care is not, of course, for everyone facing major health problems. Moreover, the Jewish demand that we seek to cure as God's agents and partners in healing makes Jews very aggressive in seeking medical cures for whatever ails them. Jews, like everyone else, know that we are all mortal, but they assume that doctors can do a great deal to overcome illness and postpone death.

For most Jews, then, hospice care is counterintuitive. By definition it involves accepting that one has a terminal, incurable disease and that the goal of medical care now is comfort rather than cure. This violates the fighting spirit that most Jews bring to their ailments.

The problem, of course, is the old Kantian dilemma: When we cannot do something, we never ask whether we should, but when we can do something, we must ask the moral question of whether we should, for there are many things that we can do that we should not do. Modern medicine now has the ability to keep many people alive who otherwise would have died. In many cases, these new medical abilities are indeed a blessing. Increasingly, though, our ability to sustain a person's life is not in the patient's best interest – when, for example, the patient is suffering from bone cancer with pain that cannot be quelled, when the patient is in a persistent vegetative state, or when the patient has experienced the failure of multiple body systems and is actively in the process of dying. In such cases, even Jews, who are accustomed to fighting diseases with whatever medicine has to offer, have come to realize that sometimes the more moral option is to alleviate suffering and let nature take its course. Rabbis – especially Orthodox rabbis – have been slower to recognize the limits of medicine, and some insist on doing everything possible to keep a person's body functioning, whether it is in the best interests of the patient or not.[56] In my mind, though, treating the patient as a person requires that we take the moral responsibility to know when to stop trying to interfere with the natural process of dying and, in the name of the welfare of the patient, provide hospice care instead.[57]

The other area where Jews are reticent to recognize the limits of medicine is infertility. Because Jews go to college and graduate school in far higher percentages than the general American population,[58] they postpone marriage until their late twenties or thirties. That is good for fulfilling the Jewish value of education – although that value also insists that Jews learn about their own heritage and not just what they will need for their career. As we have increasingly come to recognize, however, both men and women are most fertile in their late teens and twenties, and increased exposure to higher education has not changed that. As a result, a significant percentage of Jewish couples suffer from infertility, not so much as a function of Jewish genetic diseases but as the outcome of waiting too long to have children. This is clearly a problem for the couples themselves, and many who are experiencing these problems need counseling to keep their marriage intact despite the pressures and disappointments that are usually involved in facing infertility. It is also a problem for the Jewish people, as the fertility rate of American Jews now stands at 1.9, which is well below the replacement level of 2.1 and general U.S. fertility rate of 2.2.[59] Add to that assimilation and intermarriage and there are major concerns about whether the Jewish people, and the Jewish tradition, will survive in generations to come.

This makes Jews particularly interested in overcoming infertility with artificial reproductive techniques (ARTs), and rabbis have generally been supportive if they are using their own gametes and warier about using donor gametes.[60] Throughout their twenties and into their thirties, Jewish young adults assume that they will be able to have children whenever they wish, and if they have any trouble, doctors will be able to make it possible for them to procreate. Thanks to the advances in infertility treatments, this is true in a number of cases but unfortunately not so for many couples, especially those in their late thirties and beyond. One might even say that the well-publicized successes in this area of medicine, together with a firm Jewish trust in medicine, have duped Jewish young adults into thinking that medicine can do what it all too often cannot. In this area, as in end-of-life treatments, Jews need to balance their firm trust in medicine with an understanding of its limits.

## An imperative to choose life

Jewish perspectives are often different from those who go under the banner of "the right to life," but the Jewish tradition is no less respectful of God's gift of life to us. Indeed, Jewish directives on matters of medical ethics incorporate careful consideration of the best ways to preserve good health and to act as God's partners in restoring it to the sick. Therefore, when medicine is at once so promising and so morally perplexing, these famous words from the Torah have new and deep significance: "I call heaven and earth to witness against you this day: I have put before you life and death, blessing, and curse. Choose life – if you and your offspring would live – by loving the Lord your God, heeding His commands, and holding fast to Him" (Deut. 30:19–20).

## Explanation of notes

In all the following notes,

> M. = Mishnah (edited c. 200 C.E. by Rabbi Judah, President of the Sanhedrin);
> T. = Tosefta (edited c. 200 C.E. by Rabbis Ḥiyya and Oshaiya);
> B. = Babylonian Talmud (edited c. 500 C.E. by Ravina and Rav Ashi);
> M.T. = Maimonides' law code, the *Mishneh Torah* (completed in 1180 C.E.); and
> S.A. = Joseph Caro's law code, the *Shulḥan Arukh* (completed in 1565 C.E.), with glosses by Rabbi Moses Isserles to indicate where Ashkenazi (northern European) practice differed from the Sephardic (Spanish and Mediterranean) practice that Caro had recorded. There are commentaries on the *Shulḥan Arukh* that explain or expand its rulings, including the *Magen Avraham*, cited in one endnote below.

In addition, several of the notes below refer to the Rabbinic interpretations (*midrashim*; singular, *midrash*) on the books of the Bible. Some books of Rabbinic interpretation, especially on the parts of the Bible other than its laws, are entitled "the expanded [or great] Genesis, Exodus, Leviticus," and so on – which in Hebrew is designated as *Rabbah* – hence *Genesis Rabbah, Exodus Rabbah, Leviticus Rabbah*, and so on. There are also other books of Rabbinic Midrash on the non-legal verses of the Bible, some of which are cited in the notes below, such as *Midrash Shahar Tov, Tanhuma*, and *Yalkut Shemoni*. The Rabbinic Midrash on the verses of the Torah announcing laws are as follows: the *Mekhilta* on Exodus, the *Sifra* on Leviticus, and the *Sifre* on Numbers and Deuteronomy. (There is no collection of Rabbinic commentary on the laws contained in Genesis because there are only a few laws in that book.)

## Notes

1  Elliot N. Dorff, *Matters of Life and Death: A Jewish Approach to Modern Medical Ethics* (Philadelphia, PA: Jewish Publication Society, 1998). Much of the first five subsections of the second main section of this essay ("The body in Jewish sources"), some of the fourth main section ("The roles of the family and community in aiding physicians and their patients"), and the entirety of the sixth main section ("An imperative to choose life") are adapted from this book by permission of the University of Nebraska Press. Copyright 1998 by Elliot N. Dorff.

In addition, much of the fifth subsection of the second main section of this essay and much of the fourth main section are adapted from Elliot N. Dorff, *The Way into Tikkun Olam (Repairing the World)* (Woodstock, VT: Jewish Lights Publishing, 2005) and Elliot N. Dorff and Cory Willson, *The Jewish Approach to Repairing the World (Tikkun Olam): A Brief Introduction for Christians* (Woodstock, VT: Jewish Lights Publishing, 2008) by permission of Turner Publishing. Copyright 2005 and 2008 by Elliot N. Dorff.

2  See, e.g., Exod. 19:5; Deut. 10:14; Ps. 24:1.

3  Saadia Gaon, *Book of Doctrines and Beliefs*, trans. Alexander Altmann, in *Three Jewish Philosophers*, eds. Hans Lewy, Alexander Altmann, and Isaak Heinemann (New York, NY: Meridian Books, 1960), ch. VII, esp. 155–159; Moses Maimonides, *Moses Maimonides' Commentary on the Mishnah*, trans. Fred Rosner (New York, NY: Feldheim Press, 1975); Moses Maimonides, "Introduction to Perek Ha-Helek (Chapter Ten of Sanhedrin)," in *A Maimonides Reader*, trans. and ed. Isadore Twersky (New York, NY: Behrman House, 1972), 401–423.

4  For example, Rabbi Mordecai Kaplan, founder of the Reconstructionist Movement in Judaism, specifically rejects the belief in a life after death, maintaining that it undermines the conviction of Jews alive today to work to make this a better world. Mordecai Kaplan, *The Meaning of God in Modern Jewish Religion* (New York, NY: The Jewish Reconstructionist Foundation, 1937), 43–57. The Conservative Movement's official statement of its beliefs specifically says that some Conservative Jews believe in resurrection of the dead literally and some metaphorically. Commission on the Philosophy of Conservative Judaism, *Emet Ve-Emunah: Statement of Principles of Conservative Judaism* (New York, NY: Jewish Theological Seminary of America, 1988), 28–32. The liturgy of the Conservative Movement maintains the references to resurrection of the dead contained in traditional Jewish liturgy. See, e.g., *Siddur Sim Shalom: A Prayerbook for Shabbat, Festivals, and Weekdays*, ed. Jules Harlow (New York, NY: Rabbinical Assembly and United Synagogue of America, 1985), 106. The Reform rabbinate's latest platform statement of Reform beliefs states that "We trust in our tradition's promise that, although God created us as finite beings, the spirit

within us is eternal," thus denying bodily resurrection. Central Conference of American Rabbis, "A Statement of Principles for Reform Judaism," May 1999, www.ccarnet.org/rabbinic-voice/platforms/article-statement-principles-reform-judaism. This position is reflected in Reform liturgy, which in one place maintains the traditional phrase in the Hebrew rendition – *mehayyei ha-metim*, who gives life to the dead – but translates it as "who quickens those who have forgotten how to live." Chaim Stern, ed., *Gates of Prayer: The New Union Prayerbook* (New York, NY: Central Conference of American Rabbis, 1975), 255. However, this liturgy usually changes that phrase to *mehayyei ha-kol*, "who gives life to everything." See, e.g., ibid., 134.

5  *Leviticus Rabbah* 34:3. Maimonides summarizes and codifies the rules requiring proper care of the body in M.T. *Laws of Ethics (De'ot)*, chs. 3–5.

6  B. *Shabbat* 32a; B. *Bava Kamma* 15b, 80a, 91b; M.T. *Laws of Murder* 11:4-5; S.A. *Yoreh De'ah* 116:5 gloss; S.A. *Hoshen Mishpat* 427:8–10.

7  B. *Ḥullin* 10a; S.A. *Oraḥ Ḥayyim* 173:2; S.A. *Yoreh De'ah* 116:5 gloss.

8  S.A. *Yoreh De'ah* 255:2.

9  See Elliot N. Dorff and Arthur Rosett, *A Living Tree: The Roots and Growth of Jewish Law* (Albany, NY: State University of New York Press, 1988), 337–362, for a discussion of an Orthodox, a Conservative, and a Reform ruling on smoking, the latter two of which state the official position of those respective movements.

10  Gen. 9:5; M. *Semaḥot* 2:2; B. *Bava Kamma* 91b; *Genesis Rabbah* 34:19; M.T. *Laws of Murder* 2:3; M.T. *Laws of Injury and Damage* 5:1; S.A. *Yoreh De'ah* 345:1-3. See also J. David Bleich, *Judaism and Healing: Halakhic Perspectives* (New York, NY: KTAV, 1981), ch. 26.

11  This is the prohibition of *ba'al tashhit*, "Do not destroy," based on Deut. 20:19–20 and amplified in the tradition to prohibit any unnecessary destruction. M. *Bava Kamma* 8:6–7; B. *Bava Kamma* 92a, 93a; M.T. *Laws of Murder* 1:4, where Maimonides specifically invokes this theological basis for the law against suicide and applies it to property; M.T. *Laws of Injury and Damage* 5:5; S.A. *Hoshen Mishpat* 420:1, 31.

12  See also Gen. 5:1. All quotations from the Hebrew Bible are taken from the *JPS Hebrew-English Tanakh* (Philadelphia, PA: Jewish Publication Society, 1999). New Testament quotations are taken from *The Jerusalem Bible: Reader's Edition* (Garden City, NY: Doubleday, 1966).

13  Gen. 1:26–27; 3:1–7, 22–24.

14  Gen. 2:18–24; Num. 12:1–16; Deut. 22:13–19. Note also that *ha-middaber*, "the speaker," is a synonym for the human being (in comparison to animals) in medieval Jewish philosophy.

15  Moses Maimonides, *Guide of the Perplexed*, trans. Shlomo Pines (Chicago, IL: University of Chicago Press, 1963), I, ch. 1.

16  See Deut. 6:5 and Lev. 19:18, 33–34, and note that the traditional prayer book juxtaposes the paragraph that speaks of God's love for us with the first paragraph of the Shema, which commands us to love God.

17  So, for example, the Rabbis describe the human being as part divine and part animal, the latter consisting of the material aspects of the human being and the former consisting of that which we share with God. *Sifre Deuteronomy*, par. 306; 132a.

18  *Genesis Rabbah* 24:7.

19  M. *Sanhedrin* 4:5. Some manuscripts are less universalistic, speaking only of an "Israelite soul" in both clauses.

20  For a thorough discussion of this blessing and concept in the Jewish tradition, see Carl Astor, *Who Makes People Different: Jewish Perspectives on the Disabled* (New York, NY: United Synagogue of America, 1985).

21 See Rom. 6–8, especially 6:12; 7:14–24; 8:3, 10, 12–13; Gal. 5:16–24; 1 Cor. 7:2, 9, 36–38.

22 Having said that, with this volume, it has come to my attention that many Christian thinkers throughout history have explicitly resisted Greek and/or Gnostic ideas on the inferiority of the body. See, e.g., Ashley Moyse's chapter in this volume (18).

23 The Greek side of Maimonides is most in evidence in his *Guide of the Perplexed*, where he states flatly, "It is also the object of the perfect Law to make man reject, despise, and reduce his desires as much as is in his power" (III, ch. 33). For Philo's reference to "a prison house," see Philo, *Selections*, ed. Hans Lewy, in *Three Jewish Philosophers*, eds. Lewy, Altmann, and Heinemann, 72; see also 42–51, 54–55, 71–75.

24 B. *Ta'anit* 22b; *Genesis Rabbah* 14:9. The different parts that the mother, father, and God contribute to the newborn are enumerated in B. *Niddah* 31a. See also B. *Sanhedrin* 90b-91a, which asserts that the body and soul are integrated within us.

25 B. *Berakhot* 60b. This prayer appears toward the very beginning of the daily liturgy. See, for example, *Siddur Sim Shalom*, ed. Harlow, 8–11. See *Leviticus Rabbah* 18:1 (toward the end) and *Midrash Shahar Tov*, ch. 25, for the roots of this prayer.

26 The predominant view seems to be that it can (see, for example, B. *Berakhot* 18b-19a; B. *Hagigah* 12b; B. *Ketubbot* 77b). Some sources, in the meantime, assert that the soul cannot exist without the body, nor the body without the soul (e.g., *Tanhuma*, Vayikra, 11).

27 *Leviticus Rabbah* 34:3.

28 B. *Sanhedrin* 91a-91b. See also *Mekhilta, Beshalah, Shirah*, eds. H. S. Horowitz and Israel Rabin (Jerusalem, Israel: Bamberger and Wahrman, 1960), ch. 2, 125; *Leviticus Rabbah* 4:5; *Yalkut Shimoni* on Leviticus 4:2 (#464); *Tanhuma*, Vayikra 6. The very development of the term *neshamah* from solely meaning physical breath to also denoting one's inner being bespeaks Judaism's view that the physical and the spiritual are integrated.

29 M. *Pe'ah* 1:1; B. *Kiddushin* 40b.

30 M. *Avot* 2:1. See also B. *Berakhot* 35b, especially the comment of Abaye there in responding to the earlier theories of Rabbi Ishmael and Rabbi Simeon bar Yohai.

31 B. *Hagigah* 3b-4a; see also T. *Terumot* 1:3; B. *Shabbat* 105b; B. *Ketubbot* 20a; B. *Sanhedrin* 65b; B. *Niddah* 13b, 17a.

32 See, e.g., Dorff, *Matters of Life and Death*, 264–267; Levi Meir, *Jewish Values in Psychotherapy* (Lanham, MD: University Press of America, 1988); Moshe Halevi Spero, *Judaism and Psychology: Halakhic Perspectives* (New York, NY: Yeshiva University Press, 1980).

33 Num. 6:11; B. *Ta'anit* 11a; M.T. *Laws of Ethics (De'ot)* 3:1.

34 M.T. *Laws of the Sabbath* 30.

35 This is based on Exod. 21:10. See M. *Ketubbot* 5:6–7 and the later commentaries and codes based on that passage.

36 M.T. *Laws of Ethics (De'ot)* 3:3.

37 *Sifra* on Lev. 19:16; B. *Sanhedrin* 73a; M.T. *Laws of Murder* 1:14; S.A. *Hoshen Mishpat* 426.

38 On God's inflicting illness as punishment, see Lev. 26:14–16; Deut. 28:22, 27, 58–61. On God's curing, see Exod. 15:26; Deut. 32:39; Isa. 19:22, 57:18-19; Jer. 30:17, 33:6; Hos. 6:1; Pss. 103:2-3, 107:20; Job 5:18.

39 B. *Bava Kamma* 85a (on the permission to heal based on Exod. 21:19); B. *Sanhedrin* 84b (with Rashi's commentary there, s.v. *ve'ahavta* – on the permission to inflict a wound for purposes of healing based on Lev. 19:18); B. *Bava Kamma* 81b (on the obligation to heal based on Deut. 22:2). See also B. *Sanhedrin* 73a (on the use of Lev. 19:16 both to ground the obligation to save a life [e.g.,

a drowning person] and to extend the obligation to heal from one's personal efforts to hiring others to help). In fact, the Jewish tradition values saving life so much that doing so supersedes all but three prohibitions. See B. *Sanhedrin* 74a ("With regard to all transgressions in the Torah except for idolatry, sexual licentiousness, and murder, if enemies say to a person, 'Transgress and then you will not be killed,' the person must transgress and not be killed. What is the reason? 'And you shall live by them [My commandments]' [Lev. 18:5] and not that he should die by them"); see also B. *Yoma* 85b; *Sifre Deuteronomy* on Deut. 22:2; and *Leviticus Rabbah* 34:3.

40  *Midrash Temurrah* as cited in *Otzar Midrashim*, ed. J. D. Eisenstein (New York, NY: Hebrew Publishing Company, 1915), 2:580–581.

41  S.A. *Yoreh De'ah* 336:1.

42  For descriptions of the role of Jews historically in medical research, see, in chronological order of publication, Harry Friedenwald, *Jews and Medicine* (New York, NY: KTAV, 1967), 2 vols.; Natalia Berger, ed., *Jews and Medicine* (Philadelphia, PA: Jewish Publication Society, 1995); Michael A. Nevins, *The Jewish Doctor: A Narrative History* (Northvale, NJ: Jason Aronson, 1996); and Frank Heynick, *Jews and Medicine* (Hoboken, NJ: KTAV, 2002). Between 1901 and 2012, fifty-three Jews have won Nobel prizes in physiology or medicine, thirty-three in chemistry, and fifty in physics. "Jewish Nobel Prize Winners," n.d., www.jinfo.org/Nobel_Prizes.html.

43  Fruits are nutritious (B. *Eruvin* 30a) and beneficial to the eyesight (B. *Sanhedrin* 18a). Vegetables are wholesome, and one should not live in a town in which vegetables are unattainable (B. *Eruvin* 55b). On the other hand, eating raw vegetables can make the complexion pale (B. *Berakhot* 44b) and can increase bowel movements, bend the stature, and decrease eyesight (B. *Pesaḥim* 42a-42b). Meat consumption in moderation is advised (Prov. 27:27) but not in excess (Prov. 23:20–21). The Jews in the desert who demanded meat died as a result of their gluttonous overeating of quail meat (Num. 11:33), and a rebellious son, subject to stoning to death by his parents (Deut. 21:18–21), becomes liable when, among other things, he eats gluttonous amounts of meat (B. *Sanhedrin* 70a). One should eat meat only when one has a great desire for it (B. *Ḥullin* 84a). On the other hand, the Rabbis thought that meat was more nourishing than vegetables or grains (B. *Nedarim* 49b), and a pregnant woman who eats meat and drinks wine has robust children (B. *Ketubbot* 60b), both of which are contrary to contemporary medical advice!

44  B. *Bava Metzia* 85b. On patient autonomy generally, see Avram Israel Reisner, "A Halakhic Ethic of Care for the Terminally Ill," in *Responsa 1980–1990 of the Committee on Jewish Law and Standards of the Conservative Movement*, ed. David J. Fine (New York, NY: Rabbinical Assembly, 2005), 476–479, www.rabbinicalassembly.org/sites/default/files/public/halakhah/teshuvot/19861990/reisner_care.pdf.

45  M. *Yoma* 8:5.

46  B. *Yoma* 83a.

47  Cited in *Magen Avraham, Oraḥ Ḥayyim* 328:8.

48  Ibid., 618:3.

49  For a discussion of these differing emphases, see my book *To Do the Right and the Good: A Jewish Approach to Modern Social Ethics* (Philadelphia, PA: Jewish Publication Society, 2002), ch. 1.

50  Catherine E. Ross, John Mirowsky, and Karen Goldsteen, "The Impact of the Family on Health: The Decade in Review," *Journal of Marriage and the Family* 52 no. 4 (1990): 1059–1078. These authors found that single men have mortality rates 250% higher than married men. In 2001, British National Institute of Health statistics showed that single men forty-five years of age and older are 23% more likely to die an early death than married men. "Single Men 'Die Younger,'" *BBC News*, August 23, 2001, http://news.bbc.co.uk/2/hi/health/1506209.stm.

However, a September 2008 article, based on the National Health Interview Survey, suggests that the differences in the health statistics between married and single men are narrowing. Hui Liu and Debra J. Umberson, "The Times They Are a Changin': Marital Status and Health Differentials from 1972 to 2003," *Journal of Health and Social Behavior* 49 no. 3 (2008): 239–253.

51 M.T. *Laws of Mourning* 14:4; see also S.A. *Yoreh De'ah* 335.

52 Gen. 17:23–27 tells the story of how Abraham circumcised the flesh of his foreskin at ninety-nine years of age – as well as the foreskin of every other male in his clan – and immediately thereafter, in Gen. 18:1, the Torah states: "The Lord appeared to him by the terebinths of Mamre." Noting that this is the case, the Rabbis say, "Just as the Holy One visited the sick . . . so too you should visit the sick." B. *Sotah* 14a.

53 M.T. *Laws of Mourning* 14:6.

54 S.A. *Yoreh De'ah* 335:3.

55 For some examples of Jewish ethical wills from the Middle Ages and early modern period, see Israel Abrahams, ed., *Hebrew Ethical Wills* (Philadelphia, PA: Jewish Publication Society, 1926), 2 vols. For more contemporary Jewish ethical wills, see Jack Riemer and Nathaniel Stampfer, eds., *Ethical Wills and How to Prepare Them: A Guide to Sharing Your Values from Generation to Generation*, rev. ed. (Woodstock, VT: Jewish Lights Publishing, 2015).

56 For a summary of Orthodox positions, see Fred Rosner, *Modern Medicine and Jewish Ethics* (Hoboken, NJ: KTAV and New York, NY: Yeshiva University Press, 1991), 197–246. The Orthodox begin with the position, as stated by Rabbi Eliezer Waldenberg, "that physicians and others are obligated to do everything possible to save the life of a dying patient, even if the patient will only live for a brief period, and even if the patient is suffering greatly. . . . Even if the patient is beyond cure and is suffering greatly and requests that his death be hastened, one may not do so or advise the patient to do so. . . . Blood transfusions, oxygen, antibiotics, intravenous fluids, oral and parenteral nutrition, and pain-relief medications must be maintained for a terminally ill patient till the very end." Waldenberg himself, however, permits physicians to put life support machines on a timer to test whether the patient is alive or only ventilating a corpse. Ibid., 208–209.

57 See Dorff, *Matters of Life and Death*, ch. 8, which is based on a rabbinic ruling approved by the Conservative Movement's Committee on Jewish Law and Standards.

58 More than half of all Jewish adults (58%) have received a college degree, and more than a quarter (28%) have earned a graduate degree. The comparable figures for the total U.S. population are 29% and 10%. Pew Research Center, *A Portrait of Jewish Americans: Findings from a Pew Research Center Survey of U.S. Jews* (Washington, DC: Pew Research Center, 2013), 42, www.pewresearch.org/wp-content/uploads/sites/7/2013/10/jewish-american-full-report-for-web.pdf.

59 Ibid., 40.

60 See Dorff, *Matters of Life and Death*, chs. 3 and 4, which are based on a rabbinic ruling approved by the Conservative Movement's Committee on Jewish Law and Standards. Orthodox rabbis are less sanguine about using donor gametes, but most approve ARTs using the couple's own gametes. See, e.g., Emanuel Feldman and Joel B. Wolowelsky, eds., *Jewish Law and the New Reproductive Technologies* (Hoboken, NJ: KTAV, 1997). For a summary of Reform positions on ARTs, see Mark Washofsky, *Jewish Living: A Guide to Contemporary Reform Practice* (New York, NY: UAHC Press, 2001), 233–241. For a Reconstructionist approach to these issues, see David A. Teutsch, *A Guide to Jewish Practice*, vol. 1 (Wyncote, PA: Reconstructionist Rabbinical College Press, 2011), 495–497.

# 4 "The believer is never impure"

## Islam and understanding the embodied person

*Ingrid Mattson*

The Prophet Muhammad is reported to have told the following parable to his companions:

> There was a man who had never done a pious deed in his life so he said to his children, "When I die, burn me to ashes and divide the ashes into two parts: scatter one part on land and the other in the ocean. By God, if my Lord gets a hold of this body, he will punish it like never before!" When the man died, his children obeyed his instructions. But God commanded the land to gather his ashes so the land collected every particle of his ashes from itself. Then God commanded the ocean, and it too gathered all the particles even from its depths. Then He asked him, "Why did you do that?" He said, "My Lord, out of fear of you!" So God forgave him.[1]

Muslim preachers and theologians derive a number of lessons from this parable. One lesson is that God is unconstrained by human valuations and conceptions of justice, including a person's self-assessment of being utterly worthless and condemnable. Another lesson is that fear of God, when not accompanied by love of God and hope for his mercy, is a deficient form of faith but is not faithlessness, and God will respond to fear with mercy and forgiveness.

Beyond these lessons, as we consider the relationship of the self to the body in Islamic thought, our attention is drawn to the centrality of the body in this parable. The sinful man sees his body as the locus of God's judgment, which he wishes to escape, hence his desperate strategy to make his body disappear after death. However, God is fully capable of reconstituting any part of his creation, no matter how dissipated it is. God reconstructs the man's body, and with that, this person once more exists and can engage in an audience with God. The person is present when the body is present.

Fazlur Rahman, the late twentieth-century theologian, even argued that the Qur'an does not recognize the existence of a disembodied person, hence its emphasis on the resurrection of the dead to make possible not just the passing of judgment but the continued existence of a person:

> The Qur'an does not appear to subscribe to the doctrine of a radical mind-body dualism. It does not hold that a heavenly soul and an earthly

body somehow come together in an uneasy union or bond whence the soul seeks release as soon as possible. The term *nafs*, which occurs so frequently in the Qur'an and is translated into English as "soul," actually means "person" or else is a reflective pronoun meaning "itself," "himself," "herself," and so on, and not "soul," a concept that does not seem to occur in the Qur'an. A human being, for the Qur'an, is a single organism functioning in a certain fashion. A person is not just the outer body, the "physical frame," but includes an inner person which may be called "mind"; together they form one organized unit. For this reason it holds forth belief in the *revival* of the dead. Later when through the legacy of Greek philosophy the idea of a radical mind-body dualism came into Islam, belief arose in *survivalism* of the soul at death and the destruction forever of the body. But the belief did not affect orthodox doctrine, although Muslim philosophers and many Sufis held to it.[2]

Before we begin our analysis, Rahman's use of the phrase "orthodox doctrine" should be noted. He is arguing for what he considers to be the theologically correct understanding of the person in Islamic thought, arguing against the "Muslim philosophers" and "many Sufis" whom he does not exile from Islam but nevertheless deems unorthodox. There is some irony here since Rahman was accused by many of his contemporaries to hold unorthodox views. Our main dilemma in addressing the Islamic understanding of the body is apparent: there is a diversity of schools of thought that have formed in Islam around constellations of hermeneutical styles, cultural expressions, and inherited institutions. The basic understanding of the components of a person – body, soul, self, spirit, mind, and heart – and their relationship to each other are understood differently by major Islamic thinkers. If we turn our gaze away from the elites and look to the practices of ordinary Muslims, we note a variety of normative discourses, cultures, and medical systems that have shaped the ways Muslims have thought about the relationship of the body to the self.

With that said, our examination of the embodied person in this chapter begins with a deeper look at the key Islamic doctrine of the resurrection of the dead and the embodied afterlife that the majority of Muslims view with great hope and fear. Moving backward in time from a hoped-for future where the reconstituted and ensouled body exists in the Divine presence, we next discuss a variety of beliefs about the body at death and in the grave. Here we find a range of views, including those who argue that a person ceases to exist until he or she is reembodied, while traditional texts and popular teachings describe a liminal state where the soul or spirit exists separated from the body.

We take another perspective on the ontology of the person by considering, in the third section, embodied worship in the life of a Muslim. Prayer, fasting, and pilgrimage are rituals of moving and disciplining the body, and these practices generally require ritual purity to be valid. Here we find an apparent paradox, however, which is that although much emphasis is placed on performing the embodied rituals with the correct movements and postures, as well as acquiring ritual purity for worship, waivers and sub-stitutions for these rules abound. It becomes clear that the ultimate aim of ablution and embodied worship is moral or spiritual, rather than physical purification and health. The real target of purification and disciplined ritual is "the soul" or "the heart," two Qur'anic terms that are variously seen as synonymous, complementary, or metonymous. It is first and foremost through embodied worship that the heart is purified and elevated. The body is not an enemy to the soul but an ally in the struggle to become an elevated and enlightened person. By performing purification rituals and embodied worship, the Muslim imbues his or her embodied existence with meaning, purpose, and dignity.

In the fourth and final section of the chapter, we examine the impor-tance of the body in Islamic thought by considering the relationship between illness and ritual observance. In some didactic and polemical contexts in Islamicate civilization, we see assertions of a material benefit to these laws beyond the primary spiritual outcome: the person who disciplines his or her body according to the sacred law enjoys superior health to one who does not. Where any unfortunate disapprobation occurs, it does not, happily, carry over into the Islamic understanding of illness, particularly illnesses that are chronic, repulsive, and/or contagious. We shall see that the domi-nant Islamic position is that "there is no blame" on the ill for what they cannot control. A disabled or diseased body does not, in Islamic thought, degrade the value of a person or signal God's judgment upon the person.

As I examine a range of views in this chapter, unlike Rahman, I will not assert "orthodoxy," for orthodoxy is a claim, not a fact, but I will mostly focus on the religious discourses generated by the Sunni majority and show how these views contrast with those offered by others. Like Rahman, I will pay much attention to the Qur'an, which always rests at the center of Islamic thought, although it is interpreted and understood at times quite differently by various schools. Unlike Rahman, but like the Sunni major-ity, I will give significant attention to reports (*hadith*) about the Prophet Muhammad's teachings and example (the Sunna) as the most important lens through which the Qur'an is interpreted.

Of course, even for religiously observant Muslims, theology and scripture are not determinative in shaping views about the relationship of the body to the person. Islam developed within a dynamic civilization in which diverse ideas and practices about the body were exchanged and contested. Alex-andra Cuffel notes that pre-modern Near Eastern Muslims shared a com-mon "medical theory" with their Christian and Jewish neighbors.[3] In the formative period of Islamic civilization, Hellenic dualism, Galenic medicine, various physiognomic theories, and a diversity of medical systems and cul-tures influenced the trajectory of Islamic thought about the body. Ibn Sīnā (a.k.a. Avicenna; d. 1037), the most influential medical theorist in tradi-tional Islamic civilization, articulated his theories primarily through Galen's framework but also drew upon Aristotle, Chinese medicine, teachings of the

Prophet Muhammad, and his own experience and observations.[4] This leads one to ask the question, what should the medical theory that dominated classical Islamic civilization be called? The late historian Marshall Hodgson argued for the use of the term "Islamicate" rather than "Islamic" to refer to culture or knowledge produced in pre-modern Muslim societies that was not focused on religious topics per se and was also not necessarily produced by Muslims. A notable example of a non-Muslim scholar and physician whose work heavily influenced Islamicate society is the ninth-century Arab Christian Ḥunayn ibn Isḥāq, an expert in Galenic medicine who translated and commented upon a large corpus of Greek medical texts in Arabic.[5] Following Hodgson, we will call the medicine practiced by Ḥunayn, Ibn Sīnā, and those who followed them "Islamicate medicine."[6] The "Islamic" tradition, in contrast, refers to the religious teachings of Muslims, including those that address physical health and medicine. Alongside Islamicate medicine there has existed a tradition of "prophetic medicine" that explains the spiritual malaise and health of the human body, mind, and spirit, as well as the impact of unseen forces, such as jinn, the evil eye, and Satan, on human health. A distinction between the two traditions – the Islamicate and the Islamic – is neither complete nor always evident; nevertheless, it can help explain some of the diversity in the materials we encounter.

Although our focus in this chapter is on traditional Islamic thought and teachings, which continue to have had the greatest impact on Muslims' views about what is or is not normative from a religious perspective, we must nevertheless note that Islamic thought continues to evolve. New trends in science, psychology, spirituality, and medicine continue to be adopted, appropriated, and absorbed into Muslim cultures. Thus, a unique confluence of identities and influences shapes Muslims' views about the body in every place and time. These views are often understood by the Muslims of those communities to be "Islamic" and are articulated through what Josep Lluís Mateo Dieste, an anthropologist of contemporary Morocco, calls "a universalizing rhetoric which invokes total unity."[7] What this means is that while most Muslims will assert that "Islam says" this or that about a subject, such statements will often be challenged by others who assert that those views reflect a particular cultural or ideological view of Islam. In other words, while this chapter presents the dominant views of Sunni Islam and traditional Islamicate culture about the embodied person, one should not be surprised if one meets Muslims who assert other views as "Islamic."

## The resurrection of the dead

A belief in some form of life after death was widespread throughout the Near East by the time of the rise of Islam in the seventh century C.E. In some belief systems, it was only the soul or spirit of a person that lived on after the death of the body. Other systems of thought, notably Christianity, professed the resurrection of the dead and some form of re-embodiment of souls. Although some residents of the Arabian Peninsula were Christians or Jews, the majority of those to whom the Prophet Muhammad first preached were polytheists who did not believe in a personal life after death. The Qur'an refers to their objections to the resurrection of the dead: "And they say, 'After we have turned into bones and dust, are we indeed going to be resurrected as a new creation?'" (17:49).[8] The pre-Islamic Arabians experienced transcendence through identification with a greater social collective – the tribe – and not through a personal relationship with God; life could continue after death but only for the group, not for an individual. The Qur'an cites their objections: "Does [your prophet] promise you that after you have died and become dust and bones that you shall be brought forth? Far-fetched! Far-fetched indeed is what you have been promised! There is only this worldly life of ours; we die and we [as a group] live but we shall never be raised from the dead" (17:35–37).

That "dust and bones" are soon all that is left of a person's body after death was readily apparent to those who traveled their lives through hot and bleak deserts. The Qur'an responds to this apparently common-sense objection to the resurrection of the dead with the assertion that humans are arrogant to consider their re-creation impossible when they are just one small part of God's vast creation: "Are you more difficult to create than the sky which He has constructed?" (79:27). The rejection of the resurrection by the elite of Muhammad's times was not just an intellectual position but a moral position, as it entailed a refusal to accept the divine judgment that would follow the resurrection. As I have stated elsewhere, "what was most disturbing to the Meccans was the fact that this eschatology is connected with an imperative to ethical responsibility."[9]

The Qur'an describes in vivid terms the bodily and emotional pleasures of heaven and the torments of hell. Whether it is possible for a person to conceive of himself or herself existing as a disembodied spirit, the Qur'an leaves no doubt that the *person* who experiences the afterlife is the same man or woman one identifies as *self* today. Judgment, however, must precede the ultimate reward or punishment, and at this juncture, the Qur'an describes people as having a kind of dissociative experience whereby they become mute while their limbs and organs gain the ability to speak in order to serve as witnesses to one's actions. The Qur'an says, "On that day, We shall set a seal on their mouths and make their hands speak to Us and their feet will bear witness to what they have done" (36:65). In light of such passages, perhaps we could see the man in the parable who wanted his body burned and ashes scattered to have been not only hoping to avoid the bodily punishments of the afterlife for what he had done but also trying to destroy the evidence. The lesson is that the destruction of the body is not a solution to moral or emotional pain and guilt. Spiritualism, suicide, or natural death can bring about a temporary dissociation from the body but offer no permanent relief from one's self, for the self will be reembodied. Self-harm is therefore irrational and must be replaced by self-reformation.

While the promise of an embodied afterlife can give rise to fear, it also gives hope to those who have lost loved ones to death. When the living mourn the dead, it is the embodied person they used to embrace and gaze upon whom they long to see once more. The loss is felt in each of the senses: the bereaved want to hear the laugh of their beloved, to touch their body, to gaze upon their face, to smell their hair, to taste their salty skin in a kiss. They do not miss a spirit or soul; they miss an embodied person. For the Muslim, the vivid Qur'anic descriptions of reembodied persons in the after-life can be a great comfort.

## Soul, spirit, and body

We have already cited Fazlur Rahman as a strong proponent of the view that the Qur'an insists on the embodiment of the person in the afterlife. He further says, "The Qur'an, unlike Muslim philosophers, does not recognize a hereafter that will be peopled by disembodied souls – in fact, it does not rec-ognize the dualism of the soul and the body and man, for it is a unitary, living, and fully functioning organism."[10] The major scholars of Sunni Islam have always agreed that belief in the resurrection of the dead is a necessary part of faith. For this reason, the twelfth-century theologian al-Ghazālī, among oth-ers, argued that "philosophers such as al-Fārabī and Ibn Sīnā who . . . argued that only the soul survived after death should be considered unbelievers."[11]

Rahman seems to be going beyond the mainstream Sunni position, how-ever, in arguing not only that the person is embodied in the afterlife but also that the soul cannot be separated from the body; in other words, the *nafs* is not a *soul* but a *self* that is an embodied person. This appears to be a form of Aristotelian hylomorphism, except that Rahman emphasizes the importance of the resurrection of the body as a key Qur'anic belief. Rahman seems to come close to the view of the thirteenth-century Syrian physician Ibn al-Nafīs (perhaps best known for being the first to describe pulmonary cir-culation), whom historian of Islamic science Nahyan Fancy cites as saying that the soul is no more than "what a human indicates by saying 'I'."[12] Ibn al-Nafīs uses embryogenesis to explain the relationship between the body and the soul and how the resurrection is possible. He describes the origin of the individual person occurring when the soul is attached to "mixed matter" that is "generated from sperm and similar things and when the soul becomes attached to it, [this matter] takes up nourishment and creates the organs, and from that the body comes into being." Upon death, "the soul remains attached to this mixed matter, but the matter is no longer capable of nour-ishing itself, so the body decomposes." When it is time for the resurrection, "the soul stirs" and the matter "then nourishes itself by attracting stuff to itself and transforming this stuff to the nature of that matter. Thus from that the body comes into being a second time."[13]

Muslim philosophers and theologians had a range of opinions about the composition of the soul – whether it is material or immaterial – and how it relates to the body.[14] Most ordinary Muslims were unaware of these philosophical debates and simply accepted the predominant religious teaching that the *nafs* is a soul that can separate from the body. This separation is described by the Qur'an as occurring at the moment of death: "If you were to see the oppressors undergoing the agonies of death when the angels stretch out their hands [saying], 'Out with your souls [*anfusakum*]!'" (6:93).[15] Another passage suggests that it is possible for the soul to be liberated not only from the dead body but even from the living body for a time: "God takes away the souls [*anfus*] at the time of their death, and those who do not die, (he takes their souls) in their sleep. He keeps those for whom he has destined death and sends the others back for an appointed term" (Qur'an 39:42).

Generally, it could be said that the Qur'an does not define *nafs* so much as it refers to it, thereby allowing for a range of interpretations. As for the state of a person between death and the resurrection, the Qur'an displays a noticeable lack of interest. The main focus of the Qur'an, instead, is the resurrection and re-embodiment of the person since it is this that makes the divine judgment of persons possible. Islamic discourse outside of the Qur'an, in contrast, is rich with discussions of the state of the pre-resurrected dead. The literature reflects a deep level of concern about this liminal state, a concern that is widely displayed across Islamic cultures through the attention paid to burial rites as well as the contentious debate over visitation practices and the intercession of the saintly dead.[16] Among other things, the lack of consensus about what happens to the dead before the resurrection forms the context for some of the anxiety expressed by many Muslims over the handling of the dead in medical settings, transplants, and autopsies.

Islamic texts cite prophetic teachings to support the belief that the soul can separate from the body while a person is asleep. The Prophet Muhammad is reported to have taught his followers to pray: "In your name, O Lord, I lay down my side and in [your name], I raise it up. If you hold onto my soul [*nafsī*], forgive it. And if you send it back, guard it as you guard the souls of your righteous servants." Upon awakening from sleep, the believer is to pray, "Praise God who has brought me back to life after my death and to Him is the return." In another version, the Prophet says, "Praise God who has returned my spirit [*rūḥī*] and my health ['afānī] to my body [*jasadī*]."[17] In these prayers, collected by the thirteenth-century Syrian scholar Yaḥya ibn Sharaf al-Nawawī and found in popular prayer manuals still today, sleep is understood as a kind of minor death or, at a minimum, a state during which a person ("me," "my spirit," "my soul") can leave his or her body for a time.

Is "spirit" here simply another word for "soul," or is it something else? The Qur'an mentions "the spirit" in passages describing the creation of humanity as a species distinct from angels and jinn. In a two-part process, God first gathers the physical material of humanity and then infuses the spirit (or "His spirit") into this matter (Qur'an 15:29, 32:9, 38:72). Many metaphysicians see the spirit and the soul as separate entities such that a person is comprised of three elements: body, soul, and spirit. Ghazi bin Muhammad explains the traditionalist typology that informs Sufism in particular: "Human beings are composed of three main parts: the body, the soul, and the spirit. The body is individual and physical; the soul is individual but subtle (supra-physical); and the spirit is supra-individual and supra-physical."[18] The soul has faculties such as intelligence, as well as sentiments and will. The spirit is what is breathed into the body by God but is mysterious and not rationally understood; Bin Muhammad says, "one cannot hope to mentally know very much about the spirit."[19] This lack of "hope" in knowing much about the spirit comes from the Qur'an's declaration that this knowledge is circumscribed by God: "They will ask you [Muhammad] about the Spirit. Say: 'The Spirit is by the command of my Lord. You have been given very little knowledge of it'" (17:85).

The Qur'an's statement that even the Prophet knows little about the spirit has not restrained Muslim tradition from speculating about it and developing complex metaphysical theories and spiritual practices to understand or witness it. The ultimate goal for some Muslim schools of thought is to leave behind all sense of self so that only this universal spirit remains. Many Sufi texts are ambiguous about whether this is an actual loss of self or only a loss of self-perception.[20] The suggestion that any person, in life or after death, can lose their personhood and become part of an impersonal spirit whose relationship to the Divine is unclear is cause for accusations of pantheism by theological rivals.[21]

Although these metaphysical discussions about the spirit are not unrelated to our topic at hand, which is an analysis of the components of personhood, the focus of this study remains the various ways in which the body is understood to be related to the person and, subsequently, the ways in which that person and his or her body might be deemed pure or impure. To this end, we turn to understandings of the relationship of the individual soul and the body after death, another topic about which there is much speculation. Sunni theologians applied a much looser evidentiary standard to stories about the afterlife than they did to reports related to legal matters.[22] Many of these scholars considered the goal of frightening or enticing people into moral behavior as justification for allowing stories of questionable provenance to be referenced in preaching about the afterlife. (I have found no evidence that these scholars ever considered the possibility that harm could come from terrifying people about the punishments of the grave.)

From the early centuries of Islamic civilization, religious storytellers (*quṣṣāṣ*) specialized in tales about eschatology and the state of the dead in their graves. These stories were aimed primarily at people they called "the masses" (*al-ʿamma*), most of whom were probably illiterate. As an oral tradition, stories about spirits and life in the grave are not as well represented in the texts of the classical period as other topics.[23] However, books devoted to this subject are highly popular. One of the most widespread books in this genre is *Kitāb al-Rūḥ* ("The Book of the Soul") by the fourteenth-century Damascene scholar Ibn Qayyim al-Jawziyya.[24]

Ibn Qayyim explains that the term *rūḥ* can be used in a variety of ways, but in his book he is referring to the spirit as a synonym for the "soul" (*nafs*) that leaves the body at death. To avoid confusion with the way "spirit" is used in Sufism, I will translate Ibn Qayyim's *rūḥ* as "soul." According to Ibn Qayyim, although death occurs when the soul leaves the body, the separation of the two is by no means final. Ibn Qayyim describes a rather active and constantly changing union and separation of soul and body. In the first few days after death and internment especially, the soul lingers near the body. At this time, the person is questioned about his faith by two angels, and a preliminary judgment is made that this person will end up in hellfire or in paradise. The damned begin to experience some of their punishment in the grave, while the saved begin to enjoy the delights of the afterlife. Ibn Qayyim explores the range of views about whether this test and the ensuing punishment or reward is experienced by the body or by the soul and suggests that both are involved. The body remains a kind of home base for the soul, which leaves to visit other souls or to catch a glimpse of its final destination, and then returns to the grave to greet the living who come for a visit. Normally, the living do not see the souls of the dead, although Ibn Qayyim relates a number of such encounters that he considers plausible because such reports are so numerous and related by many righteous people.

In the end, the impression one gains from these descriptions of the state between death and the resurrection is utter liminality and uncertainty. One can never be quite certain where the soul is located at any particular time, nor its ultimate fate. After death, the body is less a useless shell of a person than a kind of dilapidated dwelling to which the soul returns from time to time until the resurrection. While this view of the body after death has almost no substantiation in the Qur'an, it is widespread in popular discourses and has some support from various hadith. This close identification of the person with his body even after death helps explain, beyond the legal obligations, the concern many Muslims have to ensure that the bodies of the dead are treated with tenderness and respect.

## The purity of the body

Just as there are some disagreements among Muslim scholars about the relationship between the body and soul after death, there are disagreements about the ways in which the components of the living person relate to each other. Despite these differences, there is a consensus among traditional Islamic discourses on a degree of dualism between body and soul that allows for them to exist separately in some sense in certain circumstances. This is not, in most cases, a dualism that degrades the body. Valerie Hoffman notes that, "The Qur'an does not speak of a body-spirit dichotomy as the problem behind the evils of human existence. . . . The cause of human abasement is not, in Qur'anic language, 'the flesh,' but pride in self, greed, and the deception of Satan, who 'whispers' his temptations to receptive humans."[25] The Qur'an sees no harm in taking pleasure in satisfying the needs and desires of the body for food, sex, and sensuality as long as one keeps within the limits set by the law: "O Children of Adam, wear your beautiful things at every occasion of worship and eat and drink, but do not be wasteful; God does not love the wasters" (7:30). Ascetic practices are generally interpreted as aimed to enhance spiritual awareness, not to punish an evil body. The Qur'an says that fasting during the month of Ramadan is required "so that you will become mindful of God" and if fasting is difficult because of travel or illness, then one is exempt because God "does not want you to undergo hardship" (2:183–185).

Among Islamic schools of thought and practice, Sufism has been the most inclined to take disciplining the body to an extreme, encouraging practices such as constant fasting, sleep deprivation through extended nightly worship, extreme reduction of food, and wearing of uncomfortable clothes in the manner of many pre-Islamic Near Eastern ascetics and mystics. Even among most Sufis, however, the infliction of discomfort upon the body is not done because the body is evil but because the self can only be accessed through the body. Hoffman says that "[t]he culprit in Sufi discussions is rarely the body, but rather is the *nafs* . . . [that is] each person's lower self, which must be tamed or even killed to liberate the human spirit to begin its ascent toward God. The human spirit is of divine origin and is naturally drawn toward the things of God, whereas the [*nafs*] in this sense is of earthly origin, and by nature is drawn to the things of this world. It must be tamed, annihilated, and transformed in the divine presence."[26] The main dichotomy in Islamic asceticism is articulated as between *nafs* and *rūḥ* ("self" and "spirit"), rather than between body and soul; in Sufi asceticism, pain to the body seems to be a kind of collateral damage in the struggle to overcome the self.

Such extreme forms of bodily denial to tame an evil *nafs* have not gone unchallenged in Islamic society; indeed, opposition to these practices appears to have arisen in some quarters soon after they first appeared. In her old age, 'A'isha, the widow of the Prophet Muhammad, is reported to have seen two frail young men walking languidly down the street in Medina. When she asked who they were, she was told they were ascetics. 'A'isha indignantly contrasted their behavior with that of the Prophet's companion, who later became ruler of the Islamic empire and was known for his rough and simple lifestyle; she said: "By God, when 'Umar ibn al-Khaṭṭāb spoke, he was heard, and when he walked, he hurried, and when he hit, he made it hurt, and he, by God, was the real ascetic."[27] Like 'A'isha, the majority of Muslims, including most Sufis, rejected flesh-mortifying practices as contrary to the example of the Prophet and his companions. Asceticism for the majority meant moderation and simplicity of lifestyle.

Sexual desire and intimacy, like the desire for and consumption of food, has no negative connotation in the Qur'an as long as it is pursued within the limits of the sacred law. The Qur'an has a certain frankness, even when using euphemisms, when addressing sexual intimacy, as in this passage revealed in response to a question about whether some sexual positions were forbidden: "Your wives are a tilth for you, so approach your tilth in the manner you desire, but first give them something of yourselves and be mindful of God and know that you will meet Him" (2:223).

The origin of the body from sperm and its early development in the womb is described in a matter-of-fact way and does not imply abasement. Biological development, from fetus to old age is, rather, a proof of the resurrection and a sign of God's creative power:

> O People! If you are in a state of doubt about the resurrection, [know that] We created you out of earth, then out of sperm then out of a suspended clot, then out of a piece of flesh partly formed and partly unformed to make you distinct; then we leave you in the wombs for as long as We will until an appointed time, then We bring you out as children, so some of you might reach full strength and some of you die, and some of you will be sent back to a lowly state such that you will know nothing after having been knowledgeable.
>
> (Qur'an 22:5)

Once again, we see the importance of the resurrection as a theme of the Qur'an, and we also notice how the history of the body narrated in this passage reinforces the physicality of the person. It appears the Qur'an is trying to lead the person through a series of visualizations of oneself embodied in, or arising out of, various forms. At the end of an imaginative review of the materials that have given rise to self, it should be easier to picture oneself emerging as another body at the resurrection. Here, too, no disgust is expressed toward the wombs in which humans originate; indeed, the Qur'an demands the contrary: "O people, be mindful of your Lord who created you from a single self [*nafs*] and from it created its mate and from the pair of them scattered widely many men and women. Be mindful of God through whom you make claims as well as (the relations established through) the wombs" (4:1).

These last two Qur'anic passages cited seem to show the body and soul of humanity as having been created from various substances or processes in different ways. All of humanity originates from a single soul or self, while the original substance of human bodies is dust or earth. From these origins, an individual's body is constituted from sperm and other biological matter. Dust, clay, earth – all words the Qur'an uses to describe the original matter of human beings – all are deemed to be pure by Sunni legal scholars. For this reason, they determined that the human body is substantially pure. Marion Katz cites several statements by Islamic scholars to this effect, including what is stated by the early jurist al-Shāfiʿī, that "no one who is alive from the children of Adam is substantially impure."[28]

While these passages and legal determinations seem to avoid any devaluation of the body by deeming its matter substantially pure, the Qur'an does invoke concepts of purity and impurity in the context of bodily functions and activities. We must ask then, what does impurity mean? What are the implications of a person becoming impure following urination or sexual activity or remaining impure during menstruation? Does impurity imply degradation? How does ritual washing or bathing transform a person from being in a state of impurity to being in a state of purity?

Islamic law scholar Kevin Reinhart argues against the conclusion that impurity in ritual law implies the kind of social or spiritual "danger" invoked by Mary Douglas in her famous anthropological studies. Reinhart states, "it would be a mistake to see the purity system as reflecting a logic independent of the dominant ritual logic of Islam itself. Islamic religious life is filled with ritual – daily rituals, life-cycle rituals, weekly and yearly rituals, rituals for extraordinary times. Some rite of purification precedes nearly all these rituals and purity must be explained not only independently but in its ritual context as well."[29] Further, Reinhart points out, "As a general rule, 'defiling' refers to things, never to persons."[30]

Reinhart draws his conclusions about purity from the texts of Muslim jurists whose discussions set out a (mostly implicit) "logic" of purity. The main sources of the law include a few, rather laconic Qur'an passages (primarily 5:6 and 4:43) and prophetic hadith that, unlike the former, are often colorful and emotive narratives. In one report, for example, a man explains to the Prophet that he had avoided him earlier in the day because he had been in a state of ritual impurity after having sex. The Prophet tells him that he should not have been concerned since "the believer is never impure."[31] In another report, the Prophet asks his wife 'A'isha, who is standing outside the main hall of the mosque, to hand him a prayer mat. 'A'isha says, "But I am menstruating." The Prophet responds, "The menstruation is not in your hand."[32]

In these reports, the Prophet does not treat the person who is in a state of ritual impurity as a defiled person. Impurity only means that the person cannot perform certain ritual actions without first performing ablution. Reinhart says, "Here we do not find states transformed by ritual but, rather, one act requires a ritual re-action, as if only the formal rather than the ontic notion of purity was of interest to the legist."[33] He concludes that the Islamic purification system "is not so much a denigration of the human body and its functions, as it is an exaltation of Islamic ritual."[34]

Because ritual purification is not primarily a hygienic practice, individuals who are unable to perform ablution in the usual manner are granted exemptions and substitute practices to the same effect. If water is unavailable, clean sand or dust is used to lightly wipe over the face and hands. If an individual is unable to use water because of a wound or for another medical reason, that person can perform an almost virtual washing by passing his or her hand over the dressing or even the space above the dressing. If a person has no control over the flow of urine or discharge of fecal matter, he or she remains pure for worship after the ablutions despite the discharge. While women do not perform ritual prayer while they are menstruating, other forms of vaginal bleeding do not cause impurity, and prolonged bleeding prompts a reclassification of apparent menstrual bleeding as *istiḥāḍa*, making its presence no longer a barrier to prayer. Neither the Prophet nor those around him seem to have been squeamish about or disgusted by blood. 'A'isha reported, "One of the wives of the Prophet joined him in retreat in the mosque during Ramadan (*'itikāf*) while she had prolonged vaginal bleeding. When she saw that she was bleeding she put a dish under her to catch the blood."[35] 'A'isha also describes how the Prophet's sister-in-law complained to him that she had vaginal bleeding for seven years. The Prophet told her to take a bath and then resume prayers. She took a bath in a washtub set up in her sister's room, which was attached to the mosque, and she was bleeding so much that "the redness of the blood overcame the water."[36]

Katz, in her study of the development of purity laws in the early Islamic period, shows how a variety of Near Eastern cultures that preceded Islam – particularly Judaism, Christianity, and Zoroastrianism – designated certain categories of people as substantively contaminating. These views may have influenced some early Islamic schools of thought; notable in this regard is the dominant Shi'ite view that non-Muslims are substantially impure (according to their interpretation of Qur'an 9:28). In contrast, as we have mentioned above, the dominant Sunni school makes an absolute distinction between things, which may be substantially impure, and people, who never are. Katz says, "By the outset of the classical period, Sunnī scholars had largely rejected or marginalized the doctrines that women, human corpses, or nonbelievers were substantially impure. For classical and post-classical scholars, the significance and structure of the system of ritual purity thus clearly were not generated by the category distinctions (male versus female, believer versus unbeliever, and life versus death) suggested at first glance by the Qur'ānic text."[37]

Here we arrive at an apparent paradox: the laws of ritual purity seem precise, rigorous, and focused fully on the body by setting out the material substances and bodily functions that invalidate ritual purity; at the same time, the law gives copious exemptions and waivers for the requirements to achieve ritual purity if these substances and functions cannot be managed or not without significant hardship. So, is the body important or not?

Some might say that this shows in matters of ritual law it is the "intention" that counts more than the regulation of physical actions, material substances, and bodily processes. Indeed, it is true that all rituals require a valid intention to be counted as "worship" (*'ibāda*) according to the famous prophetic hadith, "Actions are [judged] by their intentions."[38] If prayer, for example, is performed for the sake of impressing people rather than out of a sincere desire to worship God, its efficacy is questionable. Conversely, if a believer is compelled to perform a prohibited, even blasphemous action, it is not sinful if his intention is only to avert harm and not to renounce his faith. The Qur'an says if "his heart is content with faith," then coerced statements of disbelief are excused (16:106). The paradox is resolved, perhaps, when we realize that intention is not just a mental state, not just an "idea," but an act of will and is followed by the act of imagining the body in motion. For example, a bedridden person visualizes herself performing the actions of prayer – standing, bowing, prostrating – while also saying the words of the prayers. The reference to "the heart" here is also significant and needs to be explored in more detail to see how Islamic traditions understand the relationship between the person, his or her body and soul, and the extent to which that person might be considered pure or impure.

## Illness, blame, and the collective body

Ibn Qayyim, the author of the previously discussed *Book of the Soul*, also contributed to the genre of "prophetic medicine" with his book *Ṭibb al-Nabawī* ("Prophetic Medicine"). In addressing diseases of the body, prophetic medicine shares some of the theories and approaches of Islamicate medicine. Both Islamicate and prophetic medicine have what we might call a holistic approach to health. This includes not only drawing the relationship between body, heart, and mind but also connecting personal health to the environment in which one lives. Foul wind, contaminated water and soil, overeating, and lack of exercise are all factors that can affect health; this was recognized by Jewish, Christian, and Muslim physicians in Islamicate societies. Dietary laws and practices of ritual ablution were religion-specific, however; it is with these practices that we can sometimes see a nexus among beliefs about the relationship between faith, health, and a wholesome lifestyle. In other words, while the primary goal of ritual ablution is not hygiene, when done in the standard way, it does in fact clean the body. The consequence is that at certain times, such as during the medieval period when European Christians engaged neither in regular ritual ablution nor in hygienic bathing, some Muslim scholars linked their disbelief (a state of heart and mind) to their purported uncleanliness (a state of body). Similarly, since blood and carrion are impure for Muslims, the consumption of these substances by Christians is a direct act of embodying disbelief that Muslims might claim will lead to sickness. As David Freidenreich has shown, this kind of communal stigmatizing can be found among Christians, Jews, and Muslims in the medieval period in similar ways.[39]

In terms of their overall approaches, the Islamicate and prophetic medical traditions do not generally identify moral failings as the cause of physical illness – for believers or for unbelievers. It is a common misconception that there is such a link, possibly because the prayer the Prophet Muhammad taught to say to the sick is, "No harm in it; it is purification, God willing." The reference to "purification" here is striking because it seems to contradict the argument that Islamic doctrine denies that a person can be impure. A number of related hadith do not use the word "purification" with respect to illness but say that God will "rid the faults" of the person who is ill, just like "leaves are shed by a tree." Many other hadith state that it is not the most evil persons but the most righteous who suffer from illness and other trials. When the Prophet was ill, he told his visitor that "[t]he people most tested by trials are the prophets, then those who are like them." The Prophet is also reported to have said that illness can elevate a person's spiritual rank.[40] For the infallible prophets, illness provides an opportunity for spiritual elevation. For ordinary people, who are fallible, illness is an occasion for spiritual purification as well as elevation.

The Prophet's statement, "the believer is never impure," is understood in light of these other evidences to mean that no believer is ever *substantially* impure. This means that the body of that person, unlike bodily waste, pork, or alcohol, is not contaminating. The dominant Muslim tradition argues further, as we have seen, that *no* human being is substantially impure. In contrast, on the spiritual and moral level, every human being – other than prophets or other unique individuals chosen by God – sins; according to the Qur'an and the prophetic hadith, these sins leave a mark, stain, or impurity on the person. The location of the stain is sometimes called "the heart" and sometimes called "the soul"; the two terms are, for the most part, used in sources and by commentators interchangeably or are explained to be metonyms. Islamic discourses on the purification of the heart (or soul) are pervasive, with a general emphasis on how easy it is to transgress and thus cause a stain on the soul, while at the same time explaining the many opportunities to remove these stains through worship, good deeds, and patience in times of trials.[41] The goal of these actions is to affect the soul – to make it "soft," "healthy," "pure," and in "remembrance of God."[42] Thus, while moral impurities can accumulate within a person's heart or soul, there is never a complete conflation between the person and that individual's heart or soul.

The belief that a sick person may reach a level of spiritual awareness that is beyond that of healthy people, and thus be especially blessed by illness rather than cursed by it, is not generally considered a reason to avoid treatment, for the Prophet is reported to have said that God created a cure for every illness, so treatment should be sought. Nevertheless, some pious people, especially those from the mystical tradition, sought to bypass material causes in all things and to gain everything they needed, including food and healing, directly from God (in other words, "miraculously"[43]).

When individual Muslims or Muslim-majority cultures do make a direct causal relationship between illness and sinfulness, or between sickness and shame, religious authorities attempt to bring their views and practices in line with orthodoxy. For example, in some cultures, it is believed that congenital disorders are caused by transgressions of the parents. In other cultures, some view a disabled person as an ill omen signaling danger to be avoided, a superstition that finds support even in some traditionalist religious texts. Sunni scholars generally reject these views as contradictory to the Qur'an.[44]

Sometimes people are ashamed of or disgusted by their own illness or disability, especially when it prevents them from achieving ritual purity in the usual way. For example, in a study of a group of British Muslim ostomates, many reported they had abandoned acts of worship that require ritual purity. When British Muslim scholars were informed about the issue, they were able to give guidance to the ostomates about exemptions and substitutions so they would feel better about themselves and engage in communal worship.[45] In a related matter, the influential contemporary legal authority Yusuf al-Qaradawi gave a striking response when asked whether it is lawful for a Muslim who has a porcine valve transplant to circumambulate the sacred site of the Ka'ba in Mecca. Qaradawi stated that there is no problem with this since all Muslims perform their ritual duties while their bodies are filled with many impurities: blood, urine, and excrement.[46] With this graphic description, Qaradawi collapses the distinction between pure and impure bodies in a sense, no doubt giving some comfort to those Muslims who feel alienated from or disgusted by their bodies due to such procedures.[47]

In several places, the Qur'an invokes the phrase "there is no blame" when establishing an exemption for the sick and disabled from a duty (4:102, 9:91, 24:61, 48:17). Indeed, the general attitude of the Islamic tradition toward the ill is primarily one of blamelessness. The late scholar of Islamic social history, Michael Dols, demonstrates definitively in numerous studies that even during the extreme situation of the plague and in dealing with leprosy, Muslim religious authorities refrained from blaming the ill. Although there was debate among Muslims about whether lepers should be avoided because the disease was contagious (with some arguing, based on an ambiguous hadith, that contagion did not exist), the leper was not the target of official disapprobation. Instead, the leper "like other diseased persons, was afflicted by an unknowable God."[48] Islamicate medicine explained leprosy in terms of the theory of humors, also avoiding ascribing any stigma to the disease. When it came to the plague, Dols says:

> The Christian belief in plague as a divine punishment for men's sins was preached by clergymen deeply committed to the idea of original sin and man's guilt arising from his essential depravity, as well as to a fundamental contempt – both Christian and Stoic – for this world. The Black Death was the occasion for the vigorous realization of these ideas. However, there is no doctrine of original sin and of man's insuperable guilt in Islamic theology. The Muslim writers on plague did not dwell on the guilt of their co-religionists even if they did admit that plague was a divine warning against sin. Prayer was supplication and not expiation.[49]

Here we see that epidemics are not blamed on specific individuals and their sinfulness but might signal that a community has become lax in upholding the law.[50] In this context, we note that the metaphor of the community as a "body" in Islamic discourse is strong. A well-known hadith states: "The believers are like a body, when one limb hurts, the whole body aches."[51]

In the end, then, we might not be able to fully understand a Muslim's conception and experience of an embodied self without taking into consideration the collective or communal body. Where there is a communal body, concepts such as autonomy and self-sacrifice cannot be simply defined as competing interests between the individual and the group. This can have implications for medical decision making, as well as for the distribution of resources within a community during times of scarcity.

## Conclusion

In this chapter I have drawn upon the foundational religious texts and teachings of the Muslim-majority tradition to demonstrate the importance of the body in Islam. Persons are embodied in this life and in the next. The resurrection of the dead and the re-embodiment of persons is a core belief of Islam and offers great hope for the ultimate reunification of loved ones, as well an incentive to ethical behavior during one's life. The body is not the totality of a person, whose "self" includes a spirit or soul that can detach or separate from the body in certain circumstances. Islamic ritual practices of purification and embodied worship are not intended to punish or harm the body but to engage the whole person in meaningful and beneficial activities. The core-embodied ritual practices of Islam – prayer, fasting, pilgrimage, giving charity – create social benefits and engender group solidarity, strengthening feelings of belonging and attachment to a greater "body" of believers.

While the dominant Sunni tradition has been presented in this chapter, it must be emphasized that there exist other traditions within Islam, some of which hold alternative or contrary views about these same matters. In particular, there are philosophical and mystical schools that interpret religious teachings about the afterlife through the lens of metaphor and view the body as less integral or helpful to the elevation of the soul.

## Notes

1 Reported by Abū Hurayra, in *Ṣaḥīḥ Muslim*, ed. Muslim ibn al Ḥajjāj and trans. 'Abdul Hamid Siddiqi (Beirut, Lebanon: Dar Al Arabia, c. 1971), 4:1438.
2 Fazlur Rahman, *Health and Medicine in the Islamic Tradition: Change and Identity* (New York, NY: The Crossroad Publishing Co., 1987), 21.
3 Alexandra Cuffel, *Gendering Disgust in Medieval Religious Polemic* (Notre Dame, IN: University of Notre Dame Press, 2007), 106. While Cuffel has some interesting insights in her work, her attempt to include the Islamic tradition in her analysis is not particularly successful. As Kathryn Kueny notes in her review of the book, "Cuffel often sacrifices nuanced differences in the complex religious systems of purity and impurity to her larger methodological framework with its focus on gender." Kathryn Kueny, "Review of *Gendering Disgust in Medieval*

*Religious Polemic* by Alexandra Cuffel," *Bulletin of the School of Oriental and African Studies* 72 no. 1 (2009): 179.

4 For an overview of his work, see Lenn E. Goodman, *Avicenna* (New York, NY: Routledge, 1992).

5 Gotthard Strohmaier, "Ḥunayn b. Isḥāḳ al-ʿIbādī," in *Encyclopaedia of Islam*, 2nd ed., eds. Peri J. Bearman, Thierry Bianquis, Clifford Edmund Bosworth, Emeri J. van Donzel, and Wolfhart P. Heinrichs, BrillOnline, 2012, http://refer-enceworks.brillonline.com/entries/encyclopaedia-of-islam-2/hunayn-b-ishak-al-ibadi-COM_0300 (subscription required).

6 Marshall G. S. Hodgson, *The Venture of Islam: Conscience and History in a World Civilization, Vol. 1: The Classical Age of Islam* (Chicago, IL: University of Chicago Press, 1974), 57–60.

7 Josep Lluís Mateo Dieste, *Health and Ritual in Morocco: Conceptions of the Body and Healing Practices*, trans. Martin Beagles (Boston, MA: Brill, 2013), 11.

8 A wide array of translations and interpretations of the Qurʾan representing the range of schools of thought and sectarian communities can be found on the website www.altafsir.com. Most translations in this paper are my own but are often inspired by Muhammad Asad, *The Message of the Qurʾān* (Gibraltar: Dar al-Andalus, 1980).

9 Ingrid Mattson, *The Story of the Qurʾan: Its History and Place in Muslim Life*, 2nd ed. (Malden, MA: Wiley-Blackwell, 2013), 48.

10 Fazlur Rahman, *Major Themes of the Qurʾan* (Minneapolis, MN: Bibliotheca Islamica, 1980), 112.

11 Valerie Hoffman, "Islamic Perspectives on the Human Body: Legal, Social and Spiritual Considerations," in *Embodiment, Morality, and Medicine*, eds. Lisa Sowle Cahill and Margaret A. Farley (Dordrecht, The Netherlands: Kluwer Academic Publishers, 1995), 38. Ghazālī's views on the nature of the soul are found across a variety of texts written for different purposes and do not neces-sarily present a single, unified view on the topic. Timothy Gianotti suggests that Ghazālī was not always explicit about his real views, as he was concerned about negatively impacting the naïve faith of the ordinary believer. Timothy J. Gianotti, *Al-Ghazālī's Unspeakable Doctrine of the Soul: Unveiling the Esoteric Psychol-ogy and Eschatology of the Iḥyāʾ* (Boston, MA: Brill, 2001). Taneli Kukkonen, in contrast, sees Ghazālī's disagreement with the philosophers as arising from his perspective on the true nature of reality. Taneli Kukkonen, "Receptive to Real-ity: Al-Ghazālī on the Structure of the Soul," *The Muslim World* 102 nos. 3–4 (2012): 541–561.

12 Nahyan Fancy, *Science and Religion in Mamluk Egypt: Ibn al-Nafīs, Pulmonary Transit and Bodily Resurrection* (New York, NY: Routledge, 2013), 91.

13 Ibid., 99.

14 For a range of views, see Ayman Shihadeh, ed., "The Ontology of the Soul in Medieval Arabic Thought," *The Muslim World* 102 nos. 3–4 (2012).

15 Much of the wording of this translation is from Taqi Uthmani's Tafseer-e-Uthmani found on www.altafsir.com. Note that *anfus* is the plural of *nafs*.

16 Mattson, *The Story of the Qurʾan*, 175–180.

17 Yaḥya ibn Sharaf al-Nawawī, *Al-Adhkar: Al-Muntakhaba min Kalām Sayyid al-Abrār* (Cairo: Dār al-Ḥadīth, 1997), 23.

18 Ghazi bin Muhammad, *Love in the Holy Quran* (Chicago, IL: Kazi Publications, 2010), 269.

19 Ibid., 274.

20 For a discussion of the development of these doctrines, see Marshall G. S. Hodg-son, *The Venture of Islam: Conscience and History in a World Civilization, Vol. 2: The Expansion of Islam in the Middle Periods* (Chicago, IL: University of Chicago Press, 1977), 230–234. Typical expressions on this topic can be found

in *Two Who Attained: Twentieth-Century Sufi Saints: Shaykh Ahmad al-'Alawi and Fatima al-Yashrutiyya*, trans. Leslie Cadavid (Louisville, KY: Fons Vitae, 2005), 127.

21  Severe critiques of Sufi doctrines and practices in this regard are a hallmark of many modernists, including progressive reformers and their otherwise ideological rivals, the scriptural fundamentalists. An example is the American Muslim Jamaal al-Din M. Zarabozo, who devotes many pages to attacking Sufi concepts and methods in his *Purification of the Soul: Concept, Process and Means* (Denver, CO: Al-Basheer Co., 2001).

22  Jonathan A. C. Brown, *Hadith: Muhammad's Legacy in the Medieval and Modern World* (Oxford: Oneworld, 2009), 173–183.

23  Most historians identify the "classical" period of Islamic civilization as beginning around the ninth and tenth centuries C.E. For some historians, the classical period ends around the thirteenth or fourteenth century and is followed by the "post-classical" period. We will simplify the periodization for this essay and designate Islamic intellectual thought and institutions following the initial "formative" period of Islam until the sixteenth century as "classical."

24  Ibn Qayyim al-Jawziyya, *al-Rūh* (Beirut, Lebanon: al-Maktaba al-'Aṣriyya, 2008). This book has been republished in the modern era by popular religious presses and sits alongside contemporary titles drawing upon the same material.

25  Hoffman, "Islamic Perspectives," 38.

26  Ibid., 41.

27  Ingrid Mattson, "'A Believing Slave Is Better Than an Unbeliever': Status and Community in Early Islamic Society and Law" (PhD diss., University of Chicago Press, Chicago, IL, 1999), 70 (citing Muhammad Ibn Sa'd, *al-Ṭabaqāt al-Kubrā*, vol. 3 [Beirut, Lebanon: Dār al-Kutub al-'Ilmiyya, 1958], 220).

28  Marion Holmes Katz, *Body of Text: The Emergence of the Sunnī Law of Ritual Purity* (Albany, NY: State University of New York Press, 2002), 167 (citing Muḥammad ibn Idrīs al-Shāfi'ī, *Al-Umm*, vol. 1 [Cairo: Dār al-Ghadā al-'Arabī, 1989], 104).

29  Kevin A. Reinhart, "Impurity/No Danger," *History of Religions* 30 no. 1 (1990): 4.

30  Ibid., 7.

31  *Ṣaḥīḥ Muslim*, 1:203.

32  Ibid., 1:175.

33  Reinhart, "Impurity/No Danger," 23.

34  Ibid., 21.

35  *The Translation and Meanings of Ṣaḥīḥ al-Bukhārī: Arabic-English*, trans. Muhammad Muhsin Khan, vol. 1 (Riyadh, Saudi Arabia: Darussalam Publishers, 1997), 213.

36  *Ṣaḥīḥ Muslim*, 1:189.

37  Katz, *Body of Text*, 164.

38  *The Translation and Meanings of Ṣaḥīḥ al-Bukhārī*, 85.

39  David M. Freidenreich, *Foreigners and their Food: Constructing Otherness in Jewish, Christian, and Islamic Law* (Berkeley: University of California Press, 2011).

40  All hadith here are from Aḥmad ibn Ḥajar al-'Asqalānī, *Fatḥ al-Bārī fī Sharḥ Ṣaḥīḥ al-Bukhārī*, 14 vols., eds. 'Abd al-'Azīz ibn 'Abdullah ibn Baz, Muḥammad Fu'ād 'Abd al-Bāqī and Muḥibb al-Dīn, vol. 10 (Beirut, Lebanon: Dār al-Ma'ārifa, 1959–1970), 107–126.

41  For a classical Sufi treatment of the topic, see Abū Ḥāmid al-Ghazālī, *Kitāb Sharḥ 'Ajā'ib al-Qalb: The Marvels of the Heart: Book XXI of the Iḥyā' 'Ulūm al-Dīn* ("The Revival of the Religious Sciences"), trans. Walter James Skellie (Louisville,

KY: Fons Vitae, 2010); for a modern anti-Sufi treatment, see Zarabozo, *Purification of the Soul.*

42 For a discussion of this topic, see Jane Dammen McAuliffe, "Heart," in *Encyclopaedia of the Qur'ān*, ed. Jane Dammen McAuliffe, vol. 2 (Leiden, The Netherlands: Brill, 2002), 406–410.

43 An excellent study of miracles in Islamic thought is Isra Yazicioglu, *Understanding the Qur'anic Miracle Stories in the Modern Age* (University Park: Pennsylvania State University Press, 2013).

44 Souraya Sue ElHessen, "Disabilities: Arab States," in *The Encyclopedia of Women and Islamic Cultures*, ed. Suad Joseph, vol. 3 (Leiden, The Netherlands: Brill, 2006), 98–99; Mohammed M. Ghaly, "Physical and Spiritual Treatment of Disability in Islam: Perspectives of Early and Modern Jurists," *Journal of Religion, Disability and Health* 12 no. 2 (2008): 105–143.

45 Fareed Iqbal, Shafquat Zaman, Sharad Karandikar, Charles Hendrickse, and Douglas M. Bowley, "Engaging with Faith Councils to Develop Stoma-specific Fatawās: A Novel Approach to the Healthcare Needs of Muslim Colorectal Patients," *Journal of Religion and Health* 55 no. 3 (2016): 803–811.

46 Ghaly, "Physical and Spiritual Treatment," 124.

47 As one article notes, "One of the important findings often stated in empirical studies is the impact of Islamic clergy – often the local imam in Muslim immigrant settings – on the respondents' attitude towards organ donation and/or blood transfusion." Stef Van Den Branden and Bert Broeckaert, "The Ongoing Charity of Organ Donation: Contemporary English Sunni Fatwas on Organ Donation and Blood Transfusion," *Bioethics* 25 no. 3 (2011): 168.

48 Michael W. Dols, "The Leper in Medieval Islamic Society," *Speculum* 58 no. 4 (1983): 902. See also Russell Hopley, "Contagion in Islamic Lands: Responses from Medieval Andalusia and North Africa," *Journal for Early Modern Cultural Studies* 10 no. 2 (2010): 45–64; Matthew L. Long, "Leprosy in Early Islam," in *Disability in Judaism, Christianity, and Islam: Sacred Texts, Historical Traditions, and Social Analysis*, eds. Darla Schumm and Michael Stoltzfus (New York, NY: Palgrave Macmillan, 2011), 40–61.

49 Michael W. Dols, "The Comparative Communal Responses to the Black Death in Muslim and Christian Societies," *Viator* 5 (1974): 285.

50 Ibid., 277.

51 *Ṣaḥīḥ Muslim*, 4:1368.

# Part II
# Respecting the body

# 5 Reverence for the Body

## An ethical principle grounded in human experience

*Jacek L. Mostwin*

The idea of Reverence for the Body first formed at the time of my mother's death and funeral preparation. Having worked as a surgeon for many years, I had experienced many encounters with the human body. I had participated in various ways of approaching and treating the body in hospitals, operating rooms, and religious pilgrimages to the shrine at Lourdes in France. I knew Albert Schweitzer's principle of Reverence for Life well: I presented it to first-year medical students during their introductory ethics classes.[1] But it was not until 2010 that the idea of Reverence for the Body as an ethical gesture, rising even to the point of becoming an ethical principle, began to form.

My mother had died after a long illness with Parkinson's Disease. Her facial expressions, gestures, posture, gait, and indeed her entire body were gradually worn away by the disease and its many complications until it took great effort to see the person she had been (and still was). After her death, I was deeply moved by the care and gentleness with which the women of the funeral home prepared my mother's body for burial and by how much attention they gave to her hair, clothing, and overall appearance. Then, on the day of the funeral itself, the family stood behind the casket as we entered the church. It was a Catholic funeral Mass, and I was now in a privileged, if difficult, place from which to experience the liturgy. I remember the very first moments: the swift descent of the celebrants from the altar, dressed in flowing white vestments, moving quickly and silently down the central aisle to greet my mother at the church entrance. As they approached, they opened between them a billowing cloak of white linen and spread it high above her like a sail, settling gently to cover her silver casket before me. It was a tender moment, a moment that went beyond care and respect to the realm of reverence for her mortal remains, for someone who had been known and loved since the baptism of childhood, a reminder to her and all of us that the promises made then would now be fulfilled. Even before the spoken prayers of the funeral began, these tender gestures of reverence and holy embrace remained with me.

In August 2011, I was directed to an article in *The New Yorker* entitled "Big Med: Restaurant Chains Have Managed to Combine Quality Control, Cost Control, and Innovation. Can Health Care?"[2] The article was by a well-known physician writer. The title was provocative, the concept intriguing. As I read on, I found that the question he was asking could be rephrased as follows: why can't medicine be more like the Cheesecake Factory, a well-known and successful chain of casual-dining family restaurants where plentiful selections are made available and prepared freshly, and quality is assured by centralized control? The author cited his favorable experience with his own family at the Cheesecake Factory as an enticement for him to perform the research that led to his long investigative report into the structure of the company and its potential to serve as a model for some of the ailments of our health care system. It was a compelling article, intelligently presented, a prediction of what might come or at least, in the author's opinion, what should come to improve medicine. But after reading the first few paragraphs, I knew that something was missing. Regardless of how compelling or persuasive the arguments might be, of how fine a restaurant the Cheesecake Factory might be, something about the arguments did not feel right. Even though the author and I were both surgeons, my experiences had led me to see things differently. The events and memories surrounding my mother's funeral, which had taken place eighteen months earlier, remained on my mind.

Why couldn't medicine be more like this successful fast-food restaurant chain? The answer, I knew, was that it should be more like my mother's funeral. It should show the same reverence for and sensitivity to the body that was shown to her. I remembered how sincere and moving were the experiences of all that was done at this difficult time and how deeply grateful I was for these physical expressions of care for the body. Nothing could have prepared me for this experience. At the time, the idea of suggesting that medicine should be more like a funeral home seemed like an idea better left unsaid. But it was a place to start; a seed had been planted and started forming into what I thought might be an ethical principle. Familiar as I was with Schweitzer's principle of "Reverence for Life," the words "Reverence for the Body" now formed in my own mind. It was as if his ideas had undergone an incarnation through my own experiences with the body; they were now being recognized in various gestures and traditions, becoming manifest as a principle expressed in human behavior, one that might reveal to us our natural values and ethical inclinations. As an ethical principle, Reverence for the Body was showing us not only how we ought to be but also appeared to be grounded in how we actually are.

The Oxford English Dictionary defines *reverence*, the noun, as "deep respect, veneration, or admiration for someone or something, especially a person or thing regarded as sacred or holy."[3] Reverence is a religious concept, not a secular one. It should be no surprise that Albert Schweitzer, who used the term to express the ethical principle that he thought best summarized his own work and thought, was both a doctor and an ordained Christian minister. Schweitzer came to medicine later in life, after an earlier career in ministry, music, and theological scholarship. At the age of thirty-one, he decided he should change his focus in life; he went to medical school with the expressed intention of becoming a medical missionary. He would become a generalist, neither a specialist nor a scientist. He would explore the meaning, purpose, and value of life in his own way by his practice of medicine. The world of the sick would be his library and his laboratory, and his engagement with the real needs of the world would be the raw material for his life's learning. His Nobel Prize was given, not for Medicine, but for Peace.

I have often read to first-year medical students from Schweitzer's early writings about how the idea of Reverence for Life came to him. Like others who have struggled with complex ideas for many years before expressing them clearly, Schweitzer had been trying to synthesize his faith, his religious scholarship, and his deeply felt need to respond to human suffering. Here's how he describes the moment at which his unifying concept revealed itself to him:

> In that mental state, I had to take a long journey up the river. . . . Lost in thought, I sat on the deck of the barge, struggling to find the elementary and universal concept of the ethical that I had not discovered in any phi-losophy. I covered sheet after sheet with disconnected sentences merely to concentrate on the problem. Two days passed. Late on the third day, at the very moment when, at sunset, we were making our way through a herd of hippopotamuses, there flashed upon my mind, unforeseen and unsought, the phrase: "Reverence for Life." The iron door had yielded. The path in the thicket had become visible. Now I had found my way to the principle in which affirmation of the world and ethics are joined together![4]

Schweitzer's ideas may have been expressed in a complex, intellectual way, but for many years before he expressed this principle in words, it was being lived out at the bedsides of the sick for whom he cared in equato-rial Africa. The ideas were forged in that setting where his intentions were expressed by his behavior. His clinical and medical gestures were an expres-sion of this ethical principle long before he was able to express it in words. This ethical principle of Reverence for Life was articulated years before the Belmont Report,[5] from which grew our current normative canon of prin-ciple-based ethics: autonomy, non-maleficence, beneficence, and justice.[6] Despite the later addition of theories of virtue and care-based ethics, these four major ethical principles, articulated for years at the Kennedy Ethics Institute at Georgetown University, have endured as the core principles of bioethics taught to several generations of medical students and nurses. Even though religious language and principles were involved at the birth of contemporary bioethics,[7] the notion of reverence never found its way into bioethical language that is used to address the state of persons at the bed-side or those who care for them. When we speak of "persons" in bioethics today, we are generally referring to their sovereignty, their autonomy, their independence, and their decision-making capacity. In law and ethics, when we speak about the body, we usually refer to the body as property or speak about the rights of bodily ownership. This language is the legacy of law and philosophy arising from eighteenth-century libertarianism, which still provides the foundations of most current ethical discourse. This language has done much to advance our notions of ethical duties and obligations, but it has not helped us reflect much on our own historical and personal experience in encountering the body of that person whom Emmanuel Levinas has called "the Other."[8]

I wish now to describe some of the religious traditions and experiences that suggest a long-standing Reverence for the Body and then draw directly from my own experience and that of other physicians and nurses who have written or spoken about their own encounters with the body of the Other. I'd like first to present some religious considerations to suggest that there are human practices and beliefs that endure, not so much because of dogma or theological authority but rather because they address deep human needs. These practices and beliefs have been institutionalized as religious rituals and traditions, creating lasting social structures that help people endure loss and grief. They survive because they fulfill a practical, personal, and social need. They fulfill the role for religion that William James might have identified when judging the value of beliefs based on their pragmatic worth, on how they solve the problems at hand.

In his Gifford Lectures of 1901–1902, James emphasizes the importance of attending to the personal, lived experience of individuals when trying to understand religious experience. as I wish to do in this presentation. James writes:

> Religion, therefore, as I now ask you arbitrarily to take it, shall mean for us the feelings, acts, and experiences of individual men in their solitude, so far as they apprehend themselves to stand in relation to whatever they may consider the divine. Since the relation may be either moral, physical, or ritual, it is evident that out of religion in the sense in which we take it, theologies, philosophies, and ecclesiastical organizations may secondarily grow. In these lectures, however, as I have already said, the immediate personal experiences will amply fill our time, and we shall hardly consider theology or ecclesiasticism at all.[9]

Let us now consider some of those experiences, beginning with the role of Joseph of Arimathea in the deposition of Jesus from the Cross. In the Gospels of Luke and John, we read about the burial of Jesus: "Now there was a man named Joseph, a member of the Council, a good and upright man, who had not consented to their decision and action. He came from the Judean town of Arimathea, and he himself was waiting for the kingdom of God. Going to Pilate, he asked for Jesus' body. Then he took it down, wrapped it in linen cloth and placed it in a tomb cut in the rock, one in which no one had yet been laid. It was Preparation Day, and the Sabbath was about to begin" (Luke 23:50–54, New International Version). The Gospel of John adds that Joseph "was accompanied by Nicodemus, the man who earlier had visited Jesus at night. Nicodemus brought a mixture of myrrh and aloes, about seventy-five pounds. Taking Jesus' body, the two of them wrapped it, with the spices, in strips of linen. This was in accordance with Jewish burial customs" (John 19:39–40).

Joseph of Arimathea is mentioned in all four canonical Gospels. After the desecration of the body of Jesus by scourging and crucifixion and before his resurrection, we are given a description of the decency of a man who, at his own expense, took over the care of an unwanted corpse, washed it, wrapped it, and buried it in his own sepulcher in accordance with what we are told are Jewish burial customs. What are these customs and what values do they express? In the words of a guide to Jewish funeral practice, "The Jewish way of dealing with death is one part of a larger philosophy of life in which all persons are viewed with dignity and respect. Our people believe that, even after death, the body, which once held a holy human life, retains its sanctity. Our sages have compared the sacredness of the deceased to that of an impaired Torah scroll which, although no longer useable, retains its holiness. In Jewish tradition, therefore, the greatest consideration and respect are accorded the dead."[10]

In Hindu tradition, the ashes left behind after cremation are considered sacred to Shiva. I was once given such ashes during a meeting with a former Hindu priest in the Holy City of Banaras when he learned that I was returning to the United States on Ash Wednesday, which happened to be the same as the Day of Shiva for that year. He was struck by this coincidence and provided me with these small relics, wrapped in paper. He handed them to me with the words, "Please take this; it is a blessing."

There are two other familiar religious ideas expressing the sacredness of the body. The first is that man was made in the image of God: "So God created man in his own image, in the image of God he created him; male and female he created them" (Gen. 1:27). A second describes the body as the dwelling place of the Holy Spirit; it is found twice in one of St. Paul's epistles (1 Cor. 3:16–17, 6:19). These beliefs have been endorsed and developed further in a booklet published by the United States Conference of Catholic Bishops' Committee on the Liturgy:

> At the center of Christian faith is the belief that God has destined the human family for eternal life with Christ, the risen Lord. . . . For this reason, the human person, created in the image of God, has always been held in highest esteem in Catholic tradition. All creation is holy because it was brought into being at God's command. But humankind is especially cherished, since the human person, individually and in community, reflects the divine reality and is destined for eternal life. . . . The

body that lies in death recalls the personal story of faith, the past relationships, and the continued spiritual presence of the deceased person.[11]

In Christian tradition, the human body is further elevated to sacrality by the Incarnation, the religious mystery by which God assumed human form in the person of Jesus Christ: "The Word became flesh and made his dwelling among us" (John 1:14). Since the first Christmas, and for two thousand years throughout the Common Era, the Christian world has celebrated this moment of birth and Incarnation with images of the gentleness and tenderness of a mother for her newborn child. This universal experience of arriving, of being greeted and welcomed into the world, is one of the most ancient of human experiences. Then, when we reach the end of Christ's time on earth, we are confronted with the images of his final passion, death, and deposition from the cross. As part of the final account of events affecting Christ's mortal body, we have the story of Joseph of Arimathea as written down by the evangelists and the images of the sorrowful mother, immortalized in the statuary of Michelangelo's *Pietà* in St. Peter's Basilica at Rome.

The tragedy of Christ's mortal death, however, is followed by a mystical promise of life afterward, of enduring strength and protection for those who remain. The body of the risen Christ is brought into the presence of the faithful congregation when bread is consecrated as part of the mystery of faith. "This is my body," proclaims the Catholic priest when elevating the host, repeating the words of Jesus when he offered bread to his apostles at the last supper (Matt. 26:26).

When these words are repeated in the proper liturgical setting, the body of Christ is made present. This mystical presence offers a blessing for those who seek it, including the sick. Every day at the shrine of Lourdes, the sanctuary to which millions of sick come every year in hopes of deeper contact with God in times of trouble, there is a Eucharistic procession for the blessing of the sick. The sick are given places of honor before all others who may be present. The celebrant walks before them, presenting the consecrated host in a golden monstrance before him. He elevates it to bless the sick, making the sign of the cross before them as they bless themselves. Medical doctors who become members of the International Medical Association of Lourdes are invited to follow immediately behind the celebrant so that they may see the faces of the sick as they bless themselves and can attend to them if needed. When I have participated in this procession and been allowed to see the faces of the sick as they are blessed in their wheelchairs, upon their stretchers, or while sitting quietly in the general audience, I am deeply moved. I believe I am seeing, as William James must have seen, the "experiences of individual men in their solitude, so far as they apprehend themselves to stand in relation to whatever they may consider the divine." At this moment, I believe I am seeing the face of religion as it is lived and experienced: the numinous radiance of the Holy as first described by Rudolf Otto.[12]

A special form of Reverence for the Body can be found in the importance and veneration of relics as a source of healing and protection against illness, especially during the Middle Ages. The Oxford English Dictionary includes the following as one of the definitions of "relic": "In the Christian Church, esp. the Roman Catholic and Orthodox Churches: the physical remains (as the body or a part of it) of a saint, martyr, or other deceased holy person, or a thing believed to be sanctified by contact with him or her (such as a personal possession or piece of clothing), preserved as an object of veneration and often enshrined in some ornate receptacle."[13] Relics are venerated not only because of their intercessory role in bridging the distance between God and mankind, but also because they are considered to retain spiritual qualities beyond the mortal lives of their inhabitants. The Catholic Encyclopedia includes a description suggesting that the relic of a saintly body may retain spiritual powers even after death:

> St. Cyril, after referring to the miracle wrought by the body of Eliseus, declares that the restoration to life of the corpse with which it was in contact took place: "to show that even though the soul is not present a virtue resides in the body of the saints, because of the righteous soul which has for so many years tenanted it and used it as its minister." And he adds, "Let us not be foolishly incredulous as though the thing had not happened, for if handkerchiefs and aprons which are from without, touching the body of the diseased, have raised up the sick, how much more should the body itself of the Prophet raise the dead?"[14]

Humans cling to physical remnants of life. There is this sense of wanting to hold on to something of the deceased forever, that it is special, that it blesses and protects. In the Catholic tradition, there is the elevation to mystical power of a living corporal presence in the form of the consecrated host. There are these relics of saintly bodies that protect and preserve us. As the consecrated host is prepared for Communion at a Catholic Tridentine Latin Mass, the celebrant, who is the first to partake of it, says "May the body of . . . Christ preserve my soul for eternal life."

Still, we are daily confronted with the events that precede these mysteries, the reality of our human death and our attitude toward the body in death, of which Michelangelo's *Pietà* is an enduring expression. Other images of universal significance can also be found in modern times. One, a photograph made by Eugene Smith in the Japanese town of Minamata, has been called a modern *Pietà*.[15] Smith had gone to Japan with his wife Aileen (partly of Japanese parentage) to investigate cases of mercury poisoning taking place among fishing families in a village along a bay into which chemical wastes were being dumped by the Chisso Chemical Company. At great personal cost, Smith recorded images and attended meetings and demonstrations at which the townspeople sought compensation for their damages but also, and above all, recognition for the suffering that they had endured. It was here that Smith, a photographer who had long been interested in medical themes, created the image of a mother cradling the deformed body of her growing daughter in a ritual Japanese bath, at once as a condemnation of the injustices to which she had been exposed by the industrial practices of the chemical company but, more importantly, as a lasting tribute to human compassion and reverence for life and the body.

Smith is one of several photographers who have sought to record the human experience of the body in illness. Smith's mother had been a midwife, and perhaps for that reason he was drawn to the theater of illness. Two of his seminal works, "Country Doctor" and "Nurse Midwife,"[16] show practitioners as heroes and present images expressing his impressions of their care and tenderness toward the body. One experiences in these images a sense of the embodied person, not as a legal concept, an abstraction, or the center of a philosophical principle but as living flesh.

In my own experiences as a surgeon, I found myself thinking about my many years of silent experience with the body in the operating room, the person under anesthesia with whom I might spend hours at a time tethered by the very sutures I was placing into the body, committed to remaining at the side of the body from the moment of the first incision until the final wounds were closed and dressed. For a week in 1992 and ten days in 2009, I was a privileged observer with a camera in our own Regional Burn Center, examining the kind of work in which I had been involved, with the permission of the Center director and written informed consent of patients who were in photographs. I was trying to give voice to my experiences as a doctor using images and tried to identify what was important to me as I studied the photographs I took there.

I had deliberately chosen a setting in which I could see events affecting the body unfolding on a surface (the skin) that could be approached in visual ways, in silence, with a camera. Here, I was able to step back and look at others providing surgical care for wounds in the operating room and at the bedside without feeling the immediate personal obligation to participate. I realized that I was seeing what it is that I do in a different way, because usually I am so engaged by clinical obligations and concentration that I am unable to think about it while I am doing it. What I saw in the Burn Center was care for the body of the Other. There was something simple, tender, and profound in the bathing and dressing of patients in the Burn Center where the washing of wounds was central to their care and recovery. The current model of rapid, minimal intervention and quick return to work in other parts of the medical world seemed very distant from the world of the Burn Center in which patients spent weeks, months, and sometimes years in additional therapy and rehabilitation. In its approach to the body, the Burn Center seemed to express something of what I believed to be an essential quality of medicine.

Our bodies are the legacy of our entire evolutionary history. We are creatures who came from the sea, and we carry the waters of that same sea within our blood and our body fluids. Our skeletons resemble those of fish and dinosaurs. Our kidneys excrete and reabsorb wastes and water in ways that recapitulate all our origins. After we are born, our bodies bear the unique marks of our individual life's experience. It starts with the umbilicus, the first scar of separation from our mother. It carries on in childhood scrapes and bruises that leave our skin imperfect but functional. Over time, age, deformity, illness, and surgery affect our bodies further and leave their marks upon us. The joys and troubles of the mind are reflected in the eyes and on the face.

In my earliest years as a volunteer physician at Lourdes, I was seated across from an older man before he was to enter the baths of mountain spring water (considered by the faithful to be the holy waters of Lourdes) at the shrine. It is a part of familiar shrine practices and traditions for people to be immersed in the waters in hopes of reconnecting with their original baptismal vows,[17] as an act of faith and a prayer for healing. The man I sat across from had suffered a stroke; part of his face sagged, and there was a huge scar at the top of his corpulent abdomen from an older operation. Yet his face expressed both gravity and dignity. He had been a successful and powerful man for most of his professional life. Now he was revealed to me in a way that expressed his whole history, written upon his body. Sometimes men and women walk into the long stone baths, or *piscines*, of cold mountain water under their own power; at other times they may be held and escorted into these waters before praying and sitting back to immerse themselves. Sometimes, they are so disabled that they must be undressed and lowered in special chairs or gurneys.

For those of us who "work the baths," as we call it, the experience of assisting others can be very moving and profound. Those who are severely impaired are brought on stretchers or in wheelchairs, setting aside their crutches as they undress, or as we undress them, wrapping around their waist a wet towel. We see their sores, their scars, their catheters, their misshapen feet, their affected extremities. We look into their eyes and faces. We see them in their dignity and the fragility of their living flesh as they prepare for what William James described as "stand[ing] in relation to whatever they may consider the divine." We place them on special stretchers or chairs to lower them into the baths. Their bodies are unmasked before us, with all the history of their lives written upon them, just as we might see them in hospitals and clinics, but in this atmosphere of trust, faith, and reverence. It envelops us and creates a new attitude among the caretakers toward the bodies of the individual sick persons and toward the body in general. We are honored that they allow us to help them; we are moved and humbled by their faith. We experience reverence before their bodies and feel both humbled and blessed.

In 2012, the Medical Bureau at Lourdes held its first international colloquium entitled "What Does It Mean to Be Healed Today?" I facilitated a workshop in which a number of Lourdes doctor and nurse volunteers spoke of their experiences. One was Dr. Ann Solari-Twadell, who has led groups of student nurses from Loyola University in Chicago to serve for a week as attendants in the baths at Lourdes. She reported on the effect of their experience on their attitudes toward the sick. I was struck most strongly by the direct student quotations she referenced:

> I treat my patients differently.
> [I] can communicate on a deeper level than just language.
> I learned a lot about body language. The way you touch people and your attitude.
> I think about treating the disease, but ultimately I think about the person in the bed.
> Going back to touch, you can't teach that in a textbook or simulation lab. That is something you have to see and experience.
> I treat humans now as if they're someone belonging to God.[18]

There was also a general practitioner in our workshop from a small mountain town in Italy. The first time she came to Lourdes, she said it was because she was curious and had been encouraged by another doctor who was the chief of UNITALSI, the national Italian pilgrimage. She returned from Lourdes, in her words, "astonished"; she could not make sense of her own experience. It was deeply moving; at first, she found she could say nothing to anyone. Days later she realized that something had changed, and she began to see her patients differently. She started spending more time with patients and listening to their stories. When this happened, she saw that they seemed happy and, in her words, "there seemed to be less suffering." It was because the approach to the sick at Lourdes seemed to be different, she said: one considered the whole patient, not just the disease. The patient had now become a person who happened to have a certain disease. She gave us the following account, which I reproduce here from notes I took during the meeting:

> And this changed how I worked with the patient. . . . Now I listen much more to the stories of these patients about their families and things that seem to be totally unrelated to the diseases that bring them to me. The patient will say to me, "I want to tell you something. I [have] suffered inside myself." One patient said to me after having been cured of a tumor, "Doctor, please pray for me, because if you pray for me, I know I will feel better."
> They come to me as a doctor, but then they ask me something different and then they want to tell me their story. One patient was dying of cancer. The husband was caring for her. Everyone else in the family was gone. "I have no one. I have no will to go on," [he said]. And I told him, do not worry: we can do this together. Day by day we can do this.

I spent time with the husband of this patient who was dying. I told him we would do it together, day by day. Three months later she finally died. It was a Sunday. Normally we do not work on Sunday. I went to his home. I went to the room where she died. "What do we do now?," he asked. "We must wash her." "I've never done this before," he said. "I will help you." And so, we prepared the body. A few days later, he called me at my home. "I am calling because I have to thank you. Because I found something I thought I would never be able to do. During these months, I learned how to love my wife. I learned so much from her. I am happy. Now I am happy. I am closer to her than ever before."

So now I do all this in a different way. I have no studies nor do I know how to study this, but I can see the changes in people. Perhaps we are putting our resources into studying things that are rare, and we are ignoring other things that are important. It doesn't take much money to be healed. It may take a lot of money to be cured, but we can heal people without much money. Why don't we simply ask physicians who come to Lourdes to write a letter about how it has affected them? Surely, there must be many stories.

## Conclusions

One by one, these experiences, as well as my own experiences and observations, have spoken to me of a deep reverence for the bodies and the lives of the patients who had come with trust and faith that they would be protected and cared for. Our patients are spiritual beings who turn to us for help. And are we not also spiritual beings who experience them in ways that transcend the legal and materialistic language that seems so often now to confine us?

When I return to the article with which I began to ask the question, "Why can't medicine be more like the Cheesecake Factory?" I do not do so to dismiss it, but I do wonder if we limited ourselves to answering that question, what it would give us? Would that be it? Would that express the needs and the experiences that we have had with the human body as doctors, nurses, chaplains, and patients? Or do we need something more? Do our current principles of medical ethics give voice to these experiences? Do respect for persons and independence of the body as property express what we experience in those moments when we feel we have entered some deeper dimension in encountering the body of the Other?

If our ethical principles should express what it is that we are and what we actually do, as well as the duties and obligations that govern what we should do, then these questions remain as I try to decide whether Reverence for the Body could be an ethical principle that expresses who we are and what we stand for as a profession.

## Notes

1  Albert Schweitzer, "The Ethics of Reverence for Life," *Christendom* 1 no. 2 (1936): 225–239.
2  Atul Gawande, "Big Med: Restaurant Chains Have Managed to Combine Quality Control, Cost Control, and Innovation. Can Health Care?," *The New Yorker*, August 13, 2012: 52–63.
3  "Reverence," *Oxford English Dictionary Online* (Oxford University Press, 2018).
4  Albert Schweitzer, *Out of My Life and Thought: An Autobiography*, trans. Antje Bultmann Lemke (Baltimore, MD: Johns Hopkins University Press, 1998 [1949]), 154–155.
5  National Commission for the Protection of Human Subjects of Biomedical and Behavioral Research, *The Belmont Report: Ethical Principles and Guidelines for the Protection of Human Subjects of Research,* April 18, 1979, www.hhs.gov/ohrp/regulations-and-policy/belmont-report/read-the-belmont-report/index.html.
6  Tom L. Beauchamp and James F. Childress, *Principles of Biomedical Ethics*, 7th ed. (New York, NY: Oxford University Press, 2012).
7  Allen Verhey, ed., *Religion and Medical Ethics: Looking Back, Looking Forward* (Grand Rapids, MI: Wm. B. Eerdmans, 1996).
8  On the concept of "the Other," see, e.g., Emmanuel Levinas, *Totality and Infinity: An Essay on Exteriority*, trans. Alphonso Lingis (Pittsburgh, PA: Duquesne University Press, 1969).
9  William James, *The Varieties of Religious Experience: A Study in Human Nature* (New York, NY: The Modern Library, 1902), 31–32.
10  "A Basic Guide to Jewish Funeral Practice," n.d., www.chevrakadishagw.org/funeral-practices.html.
11  Jen Reed, "Upholding Reverence for the Body," *The Catholic Witness*, November 14, 2010, www.hbgdiocese.org/upholding-reverence-for-the-body (quoting United States Conference of Catholic Bishops' Committee on the Liturgy, "Reflections on the Body, Cremation, and Catholic Funeral Rites").
12  Rudolf Otto, *The Idea of the Holy: An Inquiry into the Non-Rational Factor in the Idea of the Divine and Its Relation to the Rational*, trans. John W. Harvey, 2nd ed. (New York, NY: Oxford University Press, 1958), 5–11.
13  "Relic," *Oxford English Dictionary Online* (Oxford University Press, 2018).
14  Herbert Thurston, "Relics," in *The Catholic Encyclopedia*, vol. 12 (New York, NY: Robert Appleton Company, 1911), www.newadvent.org/cathen/12734a.htm.
15  W. Eugene Smith and Aileen M. Smith, *Minamata: The Story of the Poisoning of a City, and of the People Who Chose to Carry the Burden of Courage* (New York, NY: Holt, Rinehart, and Winston, 1975).
16  Ben Maddow and W. Eugene Smith, *Let Truth Be the Prejudice: W. Eugene Smith, His Life and Photographs* (New York, NY: Aperture, 1985).
17  Christian baptism is a sacramental ritual by which a person is initiated into the Christian faith, establishing a covenant with God that pledges loyalty to God in exchange for protection in this world and the promise of eternal life in the next.
18  P. Ann Solari-Twadell, "The Formation of Student Nurses: Practical Applications in the Care of the Human Spirit," *Fons Vitae: The Bulletin of the Office of Medical Observations* 326 (2014).

# 6 Healthy legacies? Moses Maimonides and Thomas Aquinas on caring for others and ourselves

*John J. Fitzgerald*

Probably no thinker has exerted a greater influence on the Jewish philosophical and theological tradition than Moses Maimonides (c. 1138–1204). Known to his Hebrew-speaking audience as Rambam, an acronym for "Rabbi Moshe ben Maimon," he penned the fourteen-volume *Mishneh Torah* ("Repetition of the Torah"), an ambitious compendium of the law of the Bible and the Talmud; this work of his continues to be closely studied by Orthodox Jews and others today. Later in life, he wrote the *Guide of the Perplexed*; intended for a more limited audience, its philosophical ideas still provoke discussion in academic circles. A physician by trade (and influenced in this field by Hippocrates, Galen, Aristotle, and the Muslim doctors Rhazes of Persia and Ibn Zuhr), Maimonides unceasingly cared for his patients (richer and poorer, Jewish and Gentile), a rigorous practice that may have hastened his death. His many achievements are memorably summarized in the epitaph, "From Moses [in the Bible] to Moses [Maimonides], there was none like Moses."[1]

If we look for a worthy counterpart to Maimonides from Catholic Christianity, we easily arrive at a near-contemporary of his: Saint Thomas Aquinas (c. 1225–1274), also known as "the Angelic Doctor" (in the academic, not the medical, sense). Aquinas wrote dozens of works, the most well known of which is his massive three-part *Summa Theologica* ("Summary of Theology"). Like Maimonides's *Guide*, the *Summa* is profoundly influenced by Aristotle; moreover, Aquinas's masterpiece acknowledges and often relies on the views of his Jewish predecessor (whom he calls "Rabbi Moses"), citing him a total of twenty-five times.[2] In turn, Aquinas's thought has done much to shape Catholic teaching today; the *Catechism of the Catholic Church* cites him frequently, and Saint John Paul II declares that "the Church has been justified in consistently proposing Saint Thomas as a master of thought and a model of the right way to do theology."[3]

Given the significance of and similarities between these two thinkers, it is worthwhile to engage in a comparative analysis of them, as indeed many others have done. But how relevant are these medieval figures to a contemporary volume on medicine and religion? In comparing the authors' many considerations that bear on health care (a task that has been surprisingly neglected to date), I will argue that while some of them are biologically outdated or otherwise open to challenge, others can be reflected upon profitably by medical ethicists, health care professionals, and laypersons today. In particular, I will examine Maimonides's and Aquinas's thoughts regarding caring for our fellow humans, animals, and ourselves.

## Caring for our fellow humans

In the *Mishneh Torah*, Maimonides explains that Exod. 20:13 and 21:20 prohibit murder and punish it by death, and that said penalty is also justified by the fact that "the soul of the victim is . . . the property of the Holy One, blessed be He."[4] Murder is considered especially grave because it violates one's relationship not just with God but also with one's fellow human and therefore poses more of a "danger to society" than any other sin, including idolatry.[5] In addition, we have a positive duty to protect human life. On this point, Maimonides quotes Lev. 19:16, which says, "Do not stand [idly by] while your brother's blood [is at stake]."[6] However, he adds we should not attempt to rescue a "gentile idolater" or a Jew who is a habitual and unrepentant sinner, for such persons are not considered true "brothers."[7]

With regard to health care in particular, Maimonides provides a somewhat unusual justification (albeit one with Talmudic precedent) for his view that physicians are obliged to restore the health of the sick: Deut. 22:2, which calls for one to restore to one's kinsman that which the latter has lost.[8] Moreover, he believes that doctors have corresponding duties to not recklessly endanger those within their care, to tailor their treatment to individual patients, and to attend to their emotional well-being; Samuel Kottek concludes, "[c]*aring* for the personal character and wishes of the sick individual is thus set in front of the *curing* process."[9] As suggested by Lev. 18:5 ("[laws] which a person shall perform to live through them"), Maimonides says that even on the Sabbath a Jew must act to address any danger to life, whether physical or mental (and non-Jews are permitted to assist those with non-life-threatening illnesses), taking into account the advice of physicians where appropriate.[10] Although once again Rambam singles out gentile idolaters in maintaining that they must not be provided medical care, he relents and permits it if "one is afraid of the consequences or fears that ill feeling will be aroused." Maimonides – who as mentioned above did have non-Jewish patients – also qualifies here that a righteous gentile (*ger toshav*) who accepts the Seven Laws of Noah may also be treated, even for free, "since we are commanded to secure his well-being."[11]

Furthermore, as Maimonides explains in the penultimate set of laws in the *Mishneh Torah*, every Jew is obliged to visit the sick, a duty that he says is grounded in Lev. 19:18 ("Love your neighbor as yourself") and the corresponding idea that "whatever you would like other people to do for you, you should do for your comrade in the Torah and mitzvot."[12] More specifically, he contends, "Even a person of great spiritual stature should visit one of lesser stature. One may visit many times during the day. Whoever increases [the frequency of his visits] is praiseworthy provided he does not become burdensome. Whoever visits a sick person removes a portion of his sickness and relieves him. Whoever does not visit [the sick] is consider[ed] as if he shed blood."[13] Jews should also pray for the sick[14] and even make it a point to visit gentiles "for the sake of peace."[15]

As for those near the end of life, J. David Bleich points out that Maimonides indicates that a life full of suffering is still better than death. In particular, Rambam refers to an adulterous woman who possesses some merit (namely, from assisting the Torah study of her male family members), and he affirms that upon undergoing the designated punishment for adulteresses (drinking death-inducing "bitter water"), that merit enables her to live on for up to a few years, albeit only with great suffering.[16] Even an individual in his or her "death throes" is still a person, and killing him or her – or someone with a fatal illness – is punishable by earthly and/or heavenly authorities.[17]

Regarding whether we must respect those at the beginning of life, Maimonides is not so clear. Addressing a situation where a woman's life is endangered by her pregnancy, he holds that abortion is permissible and provides a rather original rationale: the fetus is like a *rodef* (i.e., pursuer or aggressor) of its mother. However, once the head of the baby has emerged, the threat it poses to the mother's life is now considered merely "the nature of the world," and the baby cannot be killed since "one life should not be sacrificed for another."[18] Such reasoning leaves the status of the fetus ambiguous. On the one hand, the *rodef* part of the argument might suggest that the fetus is (or is approaching) a *nefesh* (translated as "living soul"[19] and having connotations of biological and/or legal personhood[20]) and, therefore, that abortion is only permissible when the fetus directly aggresses against the mother's life – because if the fetus were not at all a *nefesh*, then there would be no need to invoke the *rodef* designation in the first place.[21] On the other hand, perhaps Maimonides agrees with Rashi (the great medieval Jewish commentator who preceded him) that the fetus is not nearly a *nefesh*, intends to use the term *rodef* to indicate how it should be dealt with (more specifically, as David Feldman relates, that it should be "stopped by whatever means necessary"), and believes that aborting it is permissible even in cases other than "extreme gravity."[22] Also somewhat confusing is the fact that Maimonides affirms in another place the Talmudic position that non-Jews are to be executed for committing an abortion and then states without further comment that this ruling does not apply to Jews.[23] A final point to note here is that Maimonides declares that any person who intentionally kills a one-day-old infant ought to be put to death, unless the baby is premature, in which case slaying it within thirty days is *not* punishable by death. (Rabbi Eliyahu Touger's commentary to this section suggests that " 'mercy' killings of unhealthy infants" are contemplated here, and that while the perpetrator may be spared capital punishment in the latter case, the act itself is still prohibited.)[24]

Turning to Aquinas, we find that he devotes an entire section of the *Summa Theologica* to the topic of murder. Aquinas argues that if we consider any human being in isolation, it is wrong to kill him, for "we ought to love the nature which God has made, and which is destroyed by slaying him."[25] In addition, from the perspective of the common good, it is never permissible to kill the innocent, because they promote that good. To buttress his argument, Aquinas cites Exod. 23:7, which states that "[t]he innocent and just person thou shalt not put to death."[26]

On the other hand, the protection of the common good does justify the execution of those who are guilty, for sin threatens that good. Just as it is permissible to remove a diseased body part in order to protect the whole, so too is it licit to kill a particularly dangerous person in order to safeguard society. Once again, Aquinas supports his case with reference to Scripture: "In the morning I put to death all the wicked of the land" (Ps. 101:8), and "[a] little leaven corrupteth the whole lump" (1 Cor. 5:6). In response to a potential counterargument that maintains that killing a fellow human is intrinsically evil, Aquinas responds that "[b]y sinning man departs from the order of reason, and consequently falls away from the dignity of his manhood, in so far as he is naturally free . . . and he falls into the slavish state of the beasts." Indeed, he holds that such a person is more dangerous and even "worse than a beast," and he concludes that just as an animal may be put to death, so too may a sinner.[27]

At any rate, granting that it is wrong to kill an innocent person, at what point do we attain such personhood? Like the Christian philosopher Boethius before him, Aquinas understands a person as "an individual substance of a rational nature."[28] So now the question becomes, when is this nature achieved? For Aquinas (following Aristotle), the first step involves the interaction of our father's semen with our mother's menstrual blood, which produces an embryo with a vegetative soul. As this new body develops, it becomes capable of sensation, at which point its soul is naturally replaced with an animal soul. After further growth of this structure to the point where it is able to support the activity of a rational soul, God himself infuses our human soul into it, and the preceding animal soul is eliminated.[29] For Aquinas, as for Aristotle, the point at which this last act occurs is "quickening," which they understand to be forty days after conception for males and ninety days after conception for females.[30] From this point in our mother's womb onwards, Aquinas suggests, we are human persons.[31] This provides the necessary context for understanding his brief reference to fetal killing in the *Summa Theologica*, where he explains that a man who strikes a pregnant woman is guilty of murder if either she or her "animated fetus" dies.[32] However, it is important to add that Aquinas also explicitly disapproves of the deliberate termination of a not-yet-animated fetus, on the grounds that it is a "maleficious act[] . . . against nature," even though not a homicide.[33]

One other point to note regarding the Angelic Doctor here is that he also speaks of visiting the sick as a merciful way of alleviating their misfortune. Here he has in mind Matthew 25, where Jesus indicates that he is present with and in those who are ill and others who are disadvantaged and that people who care for them are the "sheep" who go to his heavenly kingdom, while others who ignore them are the "goats" who enter into eternal fire. Aquinas adds that assisting the blind and the lame are specific forms of coming to the aid of the sick.[34]

Some of the aforementioned thoughts on caring for our fellow humans can function as valuable insights for Jewish and Christian health care ethicists and professionals (and others) today. For instance, Aquinas's claim that "we ought to love the nature which God has made" evokes the potentially helpful image of a divine artisan whose works we must generally respect. Aquinas provides further grounds for this respect when he points out that individuals can promote the common good; here one might think of how even the dying can contribute in ways large and small to their family and wider communities. Next, Maimonides's attention to Lev. 19:16 could rouse one to action on behalf of his or her neighbor; note that the partial similarity between this verse and the parable of the Good Samaritan in the New Testament (in Luke 10) might provide an opening for Jewish-Christian dialogue. As Simkha Weintraub notes, Maimonides's words for health care professionals in particular "may trigger some thought-provoking questions for our work with those who suffer," including "What loss might I restore to this person who I am trying to help/to heal?" and "Even if I cannot restore what I would like, what loss can I address, can I mollify?"[35] In addition, Maimonides encourages caring for (and not simply curing) the whole patient – a stance that echoes that of other authors in the present volume and that serves as an important reminder to health care professionals today. Finally, both Maimonides and Aquinas facilitate reflection on the goodness of visiting the sick and the gravity of failing to do so; Maimonides's reliance on a Golden Rule in this context would resonate with Christians, who have an explicit such rule in the New Testament (Matt. 7:12).

On the other hand, it is troubling to read Maimonides's affirmation that we may stand idly by when the life of an idolater or habitual sinner is at stake, as well as Aquinas's belief that sinners "fall[] away from [their] dignity," which Maimonides seems to share.[36] In a contemporary context, such statements could lead to the conclusion that those whose poor behavior leads to illness, such as smoking-related lung disease or alcohol-related liver disease, should automatically receive lower priority in the delivery of particular health care services or even be completely excluded, as a matter of fairness to others given scarce resources. While I acknowledge that people of goodwill might present a credible case for such a demotion, I would suggest that a better starting point than Maimonides and Aquinas lies within the modern-day Hippocratic Oath written by Louis Lasagna and presently utilized in many medical schools. This oath states in pertinent part: "I will prevent disease whenever I can . . . I will remember that I remain a member of society, with special obligations to all my fellow human beings, those sound of mind and body as well as the infirm."[37] Such an oath calls our attention to the equal dignity of all human beings and makes no distinction between patients with different degrees of virtue. For Jews and Christians, this all-encompassing dignity is further reinforced by Gen. 1:26–27, which maintains that humans, in general, are made in the image of God.[38]

More specifically, it is arguable that what would be truly unjust is a policy of exclusion or automatic demotion for patients who have liver disease brought on by their drinking and need an organ transplant. To begin with, one could reason that if we did commit to taking moral responsibility into account in such situations, we would end up in a problematic position no matter what. On the one hand, if we did not also consider genetic predispositions (to substance abuse and to liver problems) and any other mitigating circumstances, that would be unfair. On the other hand, if we did consider all such morally relevant factors, it would be too difficult to consistently determine the precise level of moral responsibility and assign appropriate penalties and too invasive into patients' personal lives.[39] In any case, there is also the potential slippery-slope danger of eroding doctors' commitment to treating *all* patients – including those whom they consider less ethical for whatever reason – to the best of their ability.[40] Accordingly, Catholic bioethicist Nicanor Austriaco concludes, "Medicine should be motivated, first and foremost, by the desire to treat the sickest among us who would benefit most from that treatment."[41]

Finally, of what value to us today are Maimonides's and Aquinas's thoughts pertaining to the subject of abortion? Their legacy here is not entirely clear, as each of them has been enlisted by those on different sides of the abortion debate. It seems that most (although not all) Jewish interpreters throughout history have held that Maimonides did not nearly believe the fetus to be a *nefesh* but rather used the term *rodef* for another reason and have concluded that abortion can accordingly be permissible even in cases other than "extreme gravity" (in particular, even when the fetus does not directly imperil the mother's life).[42] As for Aquinas, it appears that most of his contemporary Catholic adherents contend that had he known (as per modern biology) that the human being is substantially present at fertilization (with no fundamental change after that point), he would have accepted this datum and presumably concluded that the termination of a pregnancy is an impermissible taking of life from that moment onward. That said, a minority of these interpreters, while not accepting Aquinas's outdated biology, think that he has an enduring insight in saying that the early conceptus lacks the capacity to reason (and therefore full personhood) and allow that abortion may be permissible, at least at the beginning of a pregnancy.[43]

Putting these very technical debates aside, I would like to identify a couple of relevant points at which Maimonides and Aquinas are helpful (or not) to us today. On the one hand, in the light of modern biology, Aquinas's specific focus on the moment of quickening seems arbitrary,[44] and various people on different sides of the abortion debate would find Maimonides's language on premature infants to be problematic at least in a contemporary context, given that many such infants today do not have grim life prospects and that he does not specify any punishment for mercy-killers or even explicitly acknowledge any wrongdoing on their part.[45] Moreover, Maimonides's holding Gentiles to a higher standard than Jews on abortion is arguably inconsistent and even unfair. It is true, as Ronit Irshai shows, that the Talmud upon which he relies adds shortly thereafter that "nothing is permissible for a Jew but forbidden for a gentile." But she also states, "that maxim is not easily reconciled with various prohibitions applied to gentiles but not to Jews."[46] She and David Feldman also suggest that non-Jews may have been assigned a stricter punishment because they were seen as more inclined to kill fetuses and newborns.[47] Such a rationale should certainly be rejected today, and, even if it were true in the past, it is still troubling that some would be punished more than others for the same crime.

On the bright side, Maimonides and Aquinas do provide good resources for dealing with indirect abortion, which refers to a medical procedure (for instance, in cases of ectopic pregnancy) that intends to save the life of the mother and unintentionally results in the death of the unborn human inside her. Aquinas's idea that actions that have good and bad effects can be permissible as long as the bad one is not intended[48] (an insight that will be discussed later in this chapter and that is codified in the Principle of Double Effect[49]) might be of some use to Jewish ethical reflection on indirect abortion. And the position of the Catholic moral tradition on indirect abortion, which is that it can be justified according to said principle,[50] could be reinforced by thinking of the fetus as "like an aggressor or pursuer," wording that need not assign actual guilt to the fetus but emphasizes that it does pose a threat to the mother and may be killed at least as a side effect.[51]

## Caring for animals

Where does these authors' profound respect for human life leave animals? Maimonides initially affirms in his *Commentary to the Mishnah* that all things that God has created – whether living or not – are for the benefit of humankind.[52] However, in the later *Guide of the Perplexed*, he repudiates this idea and states that "all the other beings too have been intended for their own sakes and not for the sake of something else," on the grounds that humans could have existed without the rest of creation and that certain biblical passages (including Gen. 1:31 and Prov. 16:4) cut against any idea that other beings were specifically designed for us.[53] Still, the *Guide* goes on to assert that while human individuals are overseen by divine providence (as per biblical passages such as Pss. 8:5, 33:15, 144:3, as well as those regarding Abraham, Isaac, and Jacob), particular animals are not (as per Aristotle and Hab. 1:14–15), and indeed that it is "disgraceful" to think that animals who are killed are rewarded in an afterlife.[54]

Given the lack of divine providence over animals, Maimonides concludes that "killing them and employing them usefully, as we wish, has been permitted and even enjoined." That said, Rambam here also acknowledges Num. 22:32 (where an angel chides Balaam for beating his donkey) and concludes that in order to perfect ourselves and avoid "moral habits of cruelty," we should be kind to animals and not cause them gratuitous pain.[55] In a particularly poignant passage a bit later in the *Guide*, Maimonides explicitly prohibits killing an animal in the presence of its mother for the following reason: "For in these cases animals feel very great pain, there being no difference regarding this pain between man and the other animals. For the love and the tenderness of a mother for her child is not consequent upon reason, but upon the activity of the imaginative faculty, which is found in most animals just as it is found in man." He adds here that this is the rationale behind Deut. 22:6–7, which demands that one spare a mother bird the anguish of watching her offspring confiscated.[56] According to the *Mishneh Torah*, other pains should be avoided as well; one should promptly come to the assistance of a donkey who has fallen under its burden and avoid leaving large loads on an animal during the Sabbath.[57]

In contrast, Aquinas seems somewhat less sympathetic to the animal kingdom. He does acknowledge that God created all things good as per Gen. 1:31 (albeit with different degrees of excellence)[58] and thinks (with Augustine) that all things – including animals and human beings – are beneficently governed by the God who created them.[59] However, he also says (with reference to Psalm 8) that God rules animals for the sake of rational and free beings (namely, humans), who "come closer to the divine likeness."[60] Moreover, since animals are without reason and free will, cannot attain to heaven, and therefore "have no fellowship" with us, we need not – indeed, cannot – extend to them the neighborly love of friendship, although we can love them purely for being instrumental to God's glory and our own good.[61]

Next, to explain why "Thou shalt not kill" does not apply to animals, Aquinas uses the same reasoning (here attributed to Augustine): they have no fellowship with us. Furthermore, since that which is relatively imperfect exists for the sake of that which is more perfect, animals exist for our own good, and therefore it is licit to kill them for food. In fact, as Aquinas notes, God himself gives us explicit permission to do so in Gen. 9:3.[62] Commenting on Aquinas's views, the atheist moral philosopher Peter Singer points out that there is no space for doing wrong to animals in this framework; the *Summa Theologica* elsewhere divides sins solely into those against God, against one's (human) neighbor, and against one's self.[63] While one of Aquinas's earlier works (the *Summa Contra Gentiles*) does briefly acknowledge Deut. 22:6, even here he simply suggests that cruelty to animals is prohibited on the grounds that it can harm us, for example by making us more inclined to mistreat fellow humans.[64]

When we consider bioethical issues involving animals today, Aquinas offers us only limited assistance, so we turn to contemporary Catholic teaching. Citing the first, second, and ninth chapters of Genesis, the *Catechism of the Catholic Church* affirms that animals exist for our good and that we must not inflict gratuitous suffering on them; the latter teaching is tersely and somewhat opaquely grounded in the idea that such activity would be "contrary to *human* dignity."[65] While not explicitly rejecting Aquinas's conclusions, recent Catholic teaching also appears to speak of animals in a warmer and more appreciative way. Specifically, the *Catechism* contends that "[c]reatures exist only in dependence on each other, to complete each other, in the service of each other" and that "[t]here is a solidarity among all creatures arising from the fact that all have the same Creator and are all ordered to his glory."[66] In speaking of non-human animals in particular, it adds that "[God] surrounds them with his providential care. By their mere existence they bless him and give him glory. Thus men owe them kindness. . . . One can love animals; one should not direct to them the affection due only to persons." Cited in support of such statements are Dan. 3:79–81 and Matt. 6:26 (which speak respectively of various animals' exalting the Lord and of God's caring for birds), as well as the care for animals manifested by St. Francis of Assisi and St. Philip Neri.[67] With reference to both of these saints and to human experience in general, I would add that the love we can give to animals is more expansive than that envisioned by Aquinas; whether or not a dog is a man's best friend, the two can still enjoy a real fellowship.[68] These various considerations lead us to the *Catechism*'s conclusion that while experimentation on animals is permissible, it must "remain[] within reasonable limits and contribute[] to caring for or saving human lives."[69]

As for Maimonides, to be fair, he explicitly distinguishes only between sins against God and sins against other human beings[70] and at one point also appears to locate the primary rationale for not harming animals in concern for our own well-being rather than that of the creature itself. Still, he does well to call our attention to the biblical accounts of Balaam and the mother bird, and he also vividly outlines an important philosophical argument against the maltreatment of animals: animals are able to feel pain and desire to avoid it, and therefore they deserve our consideration. This basic rationale is accepted (and elaborated on) by thinkers of many other worldviews, including the Fourteenth Dalai Lama,[71] Singer,[72] and others.[73] Relying on it, one can share Singer's concern with animal testing geared toward finding the "median lethal dose" of a substance (which will cause at least half of them to die)[74] and agree with John Paul II that "the diminution of experimentation on animals, which has progressively been made ever less necessary, corresponds to the plan and well-being of all creation."[75] One can also hope that Jewish, Catholic, and other textbooks in health care ethics will dwell more on issues involving animals in the future.[76]

## Caring for ourselves

As with murder, Maimonides clearly disapproves of the ultimate act against one's own health: suicide. Referring to it as a "sin of bloodshed," Rambam then quotes Gen. 9:5, which reads that "of the blood of your own lives I will demand an account." This passage pertains to someone who kills himself, he declares, and the wording of it shows that the person's "judgment is in heaven's hands."[77] He adds that the person's acquaintances on earth are to neither mourn nor eulogize the person.[78] With few exceptions, a Jew ought to preserve his or her life even if it means obeying an order to violate a commandment, for Lev. 18:5 indicates that the reason for following God's commandments is to "find life through them."[79] If a person dare counter, "I will risk my life, what does this matter to others," such a person should be rewarded with a beating, Maimonides says.[80]

In general, Rambam emphasizes that we have a duty to take care of our bodies so that we can know and serve God.[81] How do we care for our physical health? Maimonides calls attention to at least eight areas on which we should focus. The first is food; we should not be gluttonous (even when it comes to generally healthy foods) but ingest only what is necessary to satiate hunger and nourish ourselves,[82] avoid cooking a wide variety of dishes for a meal and thereby encouraging gluttony,[83] and eat once a day if we are healthy.[84] In addition, we should take some meat (not pork – and preferably low-fat poultry over red meat) but only when we crave it (as per Deut. 12:20),[85] consume chicken soup to recover from illness,[86] avoid "harmful" foods (under which he includes mushrooms [seemingly in general], lentils, garlic, mustard, and certain "aged and salted" fare),[87] and refrain from indulging in sweets.[88] A Jew stranded in the desert may even eat a forbidden food if there is nothing else to eat.[89]

The second matter is drink; it is permissible for adults to imbibe wine in moderation (although not for children, since it is hazardous to their health).[90] Wine benefits the blood and different organs, assists digestion, and (like meat) is conducive to appropriate rejoicing on holidays; on the other hand, inordinate drinking leads to disease.[91] In addition, intoxication can cause a person to "lose his wisdom," become angry, engage in illicit sexual activity, and disrespect the name of God in front of others.[92] Maimonides also recommends drinking milk since it "nourishes a defective body, and revives it."[93] As for water, it should be drunk sufficiently but not excessively, and it should be avoided when polluted.[94]

Third, Rambam addresses another issue pertaining to bodily pleasures: sex. On the one hand, he affirms that sex, which should be both consensual and agreeable, can improve physical well-being (including that of the digestive and reproductive organs) and mood; indeed, he claims at one point that "[t]he indulgence in sexual intercourse is one of the requirements for the maintenance of health." On the other hand, he suggests that if a person engages in sexual relations too frequently, he will lose his strength (citing Prov. 31:3), experience gastric problems, and suffer premature aging.[95]

The right amount of sex is determined by one's profession; once a day for healthy men whose work is not taxing and who spend most of their time at home, once a week (on the Sabbath) for Torah scholars, once a month for camel drivers, and once every six months for seamen. A wife has the rights to prevent her husband from taking a long business trip or switching to a profession where sex should be more infrequent unless the husband desires to study Torah.[96]

The next three parts of Maimonides's blueprint for health deal with proper exercise, bathing, and sleep, respectively. He states that it is good to warm the body by walking before meals, that exercise helps ward off illnesses, and that the person who completely refrains from exercise "will be full of pain for all his days and his strength will fade away."[97] He also calls for people to bathe their entire bodies once a week and indicates that if one is somewhat ill one can wash oneself on the Day of Atonement.[98] With regard to sleep, eight hours a night is best, preferably not immediately after a meal.[99]

Seventh, the wider environment we live in also bears on our health, according to Maimonides. He encourages people to avoid the polluted air of the city as much as possible; on this note, it is desirable to live away from its center and ideally on a floor with good ventilation and sunshine.[100] And eighth and finally, he points out that physical well-being requires good mental health in turn. One should avoid activities that cause anxiety and thereby deleterious physical changes to the body.[101] Maimonides summarizes his thoughts on caring for oneself as follows: "Whoever conducts himself in the ways which we have drawn up, I will guarantee that he will not become ill throughout his life, until he reaches advanced age and dies. He will not need a doctor. His body will remain intact and healthy throughout his life. [One may rely on this guarantee] unless [his body] was impaired from the birth, he was accustomed to one of the harmful habits from birth, or should there be a plague or a drought in the world."[102]

Turning to Aquinas, we find that he also unequivocally condemns suicide. Beginning with a reference to Augustine's fifth-century work *City of God*, Aquinas explains that the commandment "Thou shalt not kill" applies to ourselves just as much as to others. In particular, he continues, taking one's own life is a mortal sin that contravenes the natural law (more specifically, the natural inclination to preserve life) and the virtue of charity by which we ought to love ourselves in addition to God and our neighbor. Suicide is also opposed to the virtue of justice since it is detrimental to the society of which we are part and since "life is God's gift to man, and is subject to His power, Who kills and makes to live." Just as one who murders a slave "usurps to himself judgment of a matter not entrusted to him" and, therefore, does the slave's master wrong, so one who takes his own life offends against God.[103]

Aquinas then moves to address a few possible counterarguments. Even if one's intention is to end one's suffering and transition to a more pleasant afterlife, suicide is prohibited since it involves a "greater evil" than suffering: death. Indeed, suicide is a graver evil than fornication, adultery, and even murder since "one injures oneself, to whom one owes the greatest love" and forecloses the possibility of repenting for such a sin.[104] Lastly, in response to the suggestion that since Samson killed himself (in Judges 16) and is praised in the New Testament (in Hebrews 11), suicide can be licit, Aquinas relies on Augustine's rationale that Samson's case is relatively special since the Holy Spirit "Who had wrought many wonders through him, had secretly commanded him to do this."[105]

That said, killing in self-defense is entirely licit. Here Aquinas makes a theological and a philosophical argument. The former is based on Exod. 22:1–2, which indicates that it can be permissible to mortally injure a person intruding into one's house; so, too, Aquinas observes, can it be legitimate to kill someone else to save one's very life. The latter argument notes that the act of self-defense has the good effect of preserving one's life and the bad effect of killing the aggressor, but the intention is to safeguard one's life, which is natural and good, not to kill the attacker without public authority, which would be bad. Since the intention is good and the death is only a side effect, Aquinas reasons, the act as a whole can be moral.[106]

In addition, charity generally dictates that we should love our own bodies, Aquinas says. Through doing so, we can serve God; here he relies on Rom. 6:13 ("Present . . . your members as instruments of justice unto God").[107] Presumably, this love would include proper care for our bodies, which raises the question of what exactly that would entail. Aquinas delves into some specifics in the *Summa Theologica*'s treatise on the cardinal virtue of temperance, particularly his questions on abstinence, fasting, gluttony, sobriety, and drunkenness.

Beginning with the virtue of abstinence, Aquinas understands it as the habit of forgoing food in a reasonable manner, with "gladness of heart," "due regard . . . for [one's] own person, and for the requirements of his health" (as per Augustine), and the intention of bringing glory to God.[108] Abstinence trains us to resist lust and gluttony and (as per Eccles. 2:3) helps us achieve wisdom.[109] Fasting is simply "an act of abstinence," and the one who engages in this act properly will not "refuse nature its necessary support."[110] More specifically, she should eat one meal, drink fluids moderately, and take necessary medications during the day.[111] Aquinas even excuses some people – namely children and certain pilgrims and workers for whom fasting would be a heavy burden – from the practice in the interest of safeguarding their health.[112] Consistent with his discussion of abstinence, Aquinas's analysis of fasting says that its goals include sharpening one's focus on "heavenly things," atoning for sins, and avoiding concupiscence and lust.[113]

At the other end of the spectrum, those who are guilty of gluttony (the immoderate desire for food and drink) suffer "dullness of sense in the understanding, on account of the fumes of food disturbing the brain," become vulnerable to lust and inappropriate speech, and can be distracted from the love of God.[114] They are even more culpable if through their excessive intake they physically harm themselves.[115] According to Aquinas, the sin of gluttony is distinct from the normal intake of food, which is good and important for we cannot live without it.[116] Elsewhere, he goes so far as to say that the person who does not feed and take care of himself is guilty of "murder[ing] himself."[117]

Like temperance in eating, moderation in drinking is that which is conducive to a person's health, and the appropriate amount may be determined by a physician in certain cases.[118] Regarding the virtue of sobriety, which deals primarily with moderation in drinking alcohol, Aquinas highlights Sirach 31, which says that "[s]ober drinking is health to soul and body; wine drunken with excess raiseth quarrels, and wrath and many ruins."[119] He later specifies (citing 1 Tim. 5:23) that wine can settle the stomach and ward away illnesses and adds (as per Sirach 31) that moderate wine intake is "the joy of the soul and the heart."[120] On the other hand, among the aforementioned ruins of drunkenness (an act of gluttony), Aquinas himself has in mind the loss of reason, which he suggests is even worse than that in the case of overeating food, and the consequent falling away from virtue and into vice.[121]

Despite his obvious concern that we protect our own health, the Angelic Doctor also indicates that the value of our own lives is not absolute. While it is natural for a person to love his or her life and that which maintains it, it is also natural "to do so in due measure, that is, to love these things not as placing his end therein, but as things to be used for the sake of his last end."[122] The act of martyrdom, in fact, "is the greatest proof of the perfection of charity" since the person gives up that which she cherishes the most, her very life, for the sake of God and the Christian faith.[123]

What are these medieval thinkers' respective legacies on caring for ourselves? The notions that life is God's property or gift (explicitly voiced by Maimonides and Aquinas, respectively) are often used today to justify opposition to physician-assisted suicide.[124] However, as John Mitchell shows, these justifications can be questioned. He believes that the idea that our soul is the property of God, on loan to us, does not in and of itself make it wrong to take our own life, since the soul itself is not killed but rather returns to God. In addition, since we do not have a duty to indefinitely keep gifts that those on earth give us, Mitchell suggests, why would we necessarily have an obligation to embrace the gift of life (or remain stewards of our physical bodies), particularly in circumstances where that life has irreversibly worn down? "For then it is no longer truly the gift; it is not what the giver bestowed." Therefore, he reasons, it is possible to relinquish it while continuing to express honor and gratitude toward God for granting it in the first place. As for the idea that life is "subject to [God's] power, Who kills and makes to live," which Aquinas also expresses, Mitchell poses the following question: if lifesaving medical procedures do not challenge this power, then why would shortening life necessarily do so? He concludes, "In the end, it may be better to think of God's sovereignty as concerned with the fact that man will die as opposed to when each person's time will come." Regarding Aquinas's defense of Samson's suicide on the grounds that Samson received permission to do so, Mitchell's words are again relevant: "If someone who is dying, near the end of life, existing in misery, claims that he or she spoke to God and got the go-ahead to end his or her life, who is to say it isn't true?" For Mitchell, then, these sorts of religious arguments against suicide do not demonstrate its immorality.[125]

If Mitchell's rebuttals here cannot be adequately countered, a better anti-suicide approach might be to claim that Samson directly intended the death of the Philistines but not his own,[126] and then to focus on Gen. 9:5 and the Fifth Commandment ("You shall not kill"), as Maimonides and Aquinas respectively do, as scriptural support against suicide. Mitchell claims that the Fifth Commandment was meant to deal only with "relational injuries . . . that would subvert a moral community" (given that these are the focus of all of the other commandments that do not deal with God directly),[127] although, as Augustine points out in the *City of God* passage to which Aquinas refers, there is no such qualification in the commandment itself (as there is with "You shall not bear false witness against your neighbor"), and in any case it should be read in the context of the scriptural call to "love our neighbor as ourselves."[128] In addition, Aquinas's articulation of the idea that suicide violates the natural law merits further reflection,[129] as does his understanding that this act has social consequences. One who commits physician-assisted suicide may rob herself of further opportunities to benefit others by comforting them with her words or presence, providing a courageous example in sustaining her spirits in the face of tribulation, and enabling them to grow in the virtue of charity as they care for her. For Catholics, the late Joseph Cardinal Bernardin would be an excellent example of someone who did all these things in manifesting the art of dying well.[130] On the other hand, as Jewish and Catholic thinkers have come to recognize, where suicide does take place, it is appropriate to consider mitigating psychological circumstances (which Maimonides and Aquinas appear to neglect) and mourn and offer prayers for the deceased.[131]

Of course, even those opposed to suicide (at the end of life or otherwise) need not hold that life must be preserved at all costs. The Catholic moral tradition, for instance, says that while we are morally obligated to use ordinary medical treatments to prolong our life (i.e., ones that are proportionate and likely beneficial), we are permitted to forego or discontinue extraordinary medical procedures that are inordinately burdensome. The tradition adds that palliative care may be provided even if (as in the case of morphine) this may hasten death.[132] Although they may not always explicitly distinguish between "extraordinary" and "ordinary" means, a number of modern Jewish thinkers have agreed that it can be appropriate to withhold or withdraw certain forms of medical treatment and that palliative care that accelerates death can be acceptable.[133] Some of Maimonides's and Aquinas's reflections can help show us why such life-shortening actions are permissible. As one commentator has noted, if like Maimonides we understand the physician to have a duty to restore lost health, then we can come to the conclusion that if restoration is not possible, the physician's obligation to provide treatment ceases, and she may be permitted to hold back or remove medical treatment from a patient near death.[134] Just as self-defense is licit since the death of the aggressor is not directly intended (as per Aquinas), so too eschewing extraordinary means and administering morphine are allowed since the death of the patient is not willed. Rather, the intentions of these actions can be described as "avoid[ing] needlessly prolonging life with treatment" and relieving pain, respectively; if the patient were to live on in either case (as sometimes happens after the removal of a respirator), we would not have to say that those intentions were thwarted.[135] Moreover, Aquinas's remark that we should love our lives in "due measure" and that our "last end" is most important provides further justification for this view of extraordinary and palliative care and against an inordinate vitalism.[136]

One especially worthwhile legacy that both Maimonides and Aquinas leave us is that caring for our *own* bodies is a moral task. They themselves focus on our bodies as an instrument for serving God, but one might also highlight the fact that when we are in good physical health, we are better able to love and serve our neighbors, including our family, friends, co-workers, and customers. And on the other hand, as Maimonides and Aquinas rightly point out, a lack of moderation in drink can lead to other problems, such as a loss of reason, the flaring up of anger, and sexual misconduct. Note also that both thinkers present an appealing "morality of happiness," particularly through their view that moderation in food, drink, and (according to Maimonides) sex is conducive to our physical and emotional well-being.[137] Despite the ethical implications of living moderately and caring for our own health, many recent general textbooks on medical ethics from Jewish, Catholic, and other perspectives do not allocate significant space to these matters.[138] Devoting even just a chapter to them would better reflect the priorities of Maimonides and Aquinas and provide fruitful insights.

Regarding the specifics of taking care of ourselves, many of Maimonides's recommendations reflect the outdated biology of his time. As any modern-day gourmand knows, there is nothing particularly detrimental about lentils, mustard, edible mushrooms, and garlic, save perhaps for the latter's effect on the breath![139] And there is no conclusive evidence that too-frequent or too-little sex has overall adverse health effects[140] and no firm consensus that there are significant health benefits to drinking wine (as Aquinas also seems to believe)[141] or milk[142] or to eating just once a day.[143] On the other hand, despite Maimonides's somewhat flawed understanding of the workings of the human body, a number of his insights do ring true. Recent research has indicated that overeating leads to obesity (which is the "number one cause of preventable death in the United States") and that many overconsume food that is depicted as healthy;[144] that a wide variety of foods at a meal can in fact foster overeating and obesity;[145] that substituting poultry for red meat and for pork can reduce one's chances of premature death;[146] that chicken soup may alleviate the common cold;[147] that consuming added sugar can lead to obesity, diabetes, and heart disease;[148] that imbibing too much wine can lead to heart and liver problems;[149] that exercise can guard against cancer, diabetes, cardiovascular and respiratory diseases, other maladies, and premature death;[150] that bathing once or twice a week is sufficient for good health (although perhaps not for a pleasing smell, and frequent handwashing is also important);[151] that eight hours of sleep is ideal and deficient sleep has adverse effects on our immune, cardiovascular, metabolic, and reproductive systems;[152] that air pollution can cause heart disease, lung cancer, and other serious illnesses;[153] and that anxiety can produce uncomfortable physical symptoms and perpetuate and even aggravate digestive, respiratory, and heart problems.[154] Some say that the ancient Hebrews discovered preventive medicine,[155] and Maimonides has arguably done more than any other thinker in the Jewish tradition to pass down and elaborate on their insights. In particular, his awareness that there is an ecological dimension to medical ethics – in that environmental pollution is detrimental to the protection of health, for instance – is another subject that should receive greater attention in modern texts in health care ethics from Jewish, Christian, and other perspectives.[156]

## Conclusion

While the analysis above has explored more than the tip of the iceberg of Maimonides's and Aquinas's respective legacies to bioethics, we have not nearly made it all the way down. But other tour guides can help us do so. For example, Edmund Pellegrino and David Thomasma have written a couple of books on how the cardinal virtues (temperance, fortitude, justice, and prudence) and theological virtues (faith, hope, and charity), as conceived by Aquinas and others, can inform the practice of medicine today.[157] As a parallel project, one could consider how Maimonides's general discussion of virtue in the *Mishneh Torah* might also do so. In particular, his reflections on how the virtuous person avoids anger and pride, and otherwise adheres to the mean between two extremes – for example, stinginess and irresponsible generosity, or giddiness and somberness – can provide food for thought for contemporary health care professionals and others.[158] Otherwise, David Feldman and Jason Eberl have probed the ramifications of Maimonides's and Aquinas's thought for the issues of contraception and organ donation, respectively.[159] Finally, Ronit Irshai dons a feminist lens in analyzing the legacy of Maimonides on the issues of procreation, birth control, and abortion,[160] as does Susanne DeCrane in examining how the writings of Aquinas bear on the issue of health care in the United States.[161]

But why bother comparing these two thinkers on medical matters? We can answer this question by calling attention to the various benefits of engaging in comparative ethics and inter-worldview dialogue: it can exercise and hone our critical thinking skills, lead us to (or remind us of) valuable wisdom from other traditions (or our own), inspire us to act in better ways, prompt joint action on important issues, and facilitate fulfilling personal relationships with the other.[162] For instance, as indicated at the very outset of this chapter, Maimonides and Aquinas themselves learned from those of different religions and worldviews. More recently, in his book *Introduction to Jewish and Catholic Bioethics*, Aaron Mackler further elaborates on the fact that ethical dialogue with another tradition can introduce us to new insights that are absent or muted in our own. With regard to medical ethics in particular, Mackler notes that he and other Jews who previously held vitalist tendencies have profited from exposure to Catholic reflection on how foregoing extraordinary medical procedures and entering hospice care do not intend death or violate God's will that we care for our own lives. He also states that one well-respected Catholic theologian (Lisa Sowle Cahill) has acknowledged that the Jewish conception of the fetus as a "pursuer" can support the idea that abortion is necessary if there is a danger to the mother's life. Finally, Mackler suggests that Jewish-Catholic dialogue on bioethics could lead to both sides' working together to secure a "decent minimum" of health care for all.[163]

In fact, merely comparing Maimonides and Aquinas, as I have done in this chapter, could lead to similar results since Maimonides himself articulates the "pursuer" notion and Aquinas reminds us that we should love our lives in "due measure" and that choices that may lead to a loss of life can be permissible as long as that result is not directly intended. And there are other ways in which the aforementioned benefits of dialogue might be realized via an analysis of Maimonides and Aquinas. For instance, when Catholics study Maimonides, they might be pressed to articulate not just a theological but also a philosophical rationale for respecting non-human creatures, learn various practical tips for safeguarding their health (with the caveat that his advice should be checked against the findings of modern science), realize that certain passages in the Hebrew Bible (e.g., Gen. 9:5; Lev. 18:5, 19:16; Deut. 22:2) oblige us to protect our own lives and come to the aid of the other, remember that it is important for health care professionals to strive to care for (and not simply cure) their patients, and be motivated to act more virtuously in various ways as a result. And when Jews read Aquinas, they might discover some significant arguments against suicide and find wisdom and inspiration in certain scriptural passages not in their own biblical canon (e.g., Sirach 31 on the pros and cons of drinking intoxicants, Matt. 25 on the importance of attending to the needy, and Rom. 6:13 on why we should love our own bodies). In addition, they might learn from Aquinas's philosophical theory of human action (which emphasizes that the object, intention, and circumstances of an act are all morally relevant)[164] and utilize his insights here in analyzing specific bioethical matters and acting accordingly. Finally, when Jews and Catholics ponder Aquinas's and Maimonides's reflections on caring for ourselves and others (including the healthy, the sick, and non-human animals), they might be motivated to work together not only in favor of access to adequate health care for all but also in defense of the protection of animals in biomedical research, against the legalization of physician-assisted suicide, and in promotion of preventive care measures.[165] In short, while we need not embrace everything we see on a tour of another's moral heritage, the promise of finding new gifts, collaborative opportunities, and friendships make it a trip worth taking.

## Notes

1 For details on Maimonides's life, works, and influence, see Jonathan Jacobs, "Maimonides (1138–1204)," *Internet Encyclopedia of Philosophy*, n.d., www. iep.utm.edu/maimonid; Fred Rosner, *The Medical Legacy of Moses Maimonides* (Hoboken, NJ: KTAV, 1998), 3–17; Kenneth Seeskin, "Maimonides," in *The Stanford Encyclopedia of Philosophy*, ed. Edward N. Zalta, Spring 2017 edition, https://plato.stanford.edu/archives/spr2017/entries/maimonides.

2 David Clough, "Angels, Beasts, Machines, and Men: Configuring the Human and Nonhuman in Judaeo-Christian Tradition," in *Eating and Believing: Interdisciplinary Perspectives on Vegetarianism and Theology*, eds. David Grumett and Rachel Muers (New York, NY: T&T Clark, 2008), 65 n. 36. As far as I can tell from an online search of the *Summa Theologica* (at http://newadvent.org/summa), all of Aquinas's direct references to Maimonides are to his *Guide of the Perplexed*; it is not clear whether Aquinas was familiar with the *Mishneh Torah*.

3 John Paul II, *Fides et Ratio* ("Faith and Reason") (Vatican City: Libreria Editrice Vaticana, 1998), § 43. For more specifics on Aquinas's life, writings, and legacy, see Christopher M. Brown, "Thomas Aquinas (1224/6–1274)," *Internet Encyclopedia of Philosophy*, n.d., www.iep.utm.edu/aquinas; Brian Davies, *Thomas Aquinas's Summa Theologiae: A Guide and Commentary* (New York, NY: Oxford University Press, 2014), 3–17; Ralph McInerny and John O'Callaghan, "Saint Thomas Aquinas," in *The Stanford Encyclopedia of Philosophy*, Summer 2018 edition, https://plato.stanford.edu/archives/sum2018/entries/aquinas.

4 Moses Maimonides, *Mishneh Torah: A New Translation with Commentaries and Notes*, trans. Eliyahu Touger (New York, NY: Moznaim Pub. Co., 1989–2010 [1178]) (hereinafter MT), *Sefer Nezikin* ("The Book of Damages"), *Hilchot Rotze'ach USh'mirat Nefesh* ("The Laws of Murder and of the Protection of Human Life"), 1:1, 4; 2:2. An online version of the Touger translation can be found here: www.chabad.org/library/article_cdo/aid/682956/jewish/Mishneh-Torah.htm. I am indebted to a number of sources for pointing me to many of the specific verses of the enormous *Mishneh Torah* that I cite in this chapter, namely Yechiel Michael Barilan, *Jewish Bioethics: Rabbinic Law and Theology in Their Social and Historical Contexts* (New York, NY: Cambridge University Press, 2014); Clough, "Angels, Beasts, Machines, and Men"; Elliot N. Dorff, *Matters of Life and Death: A Jewish Approach to Modern Medical Ethics* (Philadelphia, PA: Jewish Publication Society, 1998), David M. Feldman, *Birth Control in Jewish Law: Marital Relations, Contraception, and Abortion as Set Forth in the Classic Texts of Jewish Law* (Northvale, NJ: Jason Aronson Inc., 1998); Abraham Joshua Heschel, *God in Search of Man: A Philosophy of Judaism* (New York, NY: Farrar, Straus and Giroux, 1955); Fred Rosner, *Biomedical Ethics and Jewish Law* (Hoboken, NJ: KTAV, 2001); Fred Rosner, *Medicine in the Mishneh Torah of Maimonides* (Northvale, NJ: Jason Aronson Inc., 1997 [1984]); Fred Rosner, *Sex Ethics in the Writings of Moses Maimonides* (New York, NY: Bloch Publishing Co., 1974); Daniel Schiff, *Abortion in Judaism* (New York, NY: Cambridge University Press, 2002); Daniel B. Sinclair, *Jewish Biomedical Law: Legal and Extra-Legal Dimensions* (New York, NY: Oxford University Press, 2003); Avraham Steinberg, *Encyclopedia of Medical Ethics: A Compilation of Jewish Medical Law on All Topics of Medical Interest*,

3 vols., trans. Fred Rosner (Nanuet, NY: Feldheim Publishers, 2003); and Rabbi Touger's commentary in the aforementioned Moznaim English edition of the *Mishneh Torah*. That said, in the case of each of these verses I have gone back to this edition to read and reflect on them in their surrounding context (and alongside Touger's commentary), and have structured my discussion of them in an original manner.

5 MT, *Hilchot Rotze'ach*, 4:9. See also MT, *Sefer Nezikin, Hilchot Chovel UMazik* ("The Laws of Personal Injury"), 5:1, 11 (which prohibits injuring others more generally).

6 MT, *Hilchot Rotze'ach*, 1:14. All Biblical quotations from the *Mishneh Torah* are transcribed as they appear in the Moznaim English edition.

7 Maimonides adds that while such people should not be actively put to death, Jewish idolaters ought to be. His rationale is that "they cause difficulty to the Jews and sway the people away from God." On this issue and the one in the main text, see ibid., 4:10–12 (which contains the quotations in the main text); MT, *Sefer Madda* ("The Book of Knowledge"), *Hilchot Avodat Kochavim V'Chukkoteihem* ("The Laws of the Worship of Stars and their Statutes"), 10:1 (citing Deut. 7:2).

8 Rosner, *Biomedical Ethics and Jewish Law*, 42; Sinclair, *Jewish Biomedical Law*, 156–157 (both citing Moses Maimonides, *Commentary to the Mishnah, Nedarim*, 4:4).

9 Samuel Kottek, "Caring and Curing: Maimonides' Outlook," in *Moses Maimonides and His Practice of Medicine*, eds. Kenneth Collins, Samuel Kottek, and Fred Rosner (New York, NY: Maimonides Research Institute, 2013), 34–40, 43–44 (citing Moses Maimonides, *Treatise on Asthma; Regimen of Health*, 3:13, 4:15; *Commentary on the Aphorisms of Hippocrates*).

10 MT, *Sefer Zemanim* ("The Book of Seasons"), *Hilchot Shabbat* ("The Laws of the Sabbath"), 2:1–24; Rosner, *Medicine in the Mishneh Torah of Maimonides*, 115.

11 MT, *Hilchot Avodat Kochavim*, 10:2 (see also the accompanying Touger commentary). Daniel Sinclair notes that these seven laws include prohibitions of "idolatry, blasphemy, bloodshed, forbidden sexual relations, theft, [and] tearing of a limb from a living animal," along with "the positive obligation to set up a system of justice," and he contends that they "constitute a form of natural law in the Jewish tradition." Sinclair, *Jewish Biomedical Law*, 35–40, 44.

12 MT, *Sefer Shoftim* ("The Book of Judges"), *Hilchot Evel* ("The Laws of Mourning"), 14:1, 4.

13 Ibid., 14:4.

14 Ibid., 14:6.

15 Ibid., 14:12; *Sefer Shoftim, Hilchot Melachim U'Milchamoteihem* ("The Laws of Kings and Their Wars"), 10:12 (which contains the quotation in the main text).

16 MT, *Sefer Nashim* ("The Book of Women"), *Hilchot Sotah* ("The Laws Pertaining to a Woman Suspected of Infidelity"), 3:7, 15–16, 20 (see also the accompanying Touger commentary); J. David Bleich, *Bioethical Dilemmas: A Jewish Perspective* (Hoboken, NJ: KTAV, 1998), 63, 115. Upon reviewing our book manuscript (including my own chapter), Celia Deane-Drummond has called my attention to the ethically problematic and apparently sexist nature of this particular punishment, which was reserved for women. Celia Deane-Drummond, e-mail messages to author, January 7 and 8, 2019.

17 MT, *Hilchot Rotze'ach*, 2:7–8 (see also the Touger commentary here); *Hilchot Evel*, 4:5.

18 MT, *Hilchot Rotze'ach*, 1:9. Daniel Schiff shows that according to historical rabbinic commentary, Maimonides here specifically states that the fetus is "like

a *rodef*" (ke-rodef) rather than literally a *rodef.* Schiff, *Abortion in Judaism,* 82–83, 87, 91. Schiff also remarks that while Maimonides was following previous rabbinic authority in holding that the fetus could be aborted if the mother's life was endangered, his decision to use the *rodef* terminology here was "unprecedented," with no prompting from the Talmud. Finally, Schiff notes that Rambam's decision to apply this terminology to the fetus but not to the one whose head has emerged "appears to defy logic," given that in both cases this being poses a danger to the mother's life. Ibid., 59–61.

19  Schiff, *Abortion in Judaism,* 6 n. 22.

20  Sinclair, *Jewish Biomedical Law,* 13.

21  Regarding such a line of reasoning, see Feldman, *Birth Control in Jewish Law,* 279–281, 284; Ronit Irshai, *Fertility and Jewish Law: Feminist Perspectives on Orthodox Responsa Literature* (Waltham, MA: Brandeis University Press, 2012), 157–158, 161–164; Schiff, *Abortion in Judaism,* 61 n. 9 (citing Daniel Sinclair). For another passage that points to the value of the fetus, see MT, *Hilchot Shabbat,* 2:15 (stating that if a woman in labor perishes on the Sabbath, an attempt must be made to save the fetus in her womb, for "the Sabbath laws are violated even when there is only a possibility of saving a life").

22  Regarding such a rationale, see Feldman, *Birth Control in Jewish Law,* 277–278, 281, 283; Irshai, *Fertility and Jewish Law,* 139–140, 156–158, 173–175; Schiff, *Abortion in Judaism,* 87. For other passages that downplay the worth of the fetus, see Feldman, *Birth Control in Jewish Law,* 254 (citing Maimonides, *Commentary to the Mishnah, Niddah,* 5:3 as saying that the fetus "has no power of acquisition"); MT, *Sefer Nashim, Hilchot Ishut* ("The Laws of Marriage"), 21:11 (stating that a pregnant woman must not be prohibited, even out of concern for her child, from eating as much as she wants because "the physical pain the woman feels takes priority"); MT, *Sefer Shoftim, Hilchot Sanhedrin V'Haonshin Hamesurim Lahem* ("The Laws of the Courts and the Penalties Placed Under Their Jurisdiction"), 12:4 (asserting that in cases where a pregnant woman is sentenced to die and has not yet entered into labor, one does not spare the fetus but kills it first and then the woman herself); MT, *Hilchot Chovel UMazik,* 4:1, 5 (which alludes to Exod. 21:22–23 in indicating that someone who causes a miscarriage incurs a financial penalty while someone who also causes the pregnant mother to die merits execution). See also Moses Maimonides, *The Guide of the Perplexed,* trans. Shlomo Pines (Chicago: University of Chicago Press, 1963 [1190]) (hereinafter GP), II, ch. 17 (suggesting that the nature of a fetus is different from that of one who, "after having been born, achieves perfection").

23  MT, *Hilchot Melachim,* 9:4. On the Talmudic roots of this teaching, see Irshai, *Fertility and Jewish Law,* 127–128. Irshai and Feldman state that this penalty does not apply to cases of abortion for the sake of the woman's health. Ibid., 130–131; Feldman, *Birth Control in Jewish Law,* 259–261.

24  MT, *Hilchot Rotze'ach,* 2:6.

25  Thomas Aquinas, *Summa Theologica,* trans. Fathers of the English Dominican Province (New York, NY: Benziger, 1947 [c. 1274]) (hereinafter ST), II-II, q. 64, a. 6. An online version of this translation can be found here: www.newadvent. org/summa. Aquinas had not yet finished this work upon his death in 1274. Davies, *Thomas Aquinas's Summa Theologiae,* 7.

26  ST, II-II, q. 64, a. 6. All biblical quotations from the *Summa Theologica* are transcribed as they appear in the Benziger English edition.

27  ST, II-II, q. 64, a. 2 & ad. 3 (relying in part on Aristotle and Ps. 49:21). In contrast, Pope Francis and the current *Catechism of the Catholic Church* firmly hold that "the death penalty is inadmissible because it is an attack on the inviolability and dignity of the person." Congregation for the Doctrine of the Faith, "New Revision of Number 2267 of the *Catechism of the*

    *Catholic Church* on the Death Penalty – Rescriptum 'Ex Audientia SS.mi,'"
August 18, 2018, www.vatican.va/roman_curia/congregations/cfaith/documents/
rc_con_cfaith_doc_20180801_catechismo-penadimorte_en.html.

28  ST, I, q. 29, a. 1. I am indebted to Jason T. Eberl, *Thomistic Principles and Bioethics* (New York, NY: Routledge, 2006) for directing me to each of Aquinas's
passages cited in this paragraph that directly pertain to his understanding of personhood (endnotes 28 to 31). With that said, I cite directly to English editions of
the *Summa Theologica* and *Summa Contra Gentiles* since I have consulted them
for the wider context of said passages.

29  ST, I, q. 76, a. 3, ad. 3; q. 90, a. 2; q. 118, a. 2 & ad. 2.

30  Eberl, *Thomistic Principles and Bioethics*, 130 n. 10 (citing Thomas Aquinas,
*Commentary on the Sentences*, III, d. 3, q. 5, a. 2).

31  Thomas Aquinas, *Summa Contra Gentiles* ("Summary against the Gentiles"):
*Book Two: Creation*, trans. James F. Anderson (Notre Dame, IN: University of
Notre Dame Press, 1975 [1956]) (hereinafter SCG, II), ch. 59, § 17. The *Summa
Contra Gentiles* was completed around 1265; see Davies, *Thomas Aquinas's
Summa Theologiae*, 7. An online version of the translations of the *Summa Con-
tra Gentiles* that are referenced in this chapter is at http://dhspriory.org/thomas/
ContraGentiles.htm.

32  ST, II-II, q. 64, a. 8, obj. & ad. 2 (citing Exod. 21:22–23). Note that while
both Maimonides and Aquinas consider this biblical passage, the latter thinker
appears to arrive at a graver conclusion regarding it: the one who causes the
"animated fetus" to die has committed murder and is not simply financially
liable (cf. endnote 22).

33  Fabrizio Amerini, *Aquinas on the Beginning and End of Human Life*, trans.
Mark Henninger (Cambridge, MA: Harvard University Press, 2013 [2009]),
182 (quoting Aquinas, *Commentary on the Sentences*, IV, d. 31, q. 2, a. 3). See
also ibid., 7–8. In other words, Aquinas would have considered an abortion at
this point to be a kind of contraception and thereby unethical. George Dennis
O'Brien, *The Church and Abortion: A Catholic Dissent* (Lanham, MD: Row-
man & Littlefield, 2010), 74–75. Cf. Thomas Aquinas, *Summa Contra Gentiles:
Book Three: Providence, Part II*, trans. Vernon J. Bourke (Notre Dame, IN:
University of Notre Dame Press, 1975 [1956]) (hereinafter SCG, III), ch. 122,
§ 9 (holding that "arrang[ing] for the emission of semen apart from the proper
purpose of generating and bringing up children" is distinct from homicide, but
is still sinful on the grounds that it conflicts with the natural maintenance of the
species).

34  ST, II-II, q. 32, a. 2 & ad. 1–2.

35  Simkha Y. Weintraub, "*L'Mashal*: Metaphor and Meaning in Illness," in *Midrash and Medicine: Healing Body and Soul in the Jewish Interpretive Tradition*,
ed. William Cutter (Woodstock, VT: Jewish Lights Publishing, 2011), 11.

36  "As for the ignorant and disobedient, their state is despicable proportionately to
their lack of this overflow [of the divine intellect], and they have been relegated
to the rank of the individuals of all the other species of animals: *He is like the
beasts that speak not*. For this reason it is a light thing to kill them, and has even
been enjoined because of its utility." GP, III, ch. 18 (citing Ps. 49:13, 21).

37  For the full text of this oath, see Peter Tyson, "The Hippocratic Oath Today,"
*NOVA*, March 27, 2001, www.pbs.org/wgbh/nova/body/hippocratic-oath-
today.html.

38  While as indicated above Maimonides and Aquinas rely upon Ps. 49:21, it does
not clearly confirm any notion that humans can actually become beasts and
lose their dignity; this psalm simply suggests that foolish persons are like animals in that they both die without being specifically redeemed by God. To be
fair, Aquinas's infelicitous phrasing in question 64 regarding sinners is tempered

somewhat by his statement elsewhere that sinners are owed our charity, even when they are being put to death. ST, II-II, q. 25, a. 6 & ad. 2. For an analysis of both passages that concludes that Aquinas overall thinks that sinners do maintain dignity, see Peter Karl Koritansky, *Thomas Aquinas and the Philosophy of Punishment* (Washington, DC: The Catholic University of America Press, 2012), 186–190.

39 For considerations along these lines, see Nicanor Pier Giorgio Austriaco, O.P., *Biomedicine and Beatitude: An Introduction to Catholic Bioethics* (Washington, DC: The Catholic University of America Press, 2011), 190; Carl Cohen, Martin Benjamin, and the Ethics and Social Impact Committee of the Transplant and Health Policy Center, Ann Arbor, Michigan, "Alcoholics and Liver Transplantation," *Journal of the American Medical Association* 265 no. 10 (1991): 1299–1300. Others might counter that even those with such genetic predispositions are still morally responsible, for they should have taken special precautions in light of their condition. On this general point, see Dorff, *Matters of Life and Death*, 250–251. But even if it is most just to both take into account moral culpability and put these predispositions completely aside in doing so (a debatable point), again, it would seem unfair to not at least consider other potentially mitigating factors, such as the circumstances of the patient's engagement in substance abuse, and/or the patient's commitment to a morally praiseworthy lifestyle subsequent to a period of such abuse. Regarding such factors, see Alexandra Rockey Fleming, "When Drinkers Suffer Liver Disease, Should Getting a Transplant Be So Hard?," *Washington Post*, January 26, 2017, www.washingtonpost.com/national/health-science/when-drinking-ruins-someones-liver-should-they-qualify-for-a-transplant/2017/01/27/7ededff0-d1c7-11e6-9cb0-54ab630851e8_story.html.

40 For a similar line of reasoning, see Austriaco, *Biomedicine and Beatitude*, 190.

41 Ibid. For further discussion of different perspectives on the topic of the paragraph in the main text (including a reference to the aforementioned Cohen article), see Tom L. Beauchamp and James F. Childress, *Principles of Biomedical Ethics*, 7th ed. (New York, NY: Oxford University Press, 2013), 274–276 (concluding that no such patient should be assigned a lower priority automatically, but that such an assignment would be appropriate in certain instances due to moral blameworthiness, including where an alcoholic "fails to seek effective treatment for alcoholism and develops alcohol-related ESLF [end-stage liver failure]" and an organ recipient culpably fails to take the medication needed for the original transplant to succeed). This proposal of "evaluat[ion] on a case-by-case basis" may be preferable to a policy of total exclusion or automatic demotion, although it may not completely address Austriaco's concerns.

In reviewing a draft of this essay, the prominent Jewish ethicist Elliot Dorff thoughtfully suggests that an alcoholic's intemperate actions may still be grounds for denying that person a liver transplant since they can be indicia of future behavior that would reduce that person's chances of transplantation success relative to a non-alcoholic. Elliot N. Dorff, e-mail message to author, November 16, 2017; see also Dorff, *Matters of Life and Death*, 304. However, note that "practice guidelines from the liver-diseases association assert that 'only a small fraction' of ALD [alcoholic liver disease] transplant patients revert to heavy alcohol use or abuse and that 'overall survival rates are generally similar between alcohol-related and non-alcohol-related liver transplant recipients.'" Fleming, "When Drinkers Suffer Liver Disease" (citing Robert S. O'Shea, Srinivasan Dasarathy, Arthur J. McCullough, and the Practice Guideline Committee of the American Association for the Study of Liver Diseases and the Practice Parameters Committee of the American College of

Gastroenterology, "AASLD Practice Guidelines: Alcoholic Liver Disease," *Hepatology* 51 no. 1 [2010], www.aasld.org/sites/default/files/guideline_documents/Alcoholic LiverDisease1-2010.pdf). More recently, a study has found that while the short-term survival rate after transplant for those with alcohol-associated liver disease is similar to that for those without, the long-term survival rate (five or more years) for the former group is 11% lower. However, increased attention to the specific medical needs of the former group could help close this gap. Jessica Ravitz, "Alcohol Destroyed Their Livers: Now, They're Increasingly Getting New Ones," *CNN*, January 22, 2019, www.cnn.com/2019/01/22/health/alcohol-liver-transplants-study/index.html (citing Brian P. Lee, Eric Vittinghoff, Jennifer L. Dodge, Giuseppe Cullaro, and Norah A. Terrault, "National Trends and Long-term Outcomes of Liver Transplant for Alcohol-Associated Liver Disease in the United States," *JAMA Internal Medicine* [published online January 22, 2019]; Mack C. Mitchell and Willis C. Maddrey, "Changing Times in Liver Transplantation for Alcohol-Associated Liver Disease," *JAMA Internal Medicine* [published online January 22, 2019]).

42 For an overview of historical Jewish interpretations of Maimonides on abortion, see especially Feldman, *Birth Control in Jewish Law*, 276–281, 283–284, 343; Irshai, *Fertility and Jewish Law*, 139–140, 155–159, 161–164, 173–176 (Irshai herself is more sympathetic to the majority view here); Schiff, *Abortion in Judaism*, 87.

43 For modern-day Thomists in line with the majority view, see Benedict M. Ashley, O.P., "When Does a Human Person Begin to Exist?," in *The Ashley Reader: Redeeming Reason* (Naples, FL: Sapientia Press of Ave Maria University, 2006), 349–363, 368; Benedict M. Ashley, O.P., Jean deBlois, C.S.J., Kevin D. O'Rourke, O.P., *Health Care Ethics: A Catholic Theological Analysis* (Washington, DC: Georgetown University Press, 2006), 72–73; Austriaco, *Biomedicine and Beatitude*, 51–52, 59–60; Eberl, *Thomistic Principles and Bioethics*, 24–42; Anthony Fisher, *Catholic Bioethics for a New Millennium* (New York, NY: Cambridge University Press, 2012), 112, 130. (In fact, as Fisher points out, Aquinas already does acknowledge that one person did receive a human soul at his conception – Jesus. Ibid., 112; ST, III, q. 33, a. 2.) For an example of a scholar from the minority perspective, see O'Brien, *The Church and Abortion*, 69, 74–78. Fabrizio Amerini takes a balanced approach, arguing that modern biology does not necessarily shake Aquinas's support of delayed hominization, but that Aquinas's view regarding the embryo before quickening (specifically his notion that it is developing into a human being but not yet completely human) and his concern for maintaining the human species could logically lead to either very restrictive or somewhat more permissive views on abortion today. Amerini, *Aquinas on the Beginning and End of Human Life*, 212–222, 235–238.

For a further articulation of the idea that the nature and moral status of unborn (and infant) humans is different from that of full-fledged persons, see, e.g., Peter Singer, *Practical Ethics*, 3rd ed. (New York, NY: Cambridge University Press, 2011), 134–154 (recommending that "we accord the fetus no higher moral status than we give to a non-human animal at a similar level of rationality, self-consciousness, awareness, capacity to feel and so on"). For defenses of the notion that the nature and moral status of unborn and infant humans is equivalent to that of full persons, see Austriaco, *Biomedicine and Beatitude*, 50–60, 69–70; Charles C. Camosy, *Peter Singer and Christian Ethics: Beyond Polarization* (New York, NY: Cambridge University Press, 2012), 27–40; Charles C. Camosy, *Beyond the Abortion Wars: A Way Forward for a New Generation* (Grand Rapids, MI: Wm. B. Eerdmans, 2015), 41–58.

44 For one cogent criticism of quickening as a "morally significant dividing line," see Singer, *Practical Ethics*, 126, 128. Note that outside of the context of the morality of abortion, Maimonides himself identifies forty days (for males and

females) as the dividing line between an embryo or "water" on the one hand, and a fetus on the other hand. MT, *Sefer Kedushah* ("The Book of Holiness"), *Hilchot Issurei Bi'ah* ("The Laws Governing Forbidden Sexual Relationships"), 10:1; *Sefer Zeraim* ("The Book of Agricultural Ordinances"), *Hilchot Terumot* ("The Laws of Terumot"), 8:3. This notion echoes an earlier statement in the Talmud. Dorff, *Matters of Life and Death*, 128 & 364 nn. 30 & 32 (explaining that such a Talmudic line is "not based on a theory of ensoulment at a particular moment in the uterus," but that abortion is allowed for additional reasons beforehand, although even then only to safeguard the woman's life or health [citing B. *Yevamot* 69b and B. *Ḥullin* 58a, among other sources]).

45  Note that one can hold both that directly killing unhealthy premature infants is wrong and that we need not do everything in our power to save them. For instance, as I will emphasize again below, in the Catholic tradition refusing extraordinary (i.e., rather burdensome) care is morally permissible, for "[h]ere one does not will to cause death; one's inability to impede it is merely accepted." *Catechism of the Catholic Church*, rev. ed. (Vatican City: Libreria Editrice Vaticana, 1997), § 2278. If one applies this principle to the case of unhealthy premature infants, one could arrive at the same conclusion as a Jewish responsum that (while not using the language of "extraordinary care") holds that it is licit to abstain from "aggressive efforts" to rescue the lives of "severely premature" babies with no "realistic chance of survival." Rabbi Avram Israel Reisner, "Peri- and Neo-Natology: The Matter of Limiting Treatment," September 13, 1995, 355–356, www.rabbinica lassembly.org/sites/default/files/assets/public/halakhah/teshuvot/19912000/reis ner_natology.pdf. (My thanks to Elliot Dorff for directing me to this responsum.)

46  Irshai, *Fertility and Jewish Law*, 128–129.

47  Feldman, *Birth Control in Jewish Law*, 259–260; Irshai, *Fertility and Jewish Law*, 129–131.

48  ST, II-II, q. 64, a. 7.

49  Janet E. Smith and Christopher Kaczor, *Life Issues, Medical Choices: Questions and Answers for Catholics*, 2nd ed. (Cincinnati, OH: Servant, 2016), 24. This principle has four criteria: "the object [i.e., the act chosen] . . . must be morally good or at least morally indifferent or neutral," "the intention of the agent must be directed toward realizing the beneficial effect and avoiding the foreseen harmful effect of his actions," "the bad effect cannot cause the good effect," and "the beneficial effect must be equal to or greater than the foreseen harmful effects." Austriaco, *Biomedicine and Beatitude*, 25, 37–39. I briefly defend it against a couple of its critics (Tom Beauchamp and James Childress) in another essay. Beauchamp and Childress, *Principles of Biomedical Ethics*, 165–168; John J. Fitzgerald, "A Considerably Common Morality: Catholic Ethics and Secular Principlism in Dialogue," *Christian Bioethics* 25 no. 1 (2019): 114–115 n. 16. Another prominent critic is Peter Singer; see Singer, *Practical Ethics*, 176–177, 183–184. For other sources that articulate the principle and defend it as intuitive, see Austriaco, *Biomedicine and Beatitude*, 37–41; Camosy, *Peter Singer and Christian Ethics*, 67, 195–198; Mattison, *Introducing Moral Theology*, 170–173, 378–380; Smith and Kaczor, *Life Issues, Medical Choices*, 24–27.

50  Austriaco, *Biomedicine and Beatitude*, 62–65.

51  Thinking of the fetus as somewhat "like an aggressor" or "like a pursuer" is arguably softer than – and preferable to – directly equating the fetus with an "aggressor," given John Paul II's caution regarding this sort of language: "In no way could th[e] [unborn] human being ever be considered an aggressor, much less an unjust aggressor!" John Paul II, *Evangelium Vitae*, § 58. Cf. Camosy, *Beyond the Abortion Wars*, 65–70 (where Camosy similarly resists speaking of a fetus as an "aggressor," but also suggests that even though it does not will evil it may be a "mortal threat materially," which would justify a direct abortion to protect the mother's life). As I have suggested elsewhere, the sorts of abortions

Camosy has in mind here might be better described as indirect. See my "Review of *Beyond the Abortion Wars: A Way Forward for a New Generation* by Charles C. Camosy," *Studies in Christian Ethics* 29 no. 4 (2016): 491.

52 Rosner, *Biomedical Ethics and Jewish Law*, 210 (citing Maimonides, *Commentary on the Mishnah*, Introduction).

53 GP, III, ch. 13. On Maimonides's shift in thinking here, see Clough, "Angels, Beasts, Machines, and Men," 64. I am indebted to certain sources for directing me to a number of the passages of the *Guide of the Perplexed* referenced in this section and the next, namely Barilan, *Jewish Bioethics*; Clough, "Angels, Beasts, Machines, and Men"; Rosner, *Biomedical Ethics and Jewish Law*; Rosner, *Sex Ethics in the Writings of Moses Maimonides*; Steinberg, *Encyclopedia of Medical Ethics*; and Touger's commentary to the *Mishneh Torah*. However, I also have consulted these passages and their broader context in the English translation of the primary source itself.

54 GP, III, ch. 17.

55 Ibid.

56 Ibid., III, ch. 48. As Jonathan Sacks, former Chief Rabbi of the United Hebrew Congregations of Great Britain and the Commonwealth, has perceptively noted, Maimonides seems to backtrack here from his earlier statement in the *Mishneh Torah* that this was simply God's decree and not motivated by mercy. Jonathan Sacks, "Ki Tetse (5768) – Animal Welfare," September 13, 2008, http://rabbisacks. org/covenant-conversation-5768-ki-tetse-animal-welfare (citing MT, *Sefer Ahavah* ["The Book of the Love of God"], *Hilchot Tefilah and Birkat Kohanim* ["The Laws of Prayer and the Priestly Blessing"], 9:7).

57 MT, *Hilchot Rotze'ach*, 13:13; *Hilchot Shabbat*, 21:9–10, 25:26.

58 ST, I, q. 47, a. 1; a. 2 & ad. 1. I am beholden to Clough, "Angels, Beasts, Machines, and Men," for leading me to some of the passages discussed in this particular paragraph. That said, I also have analyzed these passages and their wider context in the English translations of the primary sources themselves.

59 ST, I, q. 103, a. 5 & ad. 2. In fact, on this issue he explicitly distinguishes himself from Maimonides. ST, I, q. 22, a. 2, ad. 5. Still, like Maimonides, Aquinas does not think that animals can attain to the perfect happiness of heaven. ST, I, q. 75, a. 6; I-II, q, 1, a. 8; q. 5, a. 1, ad. 1; II-II, q. 25, a. 3; III (supplement), q. 91, a. 5; SCG, II, ch. 82. After Aquinas's death, the *Summa Theologica* was completed via addition of a "supplement" compiled from his much earlier thought (possibly by his secretary); as Brian Davies notes, "it should not be assumed that Aquinas agreed with everything he said in [this prior work] by the time of his death." Davies, *Thomas Aquinas's Summa Theologiae*, 4–5, 7. For this reason, in the few places I do cite to the supplement, I also cite to at least one of Aquinas's later writings.

60 SCG, III, ch. 112, esp. §§ 1–2, 4, 11–12. Elsewhere, he suggests that among God's creatures, human beings and angels alone are in the image of God given their special ability to "know or understand." ST, I, q. 93, a. 2, a. 3 & ad. 2, a. 6. On the "irrational[ity]" of and lack of freedom in animals, see also ST, I, q. 76, a. 1; q. 83, a. 1; II-II, q. 64, a. 1 & ad. 2 (citing Augustine, *City of God*, I, ch. 20).

61 ST, II-II, q. 25, a. 3.

62 ST, II-II, q. 64, a. 1; see also SCG, III, ch. 112, § 12.

63 Singer, *Practical Ethics*, 240–241 (citing ST, I-II, q. 72, a. 4). See also ST, II-II, a. 64, a. 1, ad. 3 ("He that kills another's ox, sins, not through killing the ox, but through injuring another man in his property. Wherefore this is not a species of the sin of murder but of the sin of theft or robbery.")

64 SCG, III, ch. 112, § 13. In the *Summa Theologica*, Aquinas reiterates this ban on cruelty, with explicit reference to Maimonides: "as Rabbi Moses says [Doct. Perplex. iii], 'the Law chose that manner of slaying which was least painful to

the slain animal.' This excluded cruelty on the part of the offerers, and any man-
gling of the animals slain." ST, I-II, q. 102, a. 3, ad. 6. He goes on to say that
from the perspective of reason, "it matters not how man behaves to animals,
because God has subjected all things to man's power" (citing Ps. 8:8), although
from the perspective of emotion, "since it happens that even irrational animals
are sensible to pain, it is possible for the affection of pity to arise in a man with
regard to the sufferings of animals." Still, even this brief concession to sympathy
is followed by the suggestion that the goal of "practic[ing] pity" toward animals
and abstaining from cruelty to them is to enable one to act in this manner toward
one's fellow humans. Ibid., a. 6, ad. 8; see also ad. 1.

For an in-depth treatment of Augustine's and Aquinas's views on non-human
creation, with attention to their helpful insights as well as their "fundamental
anthropocentrism," see Daniel P. Scheid, *The Cosmic Common Good: Religious
Grounds for Ecological Ethics* (New York, NY: Oxford University Press, 2016),
45–63; on Aquinas's thought on this topic, see also Camosy, *Peter Singer and
Christian Ethics*, 111–114, 130–133.

65 *Catechism*, §§ 353, 2415, 2417–2418 (emphasis added). It would appear that
while causing such suffering may indeed be opposed to human dignity (perhaps because of its potential to deform our character, as Aquinas suggests), it
would more directly be contrary to animal dignity. While the *Catechism* does
not explicitly speak of the dignity of animals here, Charles Camosy has made the
case that a concern for it is present in the Bible, Church teaching, recent Catholic
theology, and the lives of many vegetarian saints. He adds that some animals can
properly be said to have rights to "life, liberty, and freedom from physical and
psychological torture." Camosy, *Peter Singer and Christian Ethics*, 101–102,
105, 130–133. Similarly, Daniel Scheid, relying on both historical and more
recent Catholic thought, argues in favor of dignity and rights for non-human
beings. Scheid, *The Cosmic Common Good*, 38, 61, 79, 101–116.

66 *Catechism*, §§ 340, 344 (citing St. Francis of Assisi, Canticle of the Creatures).
In discovering these two sections of the *Catechism*, I am obliged to Charles C.
Camosy and Susan Kopp, "The Use of Non-Human Animals in Biomedical
Research: Can Moral Theology Fill the Gap?," *Journal of Moral Theology* 3 no.
2 (2014): 66.

67 *Catechism*, §§ 2416, 2418.

68 In particular, Aquinas's aforementioned rationale – that animals lack reason and
free will, and cannot attain to heaven – can be challenged on each point. For
instance, the secular philosopher Tom Beauchamp and the Catholic moral theologian Charles Camosy suggest that at least some animals can possess a measure
of rationality and freedom/autonomy. See my "A Considerably Common Morality," 93, 110; Camosy, *Peter Singer and Christian Ethics,* 132–133. Also, unlike
Maimonides and Aquinas, Pope Francis appears to allow for the presence of animals in heaven. Francis, *Laudato Si'* ("Praise Be to You") (Vatican City: Libreria
Editrice Vaticana, 2015), § 243 ("Eternal life will be a shared experience of awe, in
which each creature, resplendently transfigured, will take its rightful place . . ."); 
see also ibid., §§ 100, 246 (suggesting that creatures in general "journey towards
[God's] infinite light" together and are guided by Jesus "towards fullness as
their end"). Francis does not here reference Psalm 49, which was mentioned
above and appears to suggest that animals will remain unredeemed (see especially vv. 13, 15–16, 21); perhaps he would hold that these verses need not be
read literally. Finally, Deane-Drummond has remarked to me that fellowship
with animals is significant in that it can actually promote our own well-being,
in turn. Deane-Drummond, e-mail messages to author, January 7 and March
4, 2019 (citing Deborah L. Wells, "The Effects of Animals on Human Health and
Well-Being," *Journal of Social Issues* 65 no. 3 [2009]: 523–543, which concludes

that "[a]lthough the evidence for a direct causal association between human well-being and companion animals is still not conclusive, the literature reviewed above is largely supportive of the widely held belief that 'pets are good for us'").

69 Ibid., § 2417. More recently, Pope Francis has called attention to a number of the relevant aspects of Aquinas's and the *Catechism*'s respective teachings on creation and animals, while also elaborating further on relevant biblical passages (with attention to Deut. 22:4, 6), the example of St. Francis of Assisi, and the problem of species extinction, among other issues. Francis, *Laudato Si'*, §§ 10–12, 33–35, 40–42, 66–69, 76–77, 80–81, 83–92 ("our indifference or cruelty towards fellow creatures of this world sooner or later affects the treatment we mete out to other human beings"), 96, 100, 130, 140, 221, 240, 246.

70 GP, III, ch. 35.

71 For the Fourteenth Dalai Lama, the fact that all sentient beings naturally want to be happy and not to suffer, just like we do, gives rise to our duty to respect those wishes. Dalai Lama XIV, *Ethics for the New Millennium* (New York, NY: Riverhead Books, 1999), 4–5, 28, 127, 147, 157, 164; Dalai Lama XIV, "A Tibetan Buddhist Perspective on Spirit in Nature," *Spirit and Nature: Why the Environment Is a Religious Issue: An Interfaith Dialogue*, eds. Steven C. Rockefeller and John C. Elder (Boston, MA: Beacon Press, 1992), 115, 119. On the Dalai Lama's concern for animals, see also my "Together Again, Naturally? Pope Benedict XVI and the Fourteenth Dalai Lama on Our Environmental Responsibility," *Journal of Catholic Social Thought* 11 no. 2 (2014): 479–486.

72 According to Singer, philosophers and religious thinkers throughout history have generally agreed that "[e]thics takes a universal point of view," and this perspective leads us to "the principle of equal consideration of interests," which mandates that "we give equal weight in our moral deliberations to the like interests of all those affected by our actions." This principle, in turn, requires us to attend to the interests of non-human animals among others, particularly their interest in avoiding suffering. In other words, for Singer, "[i]f a being suffers, there can be no moral justification for refusing to take that suffering into consideration." Singer, *Practical Ethics*, 10–12, 20–21, 48–60.

73 As I suggest in a new article, Beauchamp also is supportive of such a rationale. See my "A Considerably Common Morality," 110–111.

74 Singer, *Practical Ethics*, 56–58.

75 Kevin D. O'Rourke and Philip J. Boyle, *Medical Ethics: Sources of Catholic Teachings*, 4th ed. (Washington, DC: Georgetown University Press, 2011), 280 (quoting John Paul II, "Biological Experimentation," October 23, 1982).

76 For recent examples of such reflection from a Jewish and a Catholic perspective, respectively, see Rosner, *Biomedical Ethics and Jewish Law*, 413–433; Camosy and Kopp, "The Use of Non-Human Animals in Biomedical Research."

77 MT, *Hilchot Rotze'ach*, 2:2–3. See also MT, *Hilchot Chovel UMazik*, 5:1 (which prohibits injuring oneself more generally). Also, as Dorff says, the *Mishneh Torah* mandates that "we bless God for making people [with disabilities] different." Dorff, *Matters of Life and Death*, 187 & 374 n. 34 (citing MT, *Sefer Ahavah, Hilchot Berachot* ["The Laws of Blessings"], 10:12). For Dorff, this blessing "boldly reassert[s] the divine quality of such lives" and suggests that we should discourage them from committing suicide. Ibid.

78 MT, *Hilchot Evel*, 1:11.

79 MT, *Sefer Madda, Yesodei HaTorah* ("The Laws [Which Are] the Foundations of the Torah"), 5:1–3. Exceptions here include instances where the Jew is asked to pay homage to other gods, engage in prohibited sexual activity, or murder. Maimonides later explains why these three sins are singled out. Ibid., 5:7.

80 MT, *Hilchot Rotze'ach*, 11:4–5.

81  MT, *Sefer Madda, Hilchot De'ot* ("The Laws of Personality [Development]"), 3:3, 4:1. See also GP, III, ch. 27 (stating that the health of the body is necessary for the perfection of the soul). In the introduction to my chapter, I noted that Maimonides relied on the medical advice of non-Jews, but also that the *Mishneh Torah* is aimed at transmitting the law of the Bible and Talmud. In what follows, I will be discussing the *Mishneh Torah*'s medical advice, which naturally raises the question of whether that advice is grounded in Jewish or non-Jewish sources. Touger's commentary prefacing *Hilchot De'ot* 4 notes some debate on this question.

82  MT, *Hilchot De'ot*, 3:2; 4:1–2, 15; 5:1 (citing Prov. 13:25), 2; GP, III, ch. 8; Rosner, *Medical Legacy*, 24 (citing Maimonides, *Treatise on Asthma*, 5).

83  Reut Ben-Ami and Elliot M. Berry, "Maimonides on Nutrition and Lifestyle: Is His Advice Still Applicable Today?," in *Moses Maimonides and His Practice of Medicine*, 93 (citing Maimonides, *Treatise on Asthma*, 5:4); Rosner, *Medical Legacy*, 24 (citing Maimonides, *Treatise on Asthma*, 5).

84  Rosner, *Medical Legacy*, 24 (citing Maimonides, *Treatise on Asthma*, 6).

85  MT, *Hilchot De'ot*, 2:1, 3:1, 5:10; GP, III, ch. 48; Ben-Ami and Berry, "Maimonides on Nutrition and Lifestyle," 96–97 (citing Maimonides, *Treatise on Asthma*, 3:3–4).

86  Rosner, *Medical Legacy*, 242–245 (citing Moses Maimonides, *The Medical Aphorisms of Moses Maimonides*, vol. 2; Maimonides, *Treatise on Asthma*).

87  MT, *Hilchot De'ot*, 4:9, 15 (citing Prov. 21:23); Rosner, *Medical Legacy*, 202 (citing Maimonides, *Treatise on Poisons*). Touger's commentary to this part of *Hilchot De'ot* clarifies that in addressing mushrooms in this particular place of the *Mishneh Torah*, Maimonides presumably was concerned about their unhealthiness but not their potential poisonousness. Touger does not clarify here whether Maimonides thought that salt itself was generally unhealthy; in a nearby verse (4:13), Rambam actually recommends salt as a remedy for constipation.

88  Rosner, *Medicine in the Mishneh Torah of Maimonides*, 246 (citing Maimonides, *Medical Aphorisms*, 20:7).

89  MT, *Sefer Kedushah* ("The Book of Holiness"), *Hilchot Ma'achalot Assurot* ("The Laws Governing Forbidden Foods"), 14:13.

90  MT, *Hilchot De'ot*, 3:1–2, 4:12. Maimonides here is critical of nazarites who abstain from wine; on this point, he cites Num. 6:11 and Eccles. 7:16. However, Touger's commentary suggests that Rambam is addressing those who practice "abstention for the sake of abstention," for elsewhere the *Mishneh Torah* indicates that someone who foregoes wine in order to "establish his character traits and correct his conduct . . . is considered eager and praiseworthy." MT, *Sefer Hafla'ah* ("The Book of Promises"), *Hilchot Nedarim* ("The Laws of Vows"), 13:23. See also MT, *Sefer Hafla'ah, Hilchot Nezirut* ("The Laws of Nazarites"), 10:14 (commending the one who makes "a nazirite vow to God in a holy manner") (citing Num. 6:7–8; Amos 2:11); GP, III, chs. 33, 48 (citing Num. 6:4–5; Judg. 13:14; Prov. 7:26; Isa. 28:7).

91  MT, *Sefer Zemanim, Hilchot Shevitat Yom Tov* ("The Laws of Resting on the Holidays"), 6:18; Rosner, *Medical Legacy*, 25 (citing Maimonides, *Treatise on Asthma*, 7); Rosner, *Medicine in the Mishneh Torah of Maimonides*, 256–257 (citing Maimonides, *Medical Aphorisms*, 21:6).

92  MT, *Hilchot De'ot*, 5:3 (which contains the quotation in the main text); *Hilchot Shevitat Yom Tov*, 6:20–21; *Hilchot Issurei Bi'ah*, 22:21; Rosner, *Medicine in the Mishneh Torah of Maimonides*, 259 (citing Maimonides, *Medical Aphorisms*, 13:22, 17:26). On the "shameful[ness]" of inordinate drinking in involving "the corruption of the intellect and the body," see also GP, III, ch. 8.

93 Rosner, *Medicine in the Mishneh Torah of Maimonides*, 248 (quoting Maimonides, *Medical Aphorisms*, 20:39); see also Rosner, *Medical Legacy*, 64–66 (citing Maimonides, *Medical Aphorisms*, 20–22). However, he counsels those with headaches to avoid milk. Ben-Ami and Berry, "Maimonides on Nutrition and Lifestyle," 97 (citing Maimonides, *Treatise on Asthma*, 3:4).

94 MT, *Hilchot De'ot*, 4:2; *Hilchot Rotze'ach*, 11:6; Ben-Ami and Berry, "Maimonides on Nutrition and Lifestyle," 101.

95 MT, *Hilchot De'ot*, 3:2, 4:19, 5:4; Ben-Ami and Berry, "Maimonides on Nutrition and Lifestyle," 103 (citing Maimonides, *Treatise on Asthma*, 10:8); Rosner, *Medical Legacy*, 26 (citing Maimonides, *Treatise on Asthma*, 10); Rosner, *Sex Ethics*, 71–72 (which contains the quotation in the main text and cites Maimonides, *Medical Aphorisms*, 7, 9, 17). In the aforementioned passages from *Hilchot De'ot* and *Sex Ethics*, Maimonides pinpoints some particular dangers for the male body; he speaks of how ejaculation can in some instances be medically indicated, whereas too much release of sperm weakens the body and causes one's beard to grow unusually long.

96 MT, *Hilchot Ishut*, 14:1–2. Maimonides permits one who is unusually passionate about studying Torah to never marry, unless "his natural inclination overcomes him, [in which case] he is obligated to marry . . . lest he be prompted to sexual thoughts." Ibid., 15:3. Note that later, in the *Guide of the Perplexed*, Maimonides seems to take a more negative view, by not only pointing to general physical and mental dangers of indulging excessively in food, drink, and sexual activity, but also suggesting that our desires for these three things are "a disgrace to us" (citing Aristotle) and that sex should "be as infrequent as possible." GP, II, ch. 36; III, chs. 12, 33, 35, 49. However, his *Treatise on Cohabitation*, which was likely written in 1190 or 1191 (and therefore very close to the time of the *Guide*), adopts a more sex-positive tone in recommending various aphrodisiacs in response to the request of a sultan. Rosner, *Sex Ethics*, ix, 17–40. In any case, neither of these later works explicitly withdraws his previous considerations regarding the connection between moderate sex and health, the correct amount of sex for different individuals, or the wife's pertinent rights vis-à-vis her husband.

97 MT, *Hilchot De'ot*, 4:2, 4:14–15 (which contains the quotation in the main text); GP, III, ch. 25; Rosner, *Medical Legacy*, 63–64 (citing Maimonides, *Medical Aphorisms*, 18). In these latter two sources, Maimonides gives examples such as ball playing, wrestling, and boxing.

98 MT, *Hilchot De'ot*, 4:16; *Sefer Zemanim, Hilchot Shevitat Asor* ("The Laws of Resting on the Tenth [Day of Tishrei]"), 3:2.

99 MT, *Hilchot De'ot*, 4:4–5; see also Rosner, *Medical Legacy*, 54 (citing Maimonides, *Medical Aphorisms*, 7). As Touger's commentary points out, elsewhere the *Mishneh Torah* recommends resisting sleep at night in order to study Torah, although it is not entirely clear whether Maimonides intends for such study to cut into the prescribed eight hours. MT, *Sefer Madda, Talmud Torah* ("The Laws of Torah Study"), 3:12–13.

100 Rosner, *Medical Legacy*, 28, 198, 208 (citing Maimonides, *Treatise on Asthma*).

101 Rosner, *Medical Legacy*, 200–201 (citing Maimonides, *Regimen of Health; Medical Aphorisms*). For Maimonides, mental well-being is also directly necessary for knowledge of important matters. The one who is angry loses his wisdom, and the way to alleviate anger is to "train [oneself] to feel no reaction even if he is beaten or cursed." MT, *Hilchot De'ot*, 2:2, 3.

102 MT, *Hilchot De'ot*, 4:20. I am not sure whether Maimonides's aforementioned blueprint for health is meant only for men or for both sexes. In my

English translations of the pertinent passages I have referenced, Rambam often points to what a "man"/"he" ought to do, occasionally (as noted in endnote 95 above) comments on specific effects on the male body, but is silent on the health of women in particular. Dorff informs me that Maimonides (who was writing in patriarchal medieval times) probably assumed that only men would be reading his works, and that the Hebrew masculine singular pronoun used in *Hilchot De'ot* 4:20 could refer either exclusively to men or to both men and women. Dorff, e-mail messages to author, March 10, 2019. All of this is not to say that Maimonides was indifferent to the health of women; see, e.g., his remarks on menstruation and health in Rosner, *Medicine in the Mishneh Torah of Maimonides*, 137–138 (citing Maimonides, *Medical Aphorisms*, 16).

103 ST, II-II, q. 64, a. 5 & ad. 1.

104 ST, II-II, q. 64, a. 5, obj. & ad. 3. Aquinas elsewhere points out that harm to the soul is worse than harm to the body, and that bodily pain (such as that involved in the taking of "bitter medicine") can often lead to good things. ST, I-II, q. 39, a. 4, ad. 3; Eberl, *Thomistic Principles and Bioethics*, 104 (citing this article of the *Summa* along with Aquinas, *Commentary on Job*, I.20–21).

105 ST, II-II, q. 64, a. 5, obj. & ad. 4.

106 ST, II-II, q. 64, a. 7. Aquinas maintains that the intention must be good in order for an act as a whole to be good. ST, I-II, q. 18, a. 4 & ad. 3. Similarly, as Dorff notes, Judaism recognizes that killing in self-defense is licit and not a violation of the commandment "You shall not murder." Dorff, *Matters of Life and Death*, 176–177, 409.

107 ST, II-II, q. 25, a. 5.

108 ST, II-II, q. 146, a. 1 & ad. 4.

109 ST, II-II, q. 146, a. 2, ad. 2; q. 148, a. 6.

110 ST, II-II, q. 147, a. 1, ad. 2; a. 2.

111 ST, II-II, q. 147, a. 6 & ad. 2 & 3. Interestingly, a single daily meal is considered by Aquinas to be fasting, but by Maimonides to be normal dietary practice (as mentioned above).

112 ST, II-II, q. 147, a. 4, ad. 2 & 3.

113 ST, II-II, q. 147, aa. 1, 6 (citing Dan. 10; Joel 2:12; 2 Cor. 6:5–6; Augustine).

114 ST, II-II, q. 148, a. 1; a. 2, ad. 2 & 4; a. 6.

115 ST, II-II, q. 148, a. 3, ad. 3.

116 ST, II-II, q. 148, a. 5, a. 1. See also SCG, III, ch. 127, §§ 1–2, 4 (stating that "the use of food is not a sin in itself," but that ingesting an unhealthy type or amount of food can be morally wrong).

117 Eberl, *Thomistic Principles and Bioethics*, 114 (citing Thomas Aquinas, *Reportatio super Epistolam Secondam ad Thessalonicenses* ["Report on the Second Letter to the Thessalonians"], III.2).

118 ST, II-II, q. 150, a. 2, ad. 3.

119 ST, II-II, q. 149, a. 1.

120 Ibid., a. 3. Like Maimonides, Aquinas also acknowledges it can be appropriate to abstain from wine, even completely. Ibid. & ad. 1–3; q. 148, a. 6.

121 ST, II-II, q. 149, a. 2 & ad. 1; q. 150, a. 1–2.

122 ST, II-II, q. 126, a. 1. Aquinas understands this "last end" to be God, and the "acquisition of the last end" to be happiness. ST, I-II, q. 1, a. 8.

123 ST, II-II, q. 124, aa. 3–4 (citing John 15:13).

124 See also *Catechism*, § 2280 ("Everyone is responsible for his life before God who has given it to him. It is God who remains the sovereign Master of life. We are obliged to accept life gratefully and preserve it for his honor and the salvation of our souls. We are stewards, not owners, of the life God has entrusted to us. It is not ours to dispose of.")

125 John B. Mitchell, *Understanding Assisted Suicide: Nine Issues to Consider* (Ann Arbor, MI: The University of Michigan Press, 2007), 35–41. For similar

considerations, see Paul Badham, *Is There a Christian Case for Assisted Dying? Voluntary Euthanasia Reassessed* (London, UK: SPCK, 2009), 31–34, 60–62, 65–66. Alternatively, one might suggest, as Dorff does in this volume, that it is our *body* that is property on loan from God, and that therefore suicide is wrong. Mitchell attempts to reply to this line of reasoning as well; he states that it doesn't make sense to think of God loaning our body to us, since he's not going to "get it back" regardless after we die and are buried. Mitchell, *Understanding Assisted Suicide*, 37–38. However, as Dorff notes, most Jews who affirm a resurrection do believe it will be embodied, and he adds that "God should surely be trusted to resurrect us in a better body than the one in which we died," with all damaged internal parts "restore[d]." Dorff, *Matters of Life and Death*, 236–239. A physical resurrection is also upheld by Catholic teaching and Aquinas; the latter even specifically clarifies that the bodies of those in hell will be in good health, although also deficient in other ways. *Catechism*, §§ 997–998; Thomas Aquinas, *Summa Contra Gentiles: Book Four, Salvation*, trans. Charles J. O'Neil (Notre Dame, IN: University of Notre Dame Press, 1975 [1956]), chs. 85–86, 88–89; ST, III (supplement), q, 79, a. 2; q. 81, a. 1; q. 82, a. 1; q. 86, aa. 1–2. And Maimonides ultimately appears to support an embodied resurrection in a qualified way; he upholds the resurrection of the dead in his early *Commentary on the Mishnah*, confirms it in the *Mishneh Torah* while adding that there will be no bodies in the "world to come," emphasizes a spiritual afterlife in the *Guide of the Perplexed*, and finally suggests in his *Treatise on Resurrection* (in 1191) that there will be a temporary bodily resurrection that is succeeded by a purely spiritual "world to come." MT, *Sefer Madda, Hilchot Teshuvah* ("The Laws of Repentance"), 3:6, 8:2; Dorff, *Matters of Life and Death*, 237–238 & 383 n. 32 (citing GP, II, ch. 27; III, ch. 54); Fred Rosner, "Brief Description of the Treatise," in *Moses Maimonides' Treatise on Resurrection* (Northvale, NJ: Jason Aronson Inc., 1997), 15–17, 19. But Mitchell might respond to such considerations by saying that in the case of a physical resurrection, our body, like our soul, can return to God and would ultimately be unharmed.

126  For reasoning along these lines, see Fisher, *Catholic Bioethics for the New Millennium*, 256–258.

127  Mitchell, *Understanding Assisted Suicide*, 33–34.

128  Augustine, *City of God*, trans. Henry Bettenson (New York, NY: Penguin Books, 2003 [1972]), I, ch. 20. See also *Catechism*, §§ 2261, 2263, 2325 (explaining that this commandment specifically proscribes the intentional killing of the innocent [i.e., nonthreatening], as per Exod. 23:7, and concluding that "[s]uicide . . . is forbidden by the fifth commandment").

129  See also *Catechism*, § 2281. In response to natural law arguments against assisted suicide, Paul Badham suggests that intensive care or terminal sedation can be "even more unnatural." Badham, *Is There a Christian Case for Assisted Dying?* 40–42. But while extraordinary medical procedures (discussed further below) may indeed be unnatural, one could argue that it is still more natural to preserve one's life without intending to kill (e.g., through undergoing ordinary medical procedures and strong forms of palliative care) than to will death directly.

130  On Bernardin's witness, see Cathleen Kaveny, *Law's Virtues: Fostering Autonomy and Solidarity in American Society* (Washington, DC: Georgetown University Press, 2012), 141–149. Mitchell plays down any "social costs" of "the suicide of the elderly, suffering, terminally ill," claiming that "[f]amily members will surely be sad, but they will understand" and citing a Dutch study that found that "[f]amilies whose loved ones die as a result of euthanasia suffer less harrowing grief and fewer symptoms of stress than do those whose relations die of natural causes." Mitchell, *Understanding Assisted Suicide*, 48 & 178 n. 14 (quoting Nigel Hawkes, "Grief Eased for Euthanasia Families," *The Times*, July 25, 2003, www.thetimes.co.uk/article/grief-eased-for-euthanasia-families-

lztwvqpxcws). However, the authors of this study emphasize that they do not mean to promote euthanasia, and they indicate that a key problem with those experiencing greater grief and stress is "denial" and failure to openly discuss death with the patient. Hawkes, "Grief Eased for Euthanasia Families" (citing Nikkie B. Swarte, "Effects of Euthanasia on the Bereaved Family and Friends: A Cross Sectional Study," *British Medical Journal* 327 no. 7408 [2003]: 189). Hence, one wonders whether families might in fact be comforted in special ways when their loved ones die naturally after mutual acknowledgment of this impending death. But this is only speculative; a recent resolution of the American Psychological Association, which refrains from taking a stand on assisted dying, cites the same study as Mitchell does (along with other research) and concludes that "limited empirical data exist to determine the effects of assisted dying on survivors and on society." American Psychological Association, "Resolution on Assisted Dying and Justification," August 2017, www.apa.org/about/policy/assisted-dying-resolution.aspx. At any rate, in his analysis of "social costs," Mitchell does not explicitly consider all of the lost potential benefits alluded to in the main text.

131  Rosner, *Biomedical Ethics and Jewish Law*, 279–281 (mentioning one rabbi who takes extenuating factors into account and recommends that laws of mourning be observed, but also noting historical debate on the issue of mourning and eulogizing suicides); *Catechism*, §§ 2282–2283. Of course, much more could be said about the morality of physician-assisted suicide. Besides Mitchell and Badham's books, notable arguments in favor of the practice can be found in Beauchamp and Childress, *Principles of Biomedical Ethics*, 181–186; Singer, *Practical Ethics*, 169–176. In addressing Beauchamp and Childress, I summarize some key considerations against it in "A Considerably Common Morality," 107–108. For somewhat more extended arguments against physician-assisted suicide, see Austriaco, *Biomedicine and Beatitude*, 146–157; Susan Windley-Daoust, *Why You Shouldn't Kill Yourself: Five Tricks of the Heart about Assisted Suicide* (Eugene, OR: Cascade, 2018).

132  Austriaco, *Biomedicine and Beatitude*, 139–144; *Catechism*, §§ 2278–2279.

133  An Israeli draft law, written to be consistent with the values of "Judaism and democracy," states that "extraordinary medical treatment" may be withheld in cases where a person "has less than two weeks to live" and that "life-shortening palliative treatment is to be provided to all terminal patients, provided that the degree of danger posed by the treatment to the patient's life is not unduly serious." Sinclair, *Jewish Biomedical Ethics*, 271–273. For other modern Jewish authorities and thinkers who hold that it can be acceptable to withhold or withdraw certain forms of care or therapy and to administer painkillers that can accelerate death, see ibid., 193–201; Dorff, *Matters of Life and Death*, 185, 198–220; Aaron L. Mackler, *Introduction to Jewish and Catholic Bioethics: A Comparative Analysis* (Washington, DC: Georgetown University Press, 2003), 226–227 (explicitly expressing an affinity for the extraordinary/ordinary distinction); Reisner, "Peri- and Neo-Natology: The Matter of Limiting Treatment," 352, 355–356 (on the permissibility of withholding or withdrawing life-extending care from "[s]everely deformed and compromised newborns," including those born "severely premature"); Rosner, *Biomedical Ethics and Jewish Law*, 248–252, 261–267.

On the other hand, Bleich firmly rejects the extraordinary/ordinary distinction, although he does concede that it is not morally required to provide treatments that are "experimental" or "hazardous in nature and which may potentially foreshorten the life of the patient." Bleich, *Biomedical Dilemmas*, 74–75; see also ibid., 86–95. And as Dorff notes, Avram Reisner disagrees with him on life-shortening pain medication; Reisner holds that it is only acceptable to administer lower doses short of what would hasten death. Dorff, *Matters of Life and Death*, 373 nn. 27 & 31, 379 n. 76.

134 Sinclair, *Jewish Biomedical Law*, 193–195 (citing Immanuel Jakobovits, "The Law Relating to the Precipitation of the Death of a Hopeless Patient Who Is Undergoing Great Suffering" [Heb.], *Hapardes* 31 [1957]: pt. I, 28–31; pt. 3, 16–19).

135 William C. Mattison, *Introducing Moral Theology: True Happiness and the Virtues* (Grand Rapids, MI: Brazos Press, 2008), 378–379, 386–387.

136 On how Aquinas's remark that we should love our lives in "due measure" implies that forgoing certain forms of medical care can be appropriate, see Eberl, *Thomistic Principles and Bioethics*, 115. Like abortion, the Principle of Double Effect, and physician-assisted suicide, the extraordinary/ordinary care distinction is not without controversy among philosophers and theologians. While Beauchamp and Childress assert that this distinction is unhelpful, I contend elsewhere that they seem to be proposing the same general idea in different words. Beauchamp and Childress, *Principles of Biomedical Ethics*, 162–163, 195 n. 28; Fitzgerald, "A Considerably Common Morality," 106, 108–109. Another well-known critic is Peter Singer. Singer, *Practical Ethics*, 184–186. For other sources that explain the distinction and find it morally relevant, see Austriaco, *Biomedicine and Beatitude*, 141–144, 160–165; Camosy, *Peter Singer and Christian Ethics*, 57–65 (arguing that there is in fact common ground here between Singer and the Catholic tradition in that both acknowledge that life need not be "preserved at all costs"); Mattison, *Introducing Moral Theology*, 385–389; Smith and Kaczor, *Life Issues, Medical Choices*, 97–102.

137 As far as I am aware, Aquinas does not really dwell on the relationship between sex and health, although he does suggest at one point that "nocturnal pollution" removes an "excess of seminal humor" from the body and is not intrinsically sinful. ST, II-II, q. 154, a. 5.

On a "morality of happiness" as contrasted with a "morality of obligation," see Mattison, *Introducing Moral Theology*, 21–28, 33–36. For other passages in Maimonides that are suggestive of a morality of happiness and well-being, see MT, *Hilchot Teshuvah*, 8:1, 9:1 (citing Deut. 6:11–12, 22:7 in affirming that carrying out God's law will lead to well-being in this life and the next); MT, *Hilchot Shabbat*, 2:3 (quoting Lev. 18:5, which states that the person who follows God's commands will "live through them," and claiming that "[t]his teaches that the judgments of the Torah do not [bring] vengeance to the world, but rather bring mercy, kindness, and peace to the world"); MT, *Sefer Zemanim, Hilchot Shofar, Sukkah, V'Lulav* ("The Laws of Shofar, Sukkah, and Lulav"), 8:15 (citing Deut. 28:47 in speaking of the "happiness with which a person should rejoice in the fulfillment of the mitzvot and the love of God who commanded them"); MT, *Sefer Zeraim, Hilchot Matnot Aniyim* ("The Laws of Gifts to the Poor"), 10:4 (stating that only a person who gives to the poor "with a pleasant countenance and with happiness" is doing a truly good deed); MT, *Sefer Zemanim, Megillah vChanukah* ("The Laws of Reading the Megillah and of Chanukah"), 2:17 (claiming that "there is no greater and more splendid happiness than to gladden the hearts of the poor, the orphans, the widows, and the converts"); MT, *Hilchot De'ot*, 1:4, 2:7 (maintaining that one "should be quietly happy" and not "overly elated" or morose); GP, III, ch. 27 (citing Deut. 6:24 and stating that God's law is designed for the well-being of our body and soul). For further references to Aquinas that are line with a morality of happiness, see ST, I-II, q. 5, a. 7 (agreeing with Aristotle that "happiness is the reward of works of virtue"); I-II, q. 32, a. 6 (affirming, like Aristotle, that performing good deeds is "a cause of pleasure"); I-II, q. 107, a. 4 (stating that for those who are virtuous, the law of the New Testament is not burdensome, and citing Matt. 11:28 on this point); II-II, q. 28, aa. 1–2 (maintaining that loving God leads to joy); II-II, q. 141, a. 6 ("the end and rule of temperance itself is happiness").

At the same time, it is important to point out that both of these thinkers do recognize that following God's law is not always easy. See MT, *Sefer Madda, Yesodei Ha'Torah*, 5:1–3 (acknowledging that the right thing to do can result in martyrdom); Bleich, *Bioethical Dilemmas*, 135 (noting that Maimonides's *Shemonah Perakim* ["Eight Chapters"] suggests that a number of divine commandments prohibit actions which are natural and even appealing); ST, I-II, q. 107, a. 4 (conceding that someone not yet accustomed to virtue would find Christ's commandments hard to follow); and the articles cited above on Aquinas's discussion of martyrdom. Two passages that could each cut both ways are ST, I-II, q. 99, a. 6 and q. 107, a. 1, ad. 2 (reasoning that the "imperfect" had to be coaxed to follow the laws of the Old and New Testaments through the promise of earthly rewards).

138  One notable exception is Rosner, *Biomedical Ethics and Jewish Law*, which devotes chapters to "The Patient's Obligation to Seek Healing," "Suicide" (in general), "Smoking and Jewish Law," and "Managed Care: The Jewish View" (which deals with preventive care). For other extended discussions of some of these issues, see Barilan, *Jewish Bioethics*, 43–50 (on preventive care and the hazards of smoking); Dorff, *Matters of Life and Death*, 180–183 (on the prohibition of suicide), 245–252 (on preventive care and the dangers of smoking and drunkenness).

139  See, e.g., Roni Caryn Rabin, "What Is the Health and Nutritional Value of Mushrooms?," *New York Times*, January 19, 2018, www.nytimes.com/2018/01/19/well/eat/what-is-the-health-and-nutritional-value-of-mushrooms.html (on mushrooms as a "powerhouse of nutrition"); National Center for Complementary and Integrative Health, "Garlic," September 2016, https://nccih.nih.gov/health/garlic/ataglance.htm (expressing skepticism about certain supposed health benefits of garlic but concluding that it is "probably safe for most people in the amounts usually eaten in foods").

140  It is difficult to directly evaluate Maimonides's claim here, since as we have seen he thinks that the right amount of sex varies greatly according to one's profession. Regarding the supposed dangers of too-frequent sex, one recent survey of older men (between the ages of fifty-seven and eighty-five) did find that those who had sex relatively often (once a week or more) were at much higher risk of cardiovascular problems than those who were less sexually active. However, there was not a comparable risk for women who were in the same age range and just as sexually active. Hui Liu, Linda Waite, Shannon Shen, and Donna Wang, "Is Sex Good for Your Health? A National Study on Partnered Sexuality and Cardiovascular Risk Among Older Men and Women," *Journal of Health and Social Behavior* 57 no. 3 (2016): 286, 288–292, www.asanet.org/sites/default/files/attach/journals/sept16jhsbfeature.pdf. For an overview of the Liu study, see Alan Mozes, "For Older Men, Could Sex Be More Risky?," *CBS News*, September 6, 2016, www.cbsnews.com/news/sex-heart-health-older-men (which includes the thoughts of a cardiologist suggesting that more research on this topic is needed before drawing any definitive conclusions). Another study found that college students who had sex three or more times a week had a weaker immune system (i.e., lower levels of immunoglobulin A) than those who had sex less frequently. National Health Service (U.K.), "Benefits of Love and Sex," January 6, 2017, www.nhs.uk/live-well/sexual-health/benefits-of-love-sex-relationships (citing Carl J. Charnetski and Francis X. Brennan, "Sexual Frequency and Salivary Immunoglobulin A (IgA)," *Psychological Reports* 94 no. 3 [2004]: 839–844).

Other studies have indicated a positive correlation between frequent sex and health. For instance, one discovered that "[c]ompared to men with an average monthly frequency of 4–7 ejaculations, men reporting ≥21 [ejaculations per month] at ages 20–29 and 40–49 . . . had a significantly lower risk of total [prostate cancer]." Jennifer R. Rider et al., "Ejaculation Frequency and Risk of Prostate Cancer: Updated Results with an Additional Decade of Follow-Up," *European Urology* 70 no. 6 (2016): 977. For a summary of the Rider research, see Lisa Chedekel, "Ejaculation May Lower Prostate Cancer Risk," April 5, 2016, www.bu.edu/sph/2016/04/05/ejaculation-may-lower-prostate-cancer-risk (which includes a comment by Rider herself on how there could be a causal connection here). Another survey demonstrated that older men (forty and above) who had sex two or three times a week were at lower risk for cardiovascular disease than those whose frequency was once a month or less. Susan A. Hall, Rebecca Shackelton, Raymond C. Rosen, and Andre B. Araujo, "Sexual Activity, Erectile Dysfunction, and Incident Cardiovascular Events," *American Journal of Cardiology* 105 no. 2 (2010): 192, 194–196. This last study was brought to my attention by Sandee LaMotte, "Ten Health Benefits of Having More Sex," *CNN*, March 12, 2018, www.cnn.com/2018/03/01/health/health-benefits-of-sex-parallels/index.html. LaMotte also cites the aforementioned Liu study, but only regarding the relatively favorable data on older women, and LaMotte does not acknowledge the apparent tension between the two studies' findings on older men.

As for the alleged hazards of too-little sex, there is recent research indicating that at least some sex (as compared to none at all) is associated with a better immune system and blood pressure reactivity to stress. National Health Service (U.K.), "Benefits of Love and Sex" (citing Charnetski and Brennan, "Sexual Frequency and Salivary Immunoglobulin A (IgA)"; Stuart Brody, "Blood Pressure Reactivity to Stress Is Better for People Who Recently Had Penile-Vaginal Intercourse Than for People Who Had Other or No Sexual Activity," *Biological Psychology* 71 no. 2 [2006]: 214–222). The Charnetski and Brennan study, which was also referenced directly above, demonstrated that having sex once or twice a week was correlated with higher levels of immunoglobulin A than was no sex at all. Ibid. On the other hand, the aforementioned Liu study appears to have shown that older men and women who were completely sexually inactive had the lowest risk of cardiovascular disease. Liu et al., "Is Sex Good for Your Health?," 286, 288. And the National Health Service website remarks that "a life without sex is no bar to excellent health," referring to the ongoing "Nun Study," whose subjects tend to live noticeably longer than other women. National Health Service (U.K.), "Benefits of Love and Sex"; Pam Belluck, "Nuns Offer Clues to Alzheimer's and Aging," *New York Times*, May 7, 2001, www.nytimes.com/2001/05/07/us/nuns-offer-clues-to-alzheimer-s-and-aging.html.

141 For an overview of research on this topic, see Adrian Baranchuk, Bryce Alexander, and Sohaib Haseeb, "Drinking Red Wine Is Good for You – Or Maybe Not," *Washington Post*, December 2, 2017, www.washingtonpost.com/national/health-science/drinking-red-wine-is-good-for-you--or-maybe-not/2017/12/01/49f55e7a-cbd3-11e7-aa96-54417592cf72_story.html (citing various studies, including Sohaib Haseeb, Bryce Alexander, and Adrian Baranchuk, "Wine and Cardiovascular Health: A Comprehensive Review," *Circulation* 136 no. 15 [2017]: 1434–1448, www.ahajournals.org/doi/full/10.1161/CIRCULATIONAHA.117.030387). More recently, the pendulum seems to have swung more against wine, with two studies focusing on alcohol in general and concluding, respectively, that it's actually safest to drink no alcohol at all and that even light drinking more than three times a week may ultimately hasten one's death. Jamie Ducharme, "Drinking More Than Three Times a Week May Harm Your Health, Study Says," *TIME*, October 4, 2018, http://time.com/5414248/light-drinking-bad-for-you (citing GBD 2016 Alcohol Collaborators, "Alcohol Use and Burden for 195 Countries and Territories, 1990–2016: A Systematic Analysis for the Global Burden of Disease Study 2016,"

*The Lancet* 392 no. 10152 [2018]: 1015–1035, www.thelancet.com/article/ S0140-6736(18)31310-2/fulltext; Sarah M. Hartz et al., "Daily Drinking Is Associated with Increased Mortality," *Alcoholism: Clinical and Experimental Research* 42 no. 11 [2018]: 2246–2255). In an interview, Hartz remarks that recent findings are "kind of against the 'glass of red wine a day' recommendation." Ibid.

142  For a discussion of recent research, see Aaron E. Carroll, "Got Milk? Might Not Be Doing You Much Good," *The New York Times*, November 17, 2014, www.nytimes.com/2014/11/18/upshot/got-milk-might-not-be-doing-you-much-good.html; Dennis Thompson, "Too Much Milk May Be Bad for Your Health," *CBS News HealthDay*, October 29, 2014, www.cbsnews.com/news/too-much-milk-may-be-bad-for-your-health.

143  For a balanced review of one recent noteworthy book on this topic (including remarks by the British Dietetic Association), see Anna Hunter, "The 'One Meal a Day' Diet: Pros and Cons," *Get the Gloss*, September 25, 2017, www.getthegloss.com/article/the-one-meal-a-day-diet-pros-and-cons (citing Xand van Tulleken, *How to Lose Weight Well: Keep Weight Off Forever, the Healthy, Simple Way* [London, UK: Quadrille Publishing, 2016]).

144  Jacob Suher, Raj Raghunathan, and Wayne D. Hoyer, "Eating Healthy or Feeling Empty? How the 'Healthy=Less Filling' Intuition Influences Satiety," *Journal of the Association for Consumer Research* 1 no. 1 (2016): 26, 36. See also Tara Parker-Pope, "Ate Too Much? Tight Pants May Be the Smallest Worry," *New York Times*, November 20, 2007, www.nytimes.com/2007/11/20/health/nutrition/20well.html (discussing how individual "big meals can raise the risk for heart attack [and] gallbladder pain").

145  Ben-Ami and Berry, "Maimonides on Nutrition and Lifestyle," 93–94 (citing Hollie A. Raynor and Leonard H. Epstein, "Dietary Variety, Energy Regulation, and Obesity," *Psychological Bulletin* 127 no. 3 [2001]: 325–341).

146  "Cutting Red Meat – For a Longer Life," *Harvard Men's Health Watch*, June 6, 2012, www.health.harvard.edu/staying-healthy/cutting-red-meat-for-a-longer-life (citing An Pan et al., "Red Meat Consumption and Mortality: Results From 2 Prospective Cohort Studies," *Archives of Internal Medicine* 172 no. 7 [2012]: 555–563). See also Allison Aubrey, "This Diet Is Better For the Planet. But Is It Better For You, Too?," *NPR*, January 27, 2019, www.npr.org/sections/thesalt/2019/01/27/688765872/this-diet-is-better-for-the-planet-but-is-it-better-for-you-too (providing a balanced discussion of Walter Willett et al., "Food in the Anthropocene: the EAT–Lancet Commission on Healthy Diets from Sustainable Food Systems," *The Lancet* 393 no. 10170 [2019]: 447–492, which recommends limiting red meat but also poultry and dairy in order to promote human and planetary health).

147  Lisa Drayer, "Does Chicken Soup Really Help Fight a Cold?," *CNN*, March 9, 2018, www.cnn.com/2017/12/01/health/chicken-soup-food-drayer/index.html (citing Barbara O. Rennard, Ronald F. Ertl, Gail L. Gossman, Richard A. Robbins, and Stephen I. Rennard, "Chicken Soup Inhibits Neutrophil Chemotaxis In Vitro," *Chest* 118 no. 4 [2000]: 1150–1157).

148  "The Sweet Danger of Sugar," *Harvard Men's Health Watch*, May 2017, www.health.harvard.edu/heart-health/the-sweet-danger-of-sugar (subscription only, citing Quanhe Yang et al., "Added Sugar Intake and Cardiovascular Diseases Mortality Among US Adults," *JAMA Internal Medicine* 174 no. 4 [2014]: 516–524). See also Amanda Z. Naprawa, "Is Sugar Ruining Our Health?," October 12, 2017, www.berkeleywellness.com/healthy-eating/nutrition/article/sugar-ruining-our-health-experts-weigh (citing different experts); Berkeley Wellness, "Is Sugar Making Us Sick?," August 3, 2015, www.berkeleywellness.com/healthy-eating/nutrition/article/sugar-making-us-sick (citing various studies).

149 Baranchuk, Alexander, and Haseeb, "Drinking Red Wine Is Good for You – Or Maybe Not." See also Ducharme, "Drinking More Than Three Times a Week," on the health-related dangers of too much alcohol in general.

150 For an overview of pertinent research, see Jane E. Brody, "Even More Reasons to Get a Move On," *New York Times*, March 1, 2010, www.nytimes. com/2010/03/02/health/02brod.html; see also Wayne Drash, "Not Exercising Worse for your Health Than Smoking, Diabetes and Heart Disease, Study Reveals," *CNN*, January 11, 2019, www.cnn.com/2018/10/19/health/study-not-exercising-worse-than-smoking/index.html (citing Kyle Mandsager et al., "Association of Cardiorespiratory Fitness With Long-term Mortality Among Adults Undergoing Exercise Treadmill Testing," *JAMA Network Open* 1 no. 6 [2018], https://jamanetwork.com/journals/jamanetworkopen/fullarti-cle/2707428). And for contemporary psychological perspectives on how exercise boosts both health and overall happiness, see also Sonja Lyubomirsky, *The How of Happiness: A New Approach to Getting the Life You Want* (New York, NY: Penguin Books, 2007), 244–250; Martin E. P. Seligman, *Flourish: A Visionary New Understanding of Happiness and Well-Being* (New York, NY: Atria, 2011), 214–220.

151 Markham Heid, "You Asked: How Often Should I Shower?," *TIME*, March 16, 2016, http://time.com/4259559/shower-soap-hygiene.

152 Matthew Walker, *Why We Sleep: Unlocking the Power of Sleep and Dreams* (New York, NY: Scribner, 2017), 3, 164–189, and *passim*; Matthew Walker, "The Best Thing You Can Do for Your Health: Sleep Well," *The Guardian*, February 9, 2019, www.theguardian.com/lifeandstyle/2019/feb/09/best-thing-you-can-do-for-your-health-sleep-well. Note that Aquinas himself recommends both sleep and bathing as a way of banishing sorrow, and in turn of protecting the well-being of the body. ST, I-II, q. 37, a. 4 (citing Prov. 17:22, 25:20; Sir. 38:18); q. 38, a. 5 (referencing Augustine, *The Confessions*, 9:12).

153 World Health Organization, "Ambient (Outdoor) Air Quality and Health," May 2, 2018, www.who.int/news-room/fact-sheets/detail/ambient-(outdoor)-air-quality-and-health; Damian Carrington, "Air Pollution: Everything You Should Know About a Public Health Emergency," *The Guardian*, November 5, 2018, www.theguardian.com/environment/2018/nov/05/air-pollution-everything-you-should-know-about-a-public-health-emergency (citing various sources).

154 "Anxiety and Physical Illness," *Harvard Women's Health Watch*, May 9, 2018, www.health.harvard.edu/staying-healthy/anxiety_and_physical_illness. Again, it is unclear whether Maimonides's blueprint for health was meant to apply just to men or to both men and women, but in any case the various contemporary sources cited directly above suggest that many of his fundamental notions in that blueprint are substantially valid for people in general today.

155 Rosner, *Medical Legacy*, 189.

156 Some brief attention to this ecological dimension can be found in Austriaco, *Biomedicine and Beatitude*, 33–34; Dorff, *Matters of Life and Death*, 263–264; David F. Kelly, Gerard Magill, and Henk ten Have, *Contemporary Catholic Health Care Ethics*, 2nd ed. (Washington, DC: Georgetown University Press, 2013), 365, 367–368; Elio Sgreccia, *Personalist Bioethics: Foundations and Applications*, trans. John A. Di Camillo and Michael J. Miller (Philadelphia, PA: The National Catholic Bioethics Center, 2012 [2007]), 212–213, 729–730.

157 Edmund D. Pellegrino and David C. Thomasma, *The Virtues in Medical Practice* (New York, NY: Oxford University Press, 1993); Edmund D. Pellegrino and David C. Thomasma, *The Christian Virtues in Medical Practice* (Washington, DC: Georgetown University Press, 1996). More recently, Melanie Dobson has shown how Aquinas's cardinal virtues might be developed and manifested

---

in the context of promoting health for oneself and others today. Melanie L. Dobson, *Health as a Virtue: Thomas Aquinas and the Practice of Habits of Health* (Eugene, OR: Pickwick, 2014), 66–71, 73.

158 See generally MT, *Hilchot De'ot*, 1–2 (see also the Touger commentary to 2:3 on the appropriateness of striving for the opposite extreme in the cases of anger and pride).

159 Feldman, *Birth Control in Jewish Law*, 203–208 and *passim*; Eberl, *Thomistic Principles and Bioethics*, 116–126.

160 Irshai, *Fertility and Jewish Law*, chs. 1–4 *passim*.

161 Susanne M. DeCrane, *Aquinas, Feminism, and the Common Good* (Washington, DC: Georgetown University Press, 2004), *passim*.

162 Among others, Christian ethicists Charles Camosy, David Clairmont, Christine Gudorf, Charles Mathewes, and Daniel Scheid have pointed to some of these benefits. For further discussion, see John J. Fitzgerald, *The Seductiveness of Virtue: Abraham Joshua Heschel and John Paul II on Morality and Personal Fulfillment,* reprint ed. (New York, NY: T&T Clark, 2018), 185–187; John J. Fitzgerald, "A Considerably Common Morality," 89–90; Scheid, *The Cosmic Common Good*, 7–8, 120–122, 124–126, 180–182.

163 Mackler, *Introduction to Jewish and Catholic Bioethics*, 225–231, 236–237. Another relevant example here would be that Dorff learned about the Principle of Double Effect from Catholic ethics and has applied it to justify palliative care that may accelerate death. Dorff, e-mail message to author, November 16, 2017; Dorff, *Matters of Life and Death*, 185, 218–219, 373 n. 31, 379 n. 76.

164 ST, I-II, q. 18, aa. 2–4. Aquinas's action theory has been enshrined in Catholic teaching. *Catechism*, §§ 1749–1756, 1759.

165 There is relevant precedent for partnership in each of these areas. See, e.g., Arthur Jones, "Faith Groups Aim to Create Uproar for Uninsured," *National Catholic Reporter*, May 7, 2004, http://natcath.org/NCR_Online/archives2/2004b/050704/050704i.htm (describing collaboration between Jews and Catholics for "Cover the Uninsured Week"); National Coalition on Health Care, "Members and Supporters," n.d., https://nchc.org/about-us/coalition-members (listing Jewish and Catholic groups that "promot[e] a healthy population and a more effective, efficient and responsive health system that provides quality care for all"); Humane Society of the United States, "Faith Outreach," n.d., https://www.humanesociety.org/faith-outreach (detailing opportunities for members of different religions to promote the protection of animals); The Canadian Conference of Catholic Bishops and The Evangelical Fellowship of Canada, "Declaration Against Euthanasia and Assisted Suicide," June 3, 2016, http://web.archive.org/web/20180925212125/http://www.euthanasiadeclaration.ca/declaration (with Jewish and Catholic signatories); Substance Abuse and Mental Health Services Administration (SAMHSA), "About Faith-Based and Community Initiatives," April 23, 2018, www.samhsa.gov/faith-based-initiatives/about (mentioning collaborative efforts on behalf of substance abuse prevention and treatment).

# 7 Islam, medicine, and practice

## The manifestation of Islamic moral values in everyday aspects of the U.S. health care system

*Cortney Hughes Rinker*

Some of the popular media and scholarly literature before and particularly after the tragic events of September 11, 2001, has framed Islam as being static and against innovation or Western traditions. Lisa Henry notes, "Historically, critics comment, the media has treated Islam as violent and backwards and for Islam to be modern was inconceivable."[1] Lance Laird and colleagues similarly note, "Media reports, political rhetoric and legislative action . . . increasingly focus on Muslims as an out-group, promoting negative stereotypes of Muslims and Islam. Yet few sources ask how such attention affects the health of Muslims."[2] In particular, the Muslim body has become a target of greater scrutiny; in a study of Malian migrant women in France, Carolyn Sargent and Stephanie Larchanche state that the "[Muslim] body has become the site of inscription for the politics of discrimination."[3]

In response to bifurcations of Islam and Western culture, my main objective in this chapter is to present qualitative data that highlight the underlying Islamic nature of the medical practices that I discuss. I will show that, for my participants, routine and practical aspects of the United States health care system are sites of religious meaning-making. These are aspects with which patients engage most often across various spaces of care, from primary to specialized to acute. I suggest systematic practices are significant to my participants because they exemplify Islamic moral values of respecting others and taking care of bodies so that they remain healthy or return to health.

The premise for this chapter developed out of an interview I conducted with a Sunni imam in late 2013 at a mosque in a city about twenty-five miles outside of Washington, DC. The imam moved to the United States from Africa about twenty years ago, and all his children were born here. On this occasion, he and I were talking about Islam and end-of-life care in the United States and the ways that policies and medical standards in place for treating dying patients transect with Islamic beliefs and practices surrounding health, illness, and death. He discussed cases in which providers at hospitals contacted him for ethics consults and in which Muslim community members would ask him for advice about which medical services should and should not be administered according to Islam, such as a ventilator, feeding tube, or palliative care over curative medicine. The most recent example was that of a family who formerly attended the mosque but moved to the Midwest, upon which the husband ended up in the hospital after being diagnosed with a terminal illness. The wife called to discuss which treatment options the religion would or would not allow. At one point in our conversation he said to me, "In my opinion, Islamic moral values are found in the West and not in the Muslim world." I asked him to explain what he meant by this. He gave me this example:

> I was on a trip with one of my sons a few years ago. We were flying through [a country in the Middle East], which is Muslim. We missed our connecting flight and it wasn't our fault, but the airline wouldn't help us and it was late, so we had to stay in the airport overnight. This is not Islam even though I know the workers are Muslims. Making a person wait that long with no help is not Islamic. It's the same with health care. In my home country doctors don't show up for appointments and don't tell you in advance or they keep you waiting for hours, even when you're very sick. You suffer. This is not Islamic. You're not supposed to treat others like that if you're Muslim.

After giving this example, the imam stated he was a little amazed when he first went to a doctor's office in the United States several years ago, and even more so when his wife had prenatal care and delivered their first child in the hospital. He said that many of the routine practices he found – such as scheduling and keeping appointments – were not widely found in the Muslim world but exemplify Islamic values and ethics. Through this practice, the provider does not waste your time; in return, you will not waste the provider's time by actually showing up to the office and being punctual.

The imam knew that I had lived in Morocco for an extended period of time while I conducted ethnographic research on reproductive health care.[4] He asked me to reflect on the Moroccan health care system, given that its population is overwhelmingly Sunni Muslim. I told him that I had experienced and witnessed exceptional care more often than not but that I also heard stories from some of my participants about needing to pay bribes in order to see a doctor at the hospital. One blogger even writes the following about the bribery that happens in health care in Morocco: "[The system] is very hurt, because people have to go against their moral beliefs [when they pay a bribe]. And some people simply do not have the money and cannot see a doctor."[5] The imam responded, "See. Corruption isn't part of Islam. It's against Islamic values. I haven't found that here like I did at home." This is not to say that corruption does not happen in the U.S. health care system; it does in some cases, but he had not experienced it as he did in his home country or I did in Morocco.

The imam saw a link between Islamic moral values and everyday practices of the U.S. system. These practices reify Muslims' religious beliefs surrounding respect, health, and responsibility. I realize that they may also hold similar meanings for practitioners of other major world religions; these are not particularly contested values. For instance, there is some version of the Golden Rule – treat others the way you would wish to be treated – in each of these religions, including Judaism, Christianity, Islam, and others.[6] However, my main goal in this chapter is to illustrate that what may be called "mundane" practices – appointments, referrals, and sanitizing – serve as means for my Muslim participants to create religious meanings within their interactions with the health care system in the United States.

This chapter draws on research that I have conducted with Muslim communities in the Washington, DC, area and with Muslim medical providers. I discuss how keeping appointments, referring patients to specialists who are more knowledgeable about a particular disease, and washing hands and sterilizing instruments – practices that many Americans take for granted – are in line with Islamic values and even facilitate the practice of these values in daily life. I demonstrate that Islam may be used pragmatically to justify health decisions and encourage specific health practices. As Marcia Inhorn and Carolyn Sargent argue, "in the aftermath of . . . [September 11] the lack of Western understanding of Islam . . . has become abundantly apparent. . . . [Islam is] a religion that can be said to encourage the use of medicine, biotechnology, and therapeutic negotiation and agency in the face of illness and adversity."[7] In addition, other scholars working on health-related issues in Muslim communities have masterfully demonstrated that Islam is not opposed to modern medicine and that religious leaders have argued for its use.[8] I do not just want to show that Islam is compatible with biomedical practices; rather, I wish to explore how Muslims in my sample experience the U.S. health care system and make sense of religious and secular medical discourses together as they seek treatment in health care facilities.

## Theoretical orientation: belief, practice, and health care

The literature on Islam, health, and medicine spans across several disciplines, and there exists extremely valuable scholarship on Islamic medical ethics.[9] I will expand on this literature by providing insight through my ethnographic data on the experiential nature of health care and thinking through how theological points and religious ethics are turned into practice within the context of the United States. Researchers have noted that in the past decade, Muslim patients have faced "challenges in seeking and receiving medical care, including care that is judged to be religiously appropriate."[10] A female Muslim physician who practices in the Midwest reiterated this statement when she said to me over the phone, "The challenges that Muslims face these days is number one, they are concerned about even their identities as Muslims because they may not get proper care."

I recognize that there is a difference between Islamic and Muslim, including when it comes to meaning-making. Economic, social, cultural, and political circumstances may prohibit Muslims from living out what they believe are key Islamic tenets, or at least pose challenges.[11] Islam itself is not homogenous or monolithic, and multiple interpretations exist even within a single community.[12] Sead Zimeri writes of Islam, "Like any other doctrine it is subordinated to, mediated by, and lives through interpretation, which is undertaken by . . . culture-bound . . . and imperfect human beings. It is in constant dialogue to secure and play a role with the cultures that respect its moral and legal sanctions . . . how else can one understand Islam but as being historical. No matter how abstractly or timelessly it is thought to be, its historical character cannot be separated from it without at the same time misunderstanding the nature and the objective that it sought to achieve."[13] We must locate Islam "within its context of production just like the Muslims' understanding and practices have to be placed in their own contexts."[14] The Qur'an provides ethical guidelines and ways to live, but followers must consider that it was revealed at the time of the Prophet Muhammad. A "'unicultural perspective' of the Prophet's community is a view that 'severely limits its application and contradicts the stated universal purpose of the Book itself.'"[15] The content cannot be separated from the context and is open to reinterpretation and recontextualization by followers, who develop unique meanings in the process that are informed by their own situatedness. I use all of this as a starting point not to get at the "ultimate truth" or proper interpretation but rather to explore Muslims' understandings of what Islam says about particular health practices.

As a cultural anthropologist and ethnographer, I engage with the concept of "authentication" put forth by Lara Deeb in her work on gender and public piety in Shi'i Lebanon. Deeb argues that Islam is not monolithic and details "authentication" as a "process of establishing true or correct meaning, understanding or method of various religious social practices," while focusing on individual practice within historical and cultural contexts.[16] This concept allows me to "[capture] the nuances of 'truth'"[17] important for my participants and helps me to convey the fluidity of religious beliefs and meanings that surround health practices. I also find it useful to frame beliefs and practices in a way that allows for their discursive, historical, and cultural formations, rather than to assume a universal meaning. According to Minoo Moallem, Talal Asad observes that "there can be no universal definition of religion, since not only are the historical constituents of religion specific but the definition of religion is itself produced by discursive processes."[18] Accordingly, this chapter does not attempt to offer one moral framework in which Islam ought to be read or practiced, but instead it details the multiple interpretations that have developed within individuals' own ethical perspectives. In other words, rather than applying a normative framework here, as an anthropologist, I follow the discipline's call to offer a more holistic analysis and to provide insight into how faith and health must be understood only within the context of culture, politics, economics, and individual circumstances.

The literature shows that the relationship between religion and medicine is very complex. Scholars demonstrate that Islamic beliefs and practices impact people's health decisions and their health behaviors.[19] The data I present in this chapter illustrate how a new "assemblage" is produced with the religious and the medical.[20] To analyze my participants' experiences, I draw on Donna Haraway's concept of "situated knowledges,"[21] in order to understand how Muslims experience the U.S. health care system from their positions in society and through their religious beliefs. Instead of approaching health care as pre-constituted and as a process that is received by everyone in the same way, I interrogate the work that goes into making and experiencing health practices.[22] I will show that appointments, referrals, and sanitizing are much more than modern inventions and common health practices; they are also methods for living out Islamic principles and popular beliefs for my participants.

Finally, note that certain practices that I discuss in this chapter are not medical in nature per se, yet they are nevertheless integral parts of quality patient care that attends to all of the patient's needs. Diwakar Gupta and Brian Denton write, "Appointment scheduling systems lie at the intersection of efficiency and timely access to health services. Timely access is important for realizing good medical outcomes. It is also an important determinant of patient satisfaction."[23] Moreover, Kevin Grumbach et al. show that patients find referrals by their primary care providers an important part of high-quality care and that patients who do not obtain referrals with ease are less likely to trust their providers.[24]

## Notes on research methods

This chapter is based on qualitative research I conducted between 2013 and 2016.[25] I primarily draw on twenty-three formal interviews I conducted with Sunni imams, members of Muslim communities, and Muslim physicians and chaplains. Each of these participants was from the Washington, DC, area or another region of the United States.[26] These interviews were for my project on the intersection of medical discourses and standards in the health care system with individual and diverse Islamic beliefs and practices surrounding the body, pain, illness, and death. Even though the practices that I discuss here were not the principal drivers for my sampling, they were nonetheless raised by thirteen of my participants in our interviews as important parts of their experiences (as a provider, patient, or caregiver).[27]

All interviews with those located in the DC metropolitan area were conducted face-to-face; those with others located outside of the region were conducted over the phone. I used an open-ended interview guide that I designed, which allowed for flexibility in our discussions and exploration of relevant topics. I do not quote or discuss all the interviews I conducted during this time, but rather I have selected several (out of the thirteen) that raised themes and topics relevant to the ways that Islamic moral values are embodied within routine health practices in the United States. I audio-recorded interviews with my participants who agreed, and later my undergraduate research assistants at George Mason University transcribed them word for word as best as possible.[28] The transcripts and interview notes were then coded for key themes, including caregiving and patient care, the U.S. health care system in general, Islam, best practices, and policy or medical standards. They were then qualitatively analyzed using a Grounded Theory Approach.[29]

The beliefs and views of my participants recounted in this chapter are informed by their cultural and individual contexts; this is common to any study on religion in practice. All the participants I include would be considered middle class in contemporary U.S. society. This provides them particular opportunities for general education and specifically Islamic education and allows them access to certain religious resources, such as books, websites, and social media. The Muslim physicians either attended medical school in the United States or completed later stages of their training here. This certainly impacted what they learned about medical ethics and treatments. They all have practiced in the United States for the majority of their careers. Their professional experience could have shaped their own Islamic beliefs concerning health and illness. A Muslim physician at a hospital explained that caring for very sick patients who are waiting for transplants has influenced his Islamic beliefs about the body and has helped him to become more open to different interpretations and religious values. One of the imams I interviewed was a physician in his home country before coming to Northern Virginia. He was in the process of passing the required exams and obtaining the proper licenses needed to practice in the United States. Many of the members of the Muslim communities either held some type of college or professional degree or were working toward it. I acknowledge that education, training, background, home country, and socioeconomic status influenced my participants' religious beliefs and what they discussed in our interviews.

In addition to interviews, I conducted a review of literature in anthropology, public health, medicine, Islamic studies, and other fields in the social sciences and humanities as well as a textual analysis of blogs and other websites that introduce people to Islam, discuss key texts and principles, and are dedicated to Islam and health care particularly in Western contexts. Drawing on this research, I perform a more holistic analysis of how Muslims experience the U.S. health care system and how seemingly mundane practices take on different religious and cultural meanings depending upon the person experiencing them and the context. Here I have distinguished between different kinds of participants – including imams and Muslim physicians – but also call attention to areas of overlap on distinct themes.

## Religious beliefs and the practices of the U.S. health care system

In January 2014, I had the chance to interview a Muslim physician who has also taken on an administrative role at a university in the DC area.

He moved to the United States to attend medical school and then started practicing near the nation's capital. When I asked him about the overlaps or divergences between medicine in the United States and Islam in general, he stated, "The way the establishment recommends that medicine should be practiced is no different from the way Islam recommends it should be practiced. There is no difference." I want to point out here that he spoke in very general terms about Islam but recognized that sometimes culture and religion are used interchangeably, even though they can be very different. I will use his comment as a springboard and provide specific examples in the following subsections from my research to show how Islamic moral values of respect, health, and responsibility are embodied in some of the routine practices we find daily in the U.S. health care system.

### Scheduling and keeping appointments

As Gupta and Denton explain, "Scheduled patient encounters include primary and specialty care visits, as well as elective surgeries. In each of these environments, the process of scheduling appointments (assigning a specific time when the patient is scheduled to start receiving care) is different."[30] Of course, there are flaws in the system, but nonetheless appointments allow providers to dedicate a block of time to each of their patients during the day.

Islamic teachings call attention to the importance of keeping appointments, and more broadly the need to be respectful to all humans. J. Mark Halstead writes, "There are in fact three words in Arabic that are normally translated as 'education'; one emphasizing knowledge, one growth to maturity and one the development of good manners."[31] Respect is part of maturing and developing manners; in addition, it is critical in Islam that you treat everybody the way you would like to be treated.[32] Samir Ahmad Abuznaid states, "Ethics are . . . applicable to every aspect of Muslims' life."[33] He continues, "The Golden Rule requires us to do unto others as we would have others do unto us. In Islam, for example, the Hadith says: 'Smiling in the face of others is a gift, though, not obligatory.'"[34] Finally, one website I analyzed explains that "[i]n the first verse of Sūrat al-Mā'ida, Allah called upon the believers: 'O you who believe! Fulfil your promises' (Qur'an 5:1). . . . Keeping appointments is vital to our lives. Time is the most precious commodity; once wasted, it can never be recovered. If you made an appointment, whether with a friend, colleague or for business, you should do your utmost to keep this appointment." The site goes on: "Never make a promise while intending not to keep it. This is forbidden as it falls within lying and hypocrisy. . . . [Narrators state] the Prophet Muhammad said: 'Three traits single out a hypocrite, even if he prays or fasts and claims to be Muslim: If he speaks, he lies. If he makes a promise, he does not keep it. If he is entrusted, he betrays the trust.'"[35]

Being respectful of each other is a key theme that ran through my discussions about appointments at doctor's offices. In several of my interviews, a main concern was the regard for someone's time. The imam I discussed at the start of this chapter mentioned that "keeping appointments and being on time for them is Islamic because I'm being respectful of the doctor's limited time to see other patients." The Muslim physician at the university echoed this statement when he said that he believes there is an overuse of services in the United States and "this is against Islamic teachings." He stated, "A lot of physicians including Muslim physicians will say, 'Well, let me get this test because it'll be interesting to see what it's like.' Well, you know, that's not how medicine should be practiced, Islamic medicine or otherwise." The doctor suggested that Islam encourages seeing a doctor when your body is sick, but Muslims should not overuse medical services. This includes taking up too much of the physician's time, which, along with being late to appointments, causes the provider to be delayed in seeing other patients whose bodies may also be in desperate need of his or her attention.

In addition, when I spoke with a Muslim man living in Northern Virginia but originally from North Africa about his experiences with the U.S. health care system, he told me a story about finding a doctor when he first arrived in the United States. He said, "I called and I made an appointment for my first visit. I made sure to arrive early because they said I had to fill out paperwork first." As part of our conversation, we talked about the idea that Islamic moral values can be found in the U.S. health care system. He said, "I agree with that. I think it's true for the most part, at least what I've experienced." I asked him to elaborate on this. He returned to the story about finding a primary care provider in the United States: "I think he respected me. I didn't have to wait hours to be seen. I only waited maybe fifteen minutes. Not bad. We [Muslims] are supposed to respect ourselves and each other. It's like not drinking alcohol because it can damage your body. You're supposed to respect God first of course, but then each other. It's like this meeting. If I was late to the café, I wouldn't respect you, or if you were late, you wouldn't respect me. God and Islam don't look on this well. It's the same thing with the doctor." For these three individuals whom I interviewed, making and keeping appointments, and being relatively punctual and prepared for them, echo the importance of respect that Islam teaches.

### *Making referrals to specialists and other medical providers*

Seeking knowledge is an encouraged act in Islam. One online writer states, "Faith without knowledge is dangerous" and cites the verse from the Qur'an that proclaims, "My Lord, increase me in knowledge" (20:114).[36] In a hadith, the Prophet Muhammad says, "Seeking knowledge is an obligation upon every Muslim."[37] Franz Rosenthal notes, "There is no branch of Muslim intellectual life, of Muslim religious and political life, and of the daily life of the average Muslim that remained untouched by the all-pervasive attitude toward 'knowledge' as something of supreme value for Muslim being."[38] This pursuit of knowledge extends to specialty medicine, which existed early on in the Islamic world. Regarding this, Emilie Savage-Smith of the University of Oxford observes: "By the time you get to the 12th or 13th century you have a remarkable system of numerous hospitals in urban areas. Many of them, the largest ones, had wards devoted to only, say, ophthalmology, another ward to surgery."[39]

Along these lines, besides the need to be respectful of each other and of someone's time, a second point that my participants raised was the necessity for providers to refer patients to specialists and other medical providers who are knowledgeable of their particular illnesses. They need to be responsible and accountable for their patients' bodily care. One Sunni imam from Northern Virginia stressed to me in our interview that God looks with favor upon becoming an expert on a specific condition or illness. We should never stop learning and should master one thing if possible. He said, "You know, there are many hadiths that say a person who seeks knowledge, the angels spread their wings for him and God blesses him – so whatever you do you are doing for [the good of] humanity."

In addition, this imam stated that it is important for medical providers to refer patients to specialists when they do not know everything about their ailments. He stated, "It would be wrong for a Muslim doctor to have the patient return again and again when he doesn't have the answers. If there is someone who studied a particular disease for a long time and the patient has it, then he should tell them to go there instead. You need to recognize your limits." If a doctor were to continue to see patients without doing anything for them because he or she was not fully knowledgeable of their conditions, then the provider is not using his or her skills, education, and talent responsibly and as God had intended them to be used – which is to heal and provide care and comfort to others.

Similarly, a Muslim physician who works in an acute care setting commented during our interview that medical providers who are not versed in a particular illness should refer patients who suffer from it to specialists because those patients would benefit more from the specialists' knowledge. Otherwise, the providers are not using their medical knowledge to help all of humanity. This could be detrimental to the patient, putting him or her at risk for further health complications. In general, for my participants, it is important that medical providers realize it is impossible to become experts in every single disease and medical condition, and they should recognize their own limits.

According to Inhorn and Gamal Serour, "a hadith attributed to the Prophet Muhammad states that for every disease there is a remedy."[40] Several of my participants also explained that God creates every disease, and also a cure, but physicians are the facilitators of His will. One Muslim physician who works at a mosque explained to me the following when I asked what the role of the physician is in health care if God fashions every disease and cure: "Okay, there's a triangle here, this is the common concept of [non-Muslim] doctors. . . . At one angle is the doctor, at the other angle is the patient, at the other angle is the treatment, which includes the tests and drugs. If you have a good doctor, and a good patient, and if you have all of the good laboratories and everything else, the patient should be okay." But then he said,

> Whereas, for a Muslim doctor, it's not a triangle, it's a quadrant. There are four angles. There's a doctor here, and there's a patient here, there's all your treatment here, and there is *shifa* here. *Shifa* ["healing"] means it is from Allah, [who grants it through] prayer in Arabic, who allows the patient to get better or does not allow him to get better. The doctor prescribes the medicines and these medicines ask Allah, so-and-so doctor prescribed me for such-and-such patient, what are my orders? Allah says, show your best results. The patient takes the medicine. . . . My knowledge [as a doctor] tells me for this ailment this is the medicine. I know also that a lot of people taking the same medicine for the same illness get better, and a lot of people taking the same medicine for the same illness get worse. I know that. . . [God] comes through the patient and the doctor. The patient is God's patient. . . . And God is sending the mercy to him through [me as the doctor]. I'm a carrier in God's mercy, my knowledge, my knowledge. There is no way I can withhold it.

As this doctor illustrates in his comments, God works through medical providers; therefore, they should always make the best decisions based upon their patients' interests and health needs even if it means sending them to another provider. Through such an approach, they manifest appropriate respect for their patients and their bodies and can prevent causing any further physical or emotional harm. However, doctors should also realize they are not the ones who developed the disease or the cure – God did.

### Washing hands and sterilizing medical instruments

It is common to find a sink in an exam room; in more recent years, it has become typical to find waterless hand sanitizer outside of hospital rooms and sanitizer stands throughout medical buildings, both of which you can easily use as you exit the rooms or walk past. Noted scholar İbrahim Özdemir writes, "Islam considers cleanliness to be one of the fundamentals of belief. It thus makes a direct connection between belief and cleanliness. It is because of this that throughout the ages cleanliness has been one of the Muslims' most striking characteristics. In one Hadith, God's Messenger (PBUH ['peace be upon him']) says, 'Cleanliness is half of belief.' "[41] Prior to performing prayer five times a day, Muslims must wash certain parts of the body. As Abdel Raheem Odeh Yosef explains, "Before praying, Muslims wash their hands, face, head, and feet. The Prophet said to Muslims, 'Cleanse your bodies, Allah (God) will cleanse you (your hearts).' "[42] The Qur'an states, "Believers, when you rise to pray wash your faces and your hands as far as the elbow, and wipe your heads and your feet to the ankle. If you are unclean, cleanse yourselves" (5:6).[43] Without doing such ablution, the person's prayers would not be acceptable by God.[44] Özdemir contends that keeping clean means that a Muslim will "not neglect the purity of his heart and spirit and his moral purity." He goes on to show that in the end, the Qur'an makes it clear that cleanliness pleases God, citing 2:222:[45] "God loves those that turn to Him in penitence and strive to keep themselves clean."[46]

As Ingrid Mattson suggests in this volume, cleansing the body – and, I would also submit, sterilizing medical instruments – is a practice that brings together the religious and medical and is a site where Islamic imperatives come together with biomedical ones.[47] Perhaps an observation of Abdulaziz Sachedina, an academic Islamic studies expert, is also helpful here: "In Islam, medicine, hygiene, and communal health practices have religious implications as guidelines for good living according to God's will. In practice, Muslims have taken the responsibility very seriously."[48] An imam from Northern Virginia discussed how washing hands and sterilizing instruments have a strong connection to Islamic principles of cleanliness: "In Islam, God sees the importance of us [Muslims] being clean. So when doctors and nurses see their patients they have to wash their hands and the things they would use during the exam." Additionally, he referenced the need to wash bodies after death: "It's terrible [when] you have to cut the clothes from the body. . . . I have been washing the dead bodies of the Muslims for ten years and shrouding them. I've seen all kinds of things."

During a training session for medical residents, a Muslim physician at the hospital in which I conducted observations and interviews also highlighted the importance of cleanliness for Muslim patients and families. This session focused on how to provide services in religiously and culturally sensitive ways for Muslim patients as they receive palliative or hospice care. Using ablution as an analogy, he stated that since Muslims must clean their bodies before prayers, it is equally important to wash hands before touching a patient and to make sure that instruments are sanitized properly. He explained that cleanliness is a critical part of daily life for Muslims and also has health benefits since it can prevent the spread of germs.

One of the Muslim chaplains at the same hospital said in our interview that she often incorporates prayers for cleanliness into her visits with Muslim patients and families because she has found it to be a concern for those whom she sees. She said, "I pray for the doctors in making decisions. I pray for the nurses who are supposed to be compassionate and kind and clean and accurate and bring all these things up because people in the hospital worry about that stuff." When I asked her what she meant by cleanliness, she replied, "You have to wash before you go in and you have to wash before you go out. Some people are really concerned about cleanliness. I mean I've had Muslim friends who have caught disease in the hospital because of unclean habits." While being clean is a central part of health care in general, she emphasized its importance for Muslim patients and families in particular by making cleanliness an actual part of her prayers.

From my interviews with the imam and chaplain and my observations of the training session by the Muslim physician, I gathered that making sure that you are physically clean before touching another person, whether you are a patient or a provider, will not only protect bodies from harm by preventing the spread of viruses and bacteria – which is very important within the U.S. health care system – but will also be favorable in the eyes of God because you are carrying out a key Islamic principle concerning personal hygiene.

## Conclusion

This chapter has attempted to tease out some of the complex meanings surrounding practices that patients and providers utilize on a regular basis in the U.S. health care system. Practices that consumers often take for granted can take on many different meanings depending upon the person experiencing them and the context in which they take place. Arthur Kleinman reminds us, "Local cultural orientations (the patterned ways that we have learned to think about and act in our life worlds and that replicate the social structure of those worlds) organize our conventional common sense about how to understand and treat illness; thus we can say of illness experience that it is always culturally shaped."[49] Similar to Kleinman's argument concerning illness, my view is that culture and "local orientations" also inform the ways that we experience very practical aspects of the health care system that are not medical in nature but essential to quality patient care. The body is "not only shaped by physiological variables but also mediated by culture and emotional states" and is also "subject to a multiplicity of environmental assaults."[50]

Along these lines, the participants I included immigrated to the United States from both countries where Islam is the dominant religion and others where it is not. In our interviews, all noted the underlying Islamic nature of the U.S. health care system through discussions of particular practices, such as those in this chapter. Some, like the imam at the start of the chapter, hinted that their home countries lacked "Islamic-ness" in their health and social practices. However, this "lack" may have more to do with the deterioration or restructuring of the public health system through neoliberalization, development, and structural adjustment programs, even when they involve new technologies. For example, Marybeth MacPhee, in her research in Saharan Morocco, theorizes that the women in her study attributed ailments and illnesses to the introduction of certain innovations, like giving birth in a clinic. Meant to ease strain on the body and family, these innovations actually proved more difficult for women given their religious and cultural beliefs and their geographic location (i.e., they may have had to travel to the clinic over tough terrain).[51] I want to draw attention to the fact that health care's not being "Islamic-enough" may have to do with state and international policies and programs that alter health care systems and people's interactions with them.[52] These types of changes, in combination with cultural and political practices, may have eroded the underlying Islamic nature of health care in my participants' home countries, which has in turn impacted how they view the United States. They have come to place the U.S. health care system in opposition to the systems in their native homes and see their adopted home as a site in which their Islamic values can be put into practice on a regular basis more easily. Many participants favorably referenced their Muslim-majority home countries, but it was clear they felt as though the U.S. health care system has more Islamic references than what they found in the care they received before immigrating to the United States.

In conclusion, the stories and vignettes I shared show that practices like appointment scheduling, making referrals, and sanitizing can be found at the interstices of discourses of medicine and religion. Making appointments and being punctual embody respect, an integral Islamic principle – more specifically, respect for all of the sick bodies under a doctor's care. Making referrals demonstrates the importance of gaining knowledge in one particular area, while at the same time recognizing limits and attending to patients' corporal needs – this means the provider must act responsibly and know when he or she could potentially cause harm. Washing hands and sterilizing instruments help Muslims maintain physical cleanliness, which is important to both health care and the religion. While there is a vast literature on the relationship between religion and medical interventions and services, I hope to have pointed to the fact that sometimes what is not so obvious can be a fruitful site of analysis. The practices that I have discussed here may be considered mundane or even peripheral to quality patient care (although literature has demonstrated that sometimes it is the little things that can help improve care and patient satisfaction) but nonetheless can help us rethink the unique ways that Muslims in the United States experience the health care system and how religious and secular medical discourses are reconciled in their lives as they seek care across various settings.

## Notes

1 Lisa Henry, "Minorities in Canadian Media: Islam and the Case of Aqsa Parvez," *Over Dinner: The Laurier M.A. Journal of Religion and Culture* 2 (2010): 46.

2 Lance Laird, Mona M. Amer, Elizabeth D. Barnett, and Linda L. Barnes, "Muslim Patients and Health Disparities in the UK and the US," *Archives of Disease in Childhood* 92 no. 10 (2007): 922.

3 Carolyn Sargent and Stephanie Larchanche, "The Muslim Body and the Politics of Immigration in France: Popular and Biomedical Representations of Malian Migrant Women," *Body and Society* 13 no. 3 (2007): 79.

4 I lived in Morocco for a little over two years in total between 2005 and 2009. I have since made shorter research trips in the summers of 2014 and 2015.

5 Mariam Zaari Jabiri, "Corruption in the Healthcare Sector in Morocco," August 5, 2012, http://voices-against-corruption.ning.com/profiles/blogs/to-my-anticorruption-freinds-interested-in-finding-out-about (dead link).

6  Jacob Neusner and Bruce D. Chilton, eds., *The Golden Rule: The Ethics of Reciprocity in World Religions* (London, UK: Bloomsbury Publishing, 2009).

7  Marcia Inhorn and Carolyn Sargent, "Medical Anthropology in the Muslim World: Ethnographic Reflections on Reproductive and Child Health," *Medical Anthropology Quarterly* 20 no. 1 (2006): 1. Similarly, Inhorn and Gamal Serour state, "Muslims are encouraged to seek knowledge about their afflictions, and to pursue medical remedies administered by qualified healers." Marcia C. Inhorn and Gamal I. Serour, "Islam, Medicine, and Arab-Muslim Refugee Health in America after 9/11," *The Lancet* 378 no. 9794 (2011): 936.

8  See, e.g., Morgan Clarke, *Islam and New Kinship: Reproductive Technology and the Shariah in Lebanon* (New York, NY: Berghahn Books, 2009); Marcia C. Inhorn and Soraya Tremayne, eds., *Islam and Assisted Reproductive Technologies: Sunni and Shia Perspectives* (New York, NY: Berghahn Books, 2012); Susi Krehbiel Keefe, " 'Women Do What They Want': Permanent Contraception in Northern Tanzania," *Social Science & Medicine* 63 no. 2 (2006); Cortney L. Hughes, "The 'Amazing' Fertility Decline: Islam, Economics, and Reproductive Decision Making among Working-Class Moroccan Women," *Medical Anthropology Quarterly* 25 no. 4 (2011).

9  See, e.g., Jonathan E. Brockopp, ed., *Islamic Ethics of Life: Abortion, War, and Euthanasia* (Columbia: University of South Carolina Press, 2002); Jonathan E. Brockopp and Thomas Eich, eds., *Muslim Medical Ethics: From Theory to Practice* (Columbia: University of South Carolina Press, 2008); Faroque A. Khan, "Religious Teachings and Reflections on Advance Directive – Religious Values and Legal Dilemmas in Bioethics: An Islamic Perspective," *Fordham Urban Law Journal* 30 no. 1 (2002): 267–275.

10  Inhorn and Serour, "Islam, Medicine, and Arab-Muslim Refugee Health in America After 9/11," 935.

11  On such challenges, see William R. Miller and Carl E. Thoresen, "Spirituality, Religion, and Health: An Emerging Research Field," *American Psychologist* 58 no. 1 (2003): 24–35; Gerard A. Silvestri, Sommer Knittig, Paul J. Nietert, and James S. Zoller, "Importance of Faith on Medical Decisions Regarding Cancer Care," *Journal of Clinical Oncology* 21 no. 7 (2003): 1379–1382.

12  See, e.g., Ingrid Mattson's chapter in this volume.

13  Sead Zimeri, "A Prolegomena to an Emancipatory Reading of Islam," *Crisis & Critique* 2 no. 1 (2015): 101 & n.5.

14  Ibid., 105.

15  Asma Barlas, *"Believing Women" in Islam: Unreading Patriarchal Interpretations of the Qur'an* (Austin: University of Texas Press, 2002), 52 (quoting Amina Wadud, *Qur'an and Woman: Rereading the Sacred Text from a Woman's Perspective* [Oxford, UK: Oxford University Press, 1999], 6).

16  Lara Deeb, *An Enchanted Modern: Gender and Public Piety in Shi'i Lebanon* (Princeton, NJ: Princeton University Press, 2006), 20.

17  Ibid.

18  Minoo Moallem, *Between Warrior Brother and Veiled Sister: Islamic Fundamentalism and the Politics of Patriarchy in Iran* (Berkeley: University of California Press, 2005), 9 (citing Talal Asad, *Genealogies of Religion: Discipline and Reasons of Power in Christianity and Islam* [Baltimore, MD: Johns Hopkins University Press, 1993], 29).

19  Marcia Inhorn, "Middle Eastern Masculinities in the Age of New Reproductive Technologies: Male Infertility and Stigma in Egypt and Lebanon," *Medical Anthropology Quarterly* 18 no. 2 (2004): 162–182; Aasim Padela, Katie Gunter, and Amal Killawi, *Meeting the Healthcare Needs of American Muslims: Challenges and Strategies for Healthcare Settings* (Washington, DC: Institute for Social Policy and Understanding, 2011); Carolyn Sargent, "Reproductive

Strategies and Islamic Discourse: Malian Migrants Negotiate Everyday Life in Paris, France," *Medical Anthropology Quarterly* 20 no. 1 (2006): 31–49.

20 Stephen J. Collier and Aihwa Ong, "Global Assemblages, Anthropological Problems," in *Global Assemblages: Technology, Politics, and Ethics as Anthropological Problems*, eds. Stephen J. Collier and Aihwa Ong (Oxford, UK: Wiley-Blackwell, 2005), 1–21.

21 Donna Haraway, "Situated Knowledges: The Science Question in Feminism as a Site of Discourse on the Privilege of Partial Perspective," *Feminist Studies* 14 no. 3 (1988): 581, 584.

22 Here I am influenced by Joseph Dumit, "A Digital Image of the Category of the Person: PET Scanning and Objective Self-Fashioning," in *Cyborgs and Citadels: Anthropological Interventions in Emerging Sciences and Technologies*, eds. Gary Lee Downey and Joseph Dumit (Santa Fe, NM: School of American Research Press, 1997), 83–102.

23 Diwakar Gupta and Brian Denton, "Appointment Scheduling in Health Care: Challenges and Opportunities," *IIE Transactions* 40 no. 9 (2008): 800–819.

24 Kevin Grumbach, Joe V. Selby, Cheryl Damberg, Andrew B. Bindman, Charles Quesenberry, Alison Truman, and Connie Uratsu, "Resolving the Gatekeeper Conundrum: What Patients Value in Primary Care and Referrals to Specialists," *Journal of the American Medical Association* 282 no. 3 (1999): 261. Appointments and referrals have become major health policy issues in the United States particularly in regard to the Patient-Centered Medical Home (PCMH), a model that promotes high-quality, coordinated, and efficient health care for the whole person. For more on appointments and referrals within the PCMH, see Robert C. Marshall et al., "Patient-Centered Medical Home: An Emerging Primary Care Model and the Military Health System," *Military Medicine* 176 no. 11 (2011): 1253–1259; Robert J. Reid et al., "Patient-Centered Medical Home Demonstration: A Prospective, Quasi-Experimental, Before and After Evaluation," *The American Journal of Managed Care* 15 no. 9 (2009): 71–87; Thomas C. Rosenthal, "The Medical Home: Growing Evidence to Support a New Approach to Primary Care," *Journal of the American Board of Family Medicine* 21 no. 5 (2008): 427–440.

25 The George Mason University IRB approved this research. It was funded by the College of Humanities and Social Sciences, Office of Research and Economic Development, and Ali Vural Ak Center for Global Islamic Studies at George Mason University.

26 This specifically includes eight Muslim physicians, five patients or families who were going through end-of-life care at a hospital in the Washington, DC, region, three imams, four Muslim chaplains, a gerontologist, a bioethicist, and an Arabic teacher from North Africa. (I also had several informal conversations that I did not attempt to record, but I do not include them in this count.) All participants highlighted in this chapter identify as Sunni. I did not intentionally exclude Shi'a from my research. Shi'a communities may be included in the future but, given my small sample size due to the in-depth nature of the research, I drew participants only from Sunni communities. Note that I will not use individuals' names or any personal identifiers to protect the privacy of my participants.

27 Some of these practices were mentioned in relation to another practice or belief, and some of the participants and I had more detailed discussions of these practices.

28 I would like to thank my research assistants between 2012 and 2016 for their help in transcribing and coding: Serena Abdallah, Oliver Pelland, Hannah Embler, Elyse Bailey, Emily Harvey, and Jesse Roof.

29 For more on Grounded Theory in anthropological research, see H. Russell Bernard, *Research Methods in Anthropology: Qualitative and Quantitative Approaches* (Lanham, MD: AltaMira Press, 2011).

30  Gupta and Denton, "Appointment Scheduling," 800.
31  J. Mark Halstead, "An Islamic Concept of Education," *Comparative Education* 40 no. 4 (2004): 519.
32  Th. Emil Homerin, "The Golden Rule in Islam," in *The Golden Rule*, eds. Neusner and Chilton, 99–115.
33  Samir Ahmad Abuznaid, "Business Ethics in Islam: The Glaring Gap in Practice," *International Journal of Islamic and Middle Eastern Finance and Management* 2 no. 4 (2009): 278.
34  Ibid., 286. (*Hadiths* are the teachings, sayings, and actions of the Prophet Muhammad as passed down through a chain of narrators who were his companions.) There is much literature on the importance of respect in general and respect for authority in Islam in various settings, such as health care, the government, religion, and the family. See, e.g., Mina Matin and Samuel LeBaron, "Attitudes Toward Cervical Cancer Screening Among Muslim Women: A Pilot Study," *Women and Health* 39 no. 3 (2004): 63–77; Aihwa Ong, "State Versus Islam: Malay Families, Women's Bodies, and the Body Politic in Malaysia," *American Ethnologist* 17 no. 2 (1990): 258–276; Jeanette S. Jouli and Schirin Amir-Moazami, "Knowledge, Empowerment and Religious Authority Among Pious Muslim Women in France and Germany," *The Muslim World* 96 no. 4 (1994): 617–642.
35  "The Etiquette of Punctuality," October 1, 2014, https://splendidpearls.org/2014/10/01/the-etiquette-of-punctuality (quoting Shaykh Abd al-Fattah Abu Ghuddah, *Islamic Manners*).
36  Shariffa Carlo, "Faith Without Knowledge is Dangerous," January 6, 2014, http://en.islamway.net/article/20439/faith-without-knowledge-is-dangerous.
37  Fawzia Reza, *The Effects of the September 11 Terrorist Attack on Pakistani-American Parental Involvement in U.S. Schools* (London, UK: Lexington Books, 2016), 6 (quoting a hadith narrated by Ibn Majah). See also Inhorn and Serour, "Islam, Medicine, and Arab-Muslim Refugee Health in America after 9/11," 936 ("the Prophet enjoined believers to seek knowledge 'from the cradle to grave.'").
38  Franz Rosenthal, *Knowledge Triumphant: The Concept of Knowledge in Medieval Islam* (Leiden, The Netherlands: Brill, 2007), 2. On the importance of seeking knowledge in Islam, see also Halstead, "An Islamic Concept of Education."
39  Tim Radford, "Islam Had Specialist Medicine in Dark Ages," *The Guardian*, September 10, 2003, www.theguardian.com/world/2003/sep/11/health.healthandwellbeing.
40  Inhorn and Serour, "Islam, Medicine, and Arab-Muslim Refugee Health in America After 9/11," 936.
41  İbrahim Özdemir, "An Islamic Approach to the Environment," 2002, www.islamawareness.net/Nature/environment_approach.html. This website appears to be a partial English translation of one of Özdemir's books.
42  Abdel Raheem Odeh Yosef, "Health Beliefs, Practice, and Priorities for Health Care of Arab Muslims in the United States: Implications for Nursing Care," *Journal of Transcultural Nursing* 19 no. 3 (2008): 286.
43  This translation is from *The Koran: With Parallel Arabic Text*, trans. N. J. Dawood (New York, NY: Penguin Books, 1991).
44  In her chapter, Mattson notes there are certain exemptions to ablution in the usual way (75–76).
45  Özdemir, "An Islamic Approach to the Environment."
46  This is also from the Dawood translation. This passage focuses on menstruation.
47  See Mattson's chapter in this volume (77).
48  Abdulaziz Sachedina, *Islamic Biomedical Ethics: Principles and Application* (Oxford, UK: Oxford University Press, 2009), 93.

49 Arthur Kleinman, *The Illness Narratives: Suffering, Healing, and the Human Condition* (New York, NY: Basic Books, 1988), 5.
50 Hans A. Baer, Merrill Singer, and Ida Susser, *Medical Anthropology and the World System* (Westport, CT: Praeger, 2003), 3.
51 Marybeth MacPhee, "The Weight of the Past in the Experience of Health: Time, Embodiment, and Cultural Change in Morocco," *Ethos* 32 no. 3 (2004): 374–396.
52 For another example of the health system being re-structured under modernization efforts, see Ellen Amster, *Medicine and the Saints: Science, Islam, and the Colonial Encounter in Morocco, 1877–1956* (Austin: University of Texas Press, 2013).

# 8 A shared common good

## Catholic and Muslim bioethical approaches to HIV/AIDS in Kenya

*Timothy James Carey*

Bioethics, as the field of study concerned with making ethical decisions in light of advances in biomedicine, includes general issues relating to the body of the individual as well as treatment, care, and cure. This is not an exhaustive list of bioethical concerns; much has been written within the Catholic intellectual tradition regarding the relationship of the body to the soul and how metaphysical questions of pain, suffering, death, and salvation can and should be addressed by religious leaders and medical professionals. Approaching the discussion in terms of biblical narratives and the common good tradition of Catholic social teaching,[1] it is possible to focus on the place of justice and how it touches everyone within society, including those most marginalized members.

Similarly, for Islam there are certain foundational and authoritative sources, namely the Qur'an and Sunna traditions of the Prophet Muhammad, that can be consulted when confronted by questions of a bioethical nature. Islam also has a long history of ethico-legal reflection, which constitutes another rich source of pertinent material. While I do not deny the existence of certain fundamental differences between Islam and Christianity (and within each of these religions, respectively) on ethical matters and otherwise,[2] in this chapter I will point toward a promising common denominator between Catholic and Muslim approaches to bioethics: the privileged place of the common good. This common good includes not only those who are suffering from any form of disease but also the hungry and the thirsty, as scriptural accounts will illuminate. Bioethics through the lens of justice and compassion for those suffering can thus be considered an entry point for dialogue between both religions. This discussion directly ties into the theme of "respecting the body," for I will show how different religious scriptures, traditions, and practitioners are concerned with providing for the physical needs of others, including those threatened by bodily diseases.

In the first section, this chapter considers contemporary Catholic approaches to bioethics in the wake of the secular principlism of the Georgetown approach. Specifically, while cognizant of the breadth of opinion on theological bioethics from different faith traditions, I offer Lisa Sowle Cahill's approach, one that is deeply rooted in the Catholic common good tradition and involves a participatory aspect that sets a framework for a practical engagement of some major themes common to Islam and Christianity. With Cahill, I understand theology here in terms of critical reflection on the experiences, stories, and symbols of a religious tradition, including their relationship and import. In turn, as she explains, "theological ethics is the explication and defense of the personal moral and the social behavior required or idealized by a religious tradition." She adds that the input of theologians was especially helpful at the birth of bioethics, given their "long-standing traditions of reflection on life, death, and suffering" and of practical advice on such matters.[3] When reinforced by Hans Küng's emphasis on a common underlying global ethic between faith traditions of the world and Paul Knitter's attention to suffering, the vocabulary of theological bioethics can be useful in advancing a practical model for interreligious dialogue.

The second section turns to the religious tradition of Islam, more specifically the work of the Sunni Maliki jurist Abū Isḥāq Ibrāhīm al-Shāṭibī (d. 1388). I show how al-Shāṭibī develops the ethico-legal principle of *maṣlaḥa*, which is similar to the Catholic notion of the common good. Next, keeping in mind theology's attention to narratives and using the sacred scripture of both religious traditions as the foundation for a universal ethic rooted in concern for the suffering, the outcast, and those in need, I further compare Muslim and Catholic approaches to bioethics and note that their commonalities can be an opportunity for interreligious dialogue and action.

Building on the first two sections, this chapter then explores the contemporary experience of HIV/AIDS in Kenya as an example where scriptural narratives and the vocabulary of theological bioethics can underlie an interfaith response to the disease from both a Roman Catholic and a Sunni Muslim perspective. I conclude with some reflections on the relationship between universal principles and the particular contexts that are needed to realize them.

## Contemporary Catholic approaches to bioethics

Religious and ethical concerns arising from the use of medicine and the development of medical procedures have been at the forefront of theological discussion for centuries. However, the articulation of a foundational statement for secular bioethics has only occurred in the past few decades with the development of the Georgetown approach. Named for the university where its authors, Thomas Beauchamp and James Childress, were professors, the four basic principles of this method focus on the secular side of health care: autonomy, which represents respect for the individual; beneficence, or acting in the best interest of the patient; non-maleficence, doing no harm as a health care provider, a principle embodied in the Hippocratic Oath; and justice, which promotes the equality of all patients.[4]

These principles aim to uphold the inherent independence of the patient, particularly when this relates to making major decisions about one's health. Yet, the Georgetown approach emphasizes the role of the secular health care provider in caring for the patient. From this, one might conclude that health care providers attend only to the corporeal nature of human existence, while religious leaders focus exclusively on its spiritual nature. With the physiological ailments addressed and the dignity of the patient upheld, the whole person – that is, the physical and spiritual aspects of the human condition – can seemingly maintain balance.

However, such a method completely isolates the spiritual dimension of being human from the physical, and vice versa. Instead of engaging the other, the Georgetown approach holds both at bay: the religious remains the religious, and the secular remains the secular. In the words of noted Catholic ethicist Fr. James F. Keenan, S.J., "Though many claim [the principles of the Georgetown approach] to be universally applicable, in fact, they are as local in their origin as in their relevance." He continues, "They reflect a vision of bioethics, steeped in American values, that is largely focused on the professional relationship between physician and patient."[5] From such a perspective, what is necessary is a movement beyond a bioethics focused disproportionately on Western, individualistic values such as autonomy.[6] Rather, for Christians participating in bioethical discourse, an emphasis on the religious language of Catholic social teaching – including the common good and social justice – might be helpful in shifting the focus toward a bioethics that takes seriously the religious voice. According to the *Catechism of the Catholic Church*, that common good "requires the *social well-being* and *development* of the group itself," which in turn necessitates "mak[ing] accessible to each what is needed to lead a truly human life," including "food, clothing, [and] health."[7]

### *Lisa Sowle Cahill and a participatory Catholic bioethics*

Several theologians have proposed an understanding of bioethics that distances itself from the binary of the Georgetown approach, instead looking to religious language and context. Calling for bioethics to be "socially effective," Keenan writes that "[t]he new language of Catholic bioethics engages the traditional language of Catholic social justice at the same time that it makes the former more social and more attentive to issues of power and distribution of resources than was previously held."[8] In particular, Cahill asserts that anyone engaged in Catholic bioethics must be motivated by a commitment to "biblically and theologically grounded norms of justice, as the inclusion of all in the common good with a preferential option for the poor."[9] She thereby affirms the inherent dignity of all members of society – not only its Catholic contingent. In addition, she represents a marked shift in an approach to bioethics – from one that attempts to separate the secular from the spiritual to one that sees both as important to understanding the context from which questions of a bioethical nature arise.[10]

The Catholic Church also has a direct hand in shaping public policy and culture, as these concern the entire community – both religious and otherwise. Cahill indicates that a model of bioethics as participation in the common good can even prophetically support developments with "a subversive or revolutionary impact" on society, often in tandem with other religious perspectives.[11] With this model, the Church does not stand alone outside of the discussion. It is rather an active participant, holding its ground as a religious institution while promoting its aims and objectives from a theological perspective.

## A universal ethic for informing bioethical language

To articulate a model of bioethics that speaks not only to Catholics but also across religions, there must be something similar between them that allows for faithful comparison and dialogue. Swiss Catholic theologian Hans Küng maintains that there is a common global ethic between the religions of the world and that, because of this commonality, religious leaders can develop a code of behavior by which all religious believers can abide.[12] According to Küng, the ethical norms promoted by organized religion are derived from the highly complicated social and dynamic context from within which they are experienced.[13] Understanding this context is, therefore, necessary in understanding the way people act as they do. Küng stresses that "what matters in the end is that a human being should behave in a truly humane way towards fellow humans. . . . In this sense, true humanity is indeed the prerequisite of true religion, and *humanitas* is the minimum demand made of all religions."[14] From this, it would seem as though there can be similar beliefs and practices between Islam and Christianity, respectively, that promote the health and well-being of humanity. As I will demonstrate, a key commonality between these religious traditions is the notion of the common good, which can be understood as inclusive of all humanity.

This basic similarity forms the ground on which to enter the practical discussion of HIV/AIDS and the impact of the disease in Nairobi, Kenya, where religious leaders are responding to the pandemic in terms of suffering, morality, and mortality. The case of Nairobi sets the foundation for an interreligious dialogue in those communities where disease has reached an epidemic scale. However, to develop a more fully operative approach to theological bioethics and interreligious dialogue, we must first consider the place of the suffering other as it relates to this global ethic.

## Suffering and bioethics

There has been a recent trend within the field of comparative theology toward a more direct participation in interreligious dialogue. That is, while it is still important to understand the foundational texts of each religious tradition being explored, there is also the need to actually take part in the conversation to understand the religious other in their own words and on their own terms. The plight and the suffering of the least well-off, which as Paul Knitter points out "take[s] on a variety of different but interrelated faces,"[15] must be acknowledged as one of the motivating factors to engage in a discussion of bioethics based in justice and the common good.

Cahill's and Knitter's respective approaches focus on marginalized sectors of the community, as justice calls for their welfare to be taken into account by the other members of the community. Knitter considers poverty to be a kind of violence, one that can in turn be a factor in physical altercations between different ethnic and economic strata of society.[16] The idea that the suffering other is an avenue for religious traditions to understand each other is singularly promising, especially as pain takes place in real time and can be viewed, understood, and experienced. From this empathetic vantage point and using the Catholic common good tradition based in justice that affirms the inherent dignity of the individual, a practical and contextualized bioethics is not only viable but also necessary given the shared global challenges of contemporary life.

For Knitter, no interreligious interaction can proceed without consideration for those suffering on earth.[17] This is where his suffering-based ethic serves as a model of bioethics that can be applied to both Catholic and Muslim communities. For instance, my own fieldwork has shown that Muslim and Christian leaders in Nairobi have been coming together to speak of the devastating effect of HIV/AIDS on their local congregations, and they are doing so quite openly using the educated vocabulary of biomedicine. Conversations involving terms such as ART (anti-retroviral therapy), AZT (azidothymidine), and PLWHA (people living with HIV/AIDS) are being discussed in open forums between Sunni Muslim imams and Catholic priests.[18] Illuminated by Cahill's participatory bioethics and Küng's focus on *humanitas*, Knitter's ethic is at work through the compassion, communion, and collaboration between religious individuals from both faith traditions toward those suffering within their communities.

## The common good and Islamic bioethics

Regarding treatment, cure, and care of the Muslim, Islam maintains its own history of principled biomedical ethics with certain definite parallels to the basic tenets of Catholic bioethics discussed above. Based on the Qur'an and Sunna, Islamic biomedical ethics promotes a privileged place for those ignored or overlooked by much of the rest of society – the poor, orphans, widows, and the elderly. Indeed, historically, many of the first converts to Islam were among the margins of pre-Islamic Arabian society. The early Muslims, themselves faced with persecution by the Quraysh tribe in Mecca, were cognizant of the social need to take care of those who needed protection.[19]

This paradigm for how to live in society in many ways represents the ethico-legal principle of *maṣlaḥa*, which refers to providing benefit to society and avoiding the infliction of harm.[20] Attention to the common good and to public interest in the form of *maṣlaḥa* has long been a guiding principle for Sunni Muslim jurists in addressing both social and theological issues facing their society. While acknowledging the competing and often conflicting legal opinions developed by the individual *madhāhib* or schools of law throughout the centuries,[21] this chapter will focus on the reasoning of the Sunni Maliki jurist al-Shāṭibī to discern and develop an ethico-legal understanding of biomedical ethics that promotes the common good. Al-Shāṭibī's conception of *maṣlaḥa* holds a particularly significant place in the Islamic tradition; Felicitas Opwis claims that it "represents a continuation, and one may rightly say the culmination" of the conceptions of previous jurists, including al-Ghazālī.[22]

### Al-Shāṭibī, the objective of Islamic law, and the common good

Practically, Muslim physicians have long been operating within a Muslim-specific framework for treating the physiological and spiritual dimensions of human nature. Islamic moral theology, *uṣūl al-fiqh*, represents an important source of normative ethical and legal traditions that influence Muslims' views regarding life, justice, and the common good. *Uṣūl al-fiqh* is both a moral science and – given its attention to how God judges humanity – a theological discipline.[23] Accordingly, it is situated at the crossroads of Islamic law, theology, and praxis.

While an extended analysis of the history and development of *uṣūl al-fiqh* is out of the scope of this paper, in order to present the work of al-Shāṭibī, a brief overview of the normative sources common to the four Sunni *madhāhib* is in order. *Uṣūl al-fiqh* is based predominately on two sources, the Qur'an and Sunna traditions of the Prophet Muhammad. "Both of these sources are a part of the same revelatory transmission and are thus classified as divine communication (*waḥy*)," write Aasim Padela (physician and ethicist at the University of Chicago) and Omar Qureshi. Grounded in these, *uṣūl al-fiqh* "assess[es] actions along a moral gradient from obligatory to forbidden."[24]

Of particular importance in *uṣūl al-fiqh* is the Islamic ethico-legal principle of *maṣlaḥa*, loosely translated as common good. Within the Maliki School and the writings of al-Shāṭibī, particularly his four-volume work *al-Muwāfaqāt fī Uṣūl al-Sharī'a* ("Reconciliation of the Fundamentals of Islamic Law"), *maṣlaḥa* can be specifically understood as the principle aimed at preserving the best interests of the entire society. "Whenever and wherever an interest has been identified, efforts must be made to achieve and preserve it; similarly, wherever a source of harm has been determined to exist, efforts must be made to avert it and contain it even if it is not addressed by any specific legal text," remarks Ahmad al-Raysuni regarding al-Shāṭibī's conception of Islamic law. "Suffice it to note also the consensus among Muslim scholars that the most all-inclusive higher objective of the Law is to bring benefit and prevent harm both in this world and the next."[25] This understanding of *maṣlaḥa* is useful for developing an approach to Islamic bioethics based in Islamic ethico-legal reasoning with the specific aim of promoting the good for all members of society. From this standpoint, God desires that all of humanity benefit through the Islamic legal principle of *maṣlaḥa* – including those living with any form of disease or illness – not only in the physical, created world but also in the world to come.

### The benefit of preserving human life

Al-Shāṭibī holds that "[t]he Muslim community – and, indeed, all religions – are in agreement that the Law was established to preserve the five essentials, namely, religion, human life, progeny, material wealth, and the human faculty of reason." Interrelated as they are, the preservation of human life is accepted here as the second specific objective of Islamic law; accordingly, one can conclude that the legal principle of *maṣlaḥa* requires that society promote that which is beneficial (that which preserves human life) and avoid that which is harmful to humanity (that which corrupts human life).[26] Considering the Qur'an's and Sunna's stipulations to preserve life, al-Shāṭibī continues, "The preservation of human life is achieved in three ways, namely, by: (1) establishing its foundation through the legitimacy of procreation, (2) ensuring its survival after its having come into existence by providing food and drink (thereby ensuring its survival from within) and (3) providing clothing and shelter (thereby ensuring its survival from without)."[27]

These categories are helpful for establishing the foundation of an Islamic bioethics since they engage not only the theological dimensions of human life but also its practical, physical ones. Central to the present research are the second and third categories – ensuring survival from within and without – as these relate to those living with the human immunodeficiency virus in Eastern Africa. *Maṣlaḥa* mandates, as per al-Shāṭibī's commentary on the five essentials of Islamic law, that these individuals must have access to what is necessary for self-preservation, including food, water, clothing, and shelter. In this regard, *maṣlaḥa* echoes the Catholic understanding of the common good, which requires "mak[ing] accessible to each what is needed to lead a truly human life."

### Scriptural support for the common good

While the Qur'an itself does not explicitly speak of *maṣlaḥa*,[28] it does allude to aspects of it. In one instance, Abraham challenges those polytheists from the previous generation who worshiped idols, asking, "And have you considered what you have been serving, you and your fathers, the elders?" He continues on the topic of that which benefits human interests: "They are an enemy to me, except the Lord of all Being who created me, and Himself guides me, and Himself gives me to eat and drink, and, whenever I am sick, heals me, who makes me to die, then gives me life, and who I am eager shall forgive me my offence on the Day of Doom" (Qur'an 26:75–82).[29] With this supplication, Abraham addresses the physical and spiritual dimensions of being human – needing healing, life, and forgiveness – which, he makes clear, are incumbent on God's own power. In particular, Abraham cites those provisions discussed by al-Shāṭibī for human survival from within – providing food and drink – upon which the common good of society is based.

Also, a hadith in the *Ṣaḥīḥ Muslim* demonstrates an Islamic bioethics based in a common good directed toward all members of society. It reads, " 'O son of Âdam, I fell sick, and you did not visit Me.' [The man] will say: 'O Lord, how could I visit You when You are the Lord of the Worlds?' [The Lord] will say: 'Did you not know that My slave so-and-so was sick, but you did not visit him? Do you not know that if you had visited him, you would have found Me with him?' " God then goes on to challenge the believer in terms of whether he has fed or given drink to the hungry and thirsty, respectively.[30] This hadith highlights the interdependence of all humans and how God is with each of us. As per al-Shāṭibī's formulation of *maṣlaḥa*, these provisions constitute preserving life from within.

In a similar account that considers the physical nature of the human person, the Gospel of Matthew calls all Christians to perform certain corporeal works of mercy toward their fellow human beings. The parable begins with humanity's being separated on the Day of Judgment and God's welcoming the merciful with the salutation, "Come, you that are blessed by my father, inherit the kingdom prepared for you from the foundation of the world." Regarding those chosen to enter the kingdom, God acknowledges, "I was hungry and you gave me food, I was thirsty and you gave me something to drink, I was a stranger and you welcomed me, I was naked and you gave me clothing, I was sick and you took care of me, I was in prison and you visited me" (Matt. 25:34–36, New Revised Standard Version).

The Christian works of mercy address certain dimensions of being human referenced by al-Shāṭibī's second and third categories of preserving life from within and without: providing food, drink, clothing, and shelter. And, like the hadith cited above, this parable in the Gospel of Matthew calls attention to acts that illuminate the social nature of humanity. In fact, God draws a corollary between God's self and those who are hungry and thirsty, the strangers, the naked, and the imprisoned, saying, "Truly, I tell you, just as you did it to one of the least of these who are members of my family, you did it to me" (Matt. 25:40, New Revised Standard Version). As members of the human family, Christians are required to engage in acts of mercy that focus on both the physical and the social dimensions of humanity.

Therefore, the faithful, both Catholic and Muslim, are called to care for the most marginalized members of society – to visit the sick, feed the hungry, and give drink to the thirsty. For both faith communities, to overlook or ignore those members of our own societies is to deny the omnipresence of God. This idea that God is with the sick is central to Catholic and Islamic approaches to bioethics, particularly in terms of interreligious dialogue. With regard to Muslim and Catholic communities in Eastern Africa confronting the very real threat of HIV/AIDS, God's call undoubtedly includes easing the pain, stigma, and suffering associated with such a disease.

However, a Muslim approach to bioethics also puts great emphasis on the omnipotent nature of God and specifically on how diseases can only be cured by God's own grace and power. The Qur'an states that, "if God visits thee with affliction none can remove it but He; and if He visits thee with good, He is powerful over everything. He is omnipotent over His servants, and He is the All-wise, the All-aware" (6:17–18). With this quotation, the dynamics of *maṣlaḥa* as promoting benefit and avoiding harm are contingent on God's omnipotence and omniscience. Humans can only be healed from within through God's omnipotence – and so the very advances in biomedicine that call for an Islamic bioethics engage both its participatory nature (humans caring for the sick through God's call for attention to the common good as *maṣlaḥa*) and its divine nature (that affliction can only be removed by God). Thus, while humans themselves can't cure illness, they can serve in the important position of intermediaries for God's doing so. This twofold reality creates a deeper and more inclusive understanding of Islamic bioethics that can provide care for those suffering from disease, as well as account for the omnipotence of God.[31]

Accordingly, rooted in Islamic scripture as the legitimate source of God's final revelation to mankind, as well as in al-Shāṭibī's legal reasoning, an Islamic bioethics necessarily attends to the suffering other. Certainly, there are similar trends within both Christianity and Islam that can be seen as operating under the directive to assuage the fear, pain, and anguish of other living beings. When this rule is applied to the case of HIV/AIDS, the result is an interreligious dialogue that acts to affirm the inherent dignity of the suffering individual. As a national epidemic, HIV/AIDS in Kenya represents a common challenge and opportunity for members of different faith traditions to come together to provide the care that those living with the disease so urgently need.

## HIV/AIDS in Kenya

To provide a practical account of contextualized interreligious dialogue and continue from the above discussion of Catholic and Islamic bioethics based in the common good and empathy for the suffering other, this chapter next focuses on how individuals living in Kenya attempt to make sense of HIV/AIDS in terms of their religious understandings of morality and mortality. Recently, HIV infection rates have leveled off at 6.1% among the adult population of Kenya.[32] This means that over 1.6 million members of this population are HIV-positive, of which the preponderance are women and young adults. With such a high level of people dying prematurely, questions of morality often plague their legacy. Many religious individuals consider the disease to be the result of certain culturally perceived immoral or evil actions – such as promiscuity, shirking of familial responsibilities, and acceptance of urbanity and modernity.[33] Others blame the illness on the practice of the indigenous belief most readily understood as witchcraft or sorcery.[34] In each of the above understandings of the disease, there is an implicit dimension of African traditional religion at work.

Understanding the human context – that is, the social, anthropological, indigenous religious, and cultural influences – of any response to HIV/AIDS in Nairobi is singularly important since these responses are not operating in isolation. Religious and lay leaders must engage with the present pandemic and view the disease in human terms, with human faces and incorporating realistic human behavior, and consider the broader social circumstances.[35] Moreover, Christian and Muslim communities must not stand apart but must self-consciously consider how a language of theological bioethics can represent an opening for dialogue through the threat of this disease.

## Catholic bioethical responses

A pivotal aspect of the religious response to HIV/AIDS in Kenya involves those Catholic religious figures working in the field of HIV/AIDS prevention, education, and de-stigmatization. In fact, the Catholic Church provides a significant portion of HIV/AIDS health care and treatment worldwide, by some Vatican estimates up to 45%.[36] The Church thus finds itself at a unique crossroads between attending to the spirit as well as the body. Accordingly, medical practitioners and religious believers can engage each other in terms that convey the importance of the spiritual and physiological aspects of humanness.

One major ethical dilemma regarding the HIV/AIDS pandemic in Kenya is that in many cases, it makes the most marginalized poor even poorer. Even in light of government subsidies, the cost of anti-retroviral drugs (ARVs) remains prohibitive for the poorest, notwithstanding that these drug therapy regimens must be taken with food to be effective. This vicious cycle acts to detract from the autonomy of those suffering from such a debilitating and socially stigmatized disease.[37] Going further, in the later stages of the disease, men and women are so weak that they can no longer work, resulting in a loss of family income that places the stress of care on other family members. From a Catholic bioethical position, the poor living with HIV/AIDS in Kenya must never be excluded from the common good of society. This perception of the pandemic reflects the influence of Cahill, Küng, and Knitter, in that justice must be humanely directed toward the neediest members of society.

Indeed, the Catholic Bishops of Kenya have explicitly set out strategic objectives regarding prevention initiatives – from blood safety to preventing mother-to-child-transmission (MTCT) to voluntary counseling and testing (VCT).[38] "We urge the members of the Church in our countries, laity and clergy, cooperating where possible with already existing organizations to search for the most effective means of help," the Bishops of the

Kenyan Episcopal Conference entreat, "and we ask our Bishops to give their active support to this work of Christ: for it is His Body which has AIDS."[39] The imagery employed here highlights some of the pressing and very real issues facing the Church in Kenya. In terms of prevention and health care, the Roman Catholic Church inhabits a distinct position of treating both spiritually and physically those living with the disease. In other words, "The Church cares pastorally and often medically for the sick, advocating their access to treatment. A large proportion of health care and medical treatment is already offered by Catholic clinics, hospitals, parishes and other institutions, and we renew our commitment to make as many resources available as possible," the Kenya Episcopal Conference adds. "But let everything be done, not only with efficiency and professional competence, but also with the hands and mind and heart of Jesus – not just excellent but clearly Christian."[40]

Further, one major Catholic figure working in this field, Fr. A. E. Orobator, S.J., Jesuit Provincial for East Africa in Nairobi, argues that the HIV/AIDS pandemic in sub-Saharan Africa represents a twofold reality for religious individuals offering pastoral care to those infected with the disease: on the one hand, it represents a crisis – a period of intense danger or trouble; on the other, it points to a moment of *kairos* – or the appointed time for God's presence and action. When understood in this way, *kairos* "implies that God dwells in the reality under consideration, which presence stimulates a new understanding of and a positive individual and collective response to that reality."[41]

By acknowledging this dual identity of HIV/AIDS, Orobator calls for the Catholic Church to move beyond focusing purely on the negative aspects of the epidemic, instead calling for an emphasis on the salvific nature of the Church's living and operating throughout sub-Saharan Africa. According to Orobator, it is only through a paradigm shift from darkness to light that will allow the Catholic Church to act as the sign and instrument of a compassionate God that redeems and fulfills humanity, even through this devastating disease.[42] As a community of believers, the Church defines and fulfills its mission within the contextual society, yet as health care provider it additionally serves the physiological needs of the congregation.[43]

## Muslim bioethical responses

In the context of HIV/AIDS, Muslim doctors in Kenya are already implementing *maṣlaḥa*, and specifically promoting survival from within, through the recommendation of a proper diet and medicine. For instance, during my own fieldwork, one imam in Nairobi told me that

> In Islam, we respond to HIV and AIDS as the way we respond to any other disease. If you have been infected by HIV, you are advised to go to your doctor, and he will guide you on how to take care of your body, or on hygienic issues – what to eat, what not to eat. Like any other disease, you don't just say that because you are a Muslim now you don't have to

go to [the] hospital. We even encourage people to use these ARVs to keep themselves fit. So we don't only rely on spiritual advice. We also have to work hard with the doctors to make sure that the treatment fits well.[44]

An additional major practical responsibility incumbent upon Muslim as well as Christian communities lies in disseminating factual information about HIV/AIDS to religious leaders, who can then dispense this information to their local congregations. One complicating factor here is that the illness has been associated with those who have broken the religious rules of Islam (homosexuals, drug-users, the sexually promiscuous).[45] The challenge facing its leaders, then, is to sensitize Muslims toward their fellow infected congregation members. This task can be realized, in part, by using the scriptural teachings of Islam to understand how Muslims are meant to make sense of diseases such as HIV/AIDS. Certain Qur'anic passages stress that the true believer must be patient in times of sickness as well as good health. For example, the Qur'an states, when the believer is confronted with fear, hunger, and the "diminution of goods and lives and fruits," God will "give good tidings unto the patient who, when they are visited by an affliction, say, 'Surely we belong to God and to Him we return'; upon those rest blessings and mercy from their Lord, and those – they are the truly guided" (2:155–157). Even when afflicted by the harsh realities of life, such as scourge and disease, the patient believer will be rewarded with eternal life in Paradise.

In another account, God distinguishes between the true believers and the unbelievers by physically testing their human bodies. When struck with a wound, the believer is comforted by the divine sanction that "such days We deal out in turn among men, and that God may know who are the believers, and that He may take witnesses from among you; and God loves not the evildoers; and that God may prove the believers, and blot out the unbelievers." The scripture continues interrogatively, "Or did you suppose you should enter Paradise without God know who of you have struggled and who are patient?" (Qur'an 3:140–142). Once again, there exists a dimension of perseverance in the face of the struggles one encounters in life, including disease and suffering. Through them, believers are purified so that they can more fully understand God's divine presence in their own lives. When framed in scriptural terms, Islamic bioethics not only calls religious leaders and lay practitioners to serve the interests of HIV/AIDS patients (including from within and without)[46] but also provides all involved with a new understanding of such diseases.[47]

## Interreligious bioethical responses

African Catholic, Sunni Muslim, and other religious leaders have together been generating vocabularies and structures for dealing with the HIV/AIDS pandemic, an effort that represents an advance in biomedical ethics for both faith traditions. In addition to the conversations between Muslim and Catholic religious leaders that I mentioned above, many other efforts can be documented. In 1999, the Supreme Council of Kenya Muslims (SUPKEM) and the Kenya Catholic Secretariat, along with other religious organizations, worked with the Kenya Institute of Education on an AIDS education/prevention syllabus geared toward primary schools, secondary schools, and teacher training colleges.[48] In 2002, the first African Religious Leaders Assembly on HIV/AIDS and Children brought together Muslims, Catholics, and others in Nairobi to confer about the funding of prevention efforts and the problem of stigmatization of those with the disease.[49] During the next year, members of the 13th International Conference on AIDS and Sexually Transmitted Infections in Africa (ICASA), including representatives from SUPKEM and the Catholic Symposium of the Episcopal Conferences of Africa and Madagascar (SECAM), also met in Nairobi to discuss "The Role of Religious Leaders in Reducing Stigma and Discrimination Related to HIV/AIDS."[50] More recently, Catholic, Muslim, and other faith-based organizations working under the umbrella of the National AIDS Control Council of Kenya have produced an action plan that incorporates the vocabulary of biomedicine (e.g., AZT and PLHIV [PLWHA]) and aims to realize " 'A Kenya Free of HIV Infections, Stigma and AIDS related Deaths' . . . by 2030."[51] These developments, which manifest a participatory and interreligious bioethics in service of the common good, are also a form of interdisciplinary dialogue since both medicine and religion are finding common ground.

## Conclusion: of the universal and the particular

Practically speaking, then, the common good and *maṣlaḥa* can be served by providing food, drink, medicine, clothing, and shelter to those with HIV/AIDS, and Muslim and Catholic leaders have in fact been implementing the call to promote human interests, preserve human life, and safeguard human fulfillment by supporting prevention, treatment, and de-stigmatization efforts – often through interreligious collaboration.[52] In closing, I want to emphasize that the universally applicable theological and ethical principles of *maṣlaḥa* and the common good are incomplete without reference to particular humans and human institutions – and vice versa. Al-Shāṭibī writes on the relationship between the particular and the universal as it relates to Islamic law: "The rulings of the Law encompass a universal interest, as well as a particular interest peculiar to each specific case. The particular interest is indicated by each piece of evidence as it relates to this or that case or circumstance; as for the universal interest, it is for every human being to be answerable to some specific precept of the Law in all of his movement. Otherwise, he remains like a dumb beast left to roam at will until he is reined in by the Law."[53] And Lisa Sowle Cahill stresses that a theological bioethics must be not just a theory but an actual engagement with the community within which ethical decisions are made, with attention to both "transcendent" principles and particular context.[54]

More specifically, Sunni Muslim and Roman Catholic bioethical responses to HIV/AIDS take place in human society, inhabiting elements of the divine and the mundane. On the one hand, this crisis is the perfect time for God's presence and action – returning to the concept of *kairos*, to use specifically Christian terminology. On the other hand, notwithstanding their different faith commitments and motives, religious leaders and groups who share a commitment to the common good are called to work alongside each other in addressing and alleviating the pain of those suffering from such diseases as HIV/AIDS, from within and from without. Indeed, from a Catholic perspective, the papal exhortation *Evangelii Gaudium* advises: "For the Church today, three areas of dialogue stand out where she needs to be present in order to promote full human development and to pursue the common good: dialogue with states, dialogue with society – including dialogue with cultures and the sciences – and dialogue with other believers who are not part of the Catholic Church."[55]

To sum up, a participatory theological bioethics concerns universal themes – such as justice, the common good, and a preferential option for the poor[56] – as well as the "practical realities that . . . offer the chance for visions and theories to make a difference in the way the real world is imagined and engaged," in Cahill's words. She continues, "This nexus of ideas, concerns, and actions is also a place in which different, even seemingly opposed, worldviews and theories find common ground in addressing mutual problems."[57] Accordingly, theological bioethics can be a transformative presence in the lives of those with HIV/AIDS infection and an avenue for interreligious dialogue and mutual self-discovery in the face of such a debilitating disease.

## Notes

1 The *Catechism of the Catholic Church* defines the common good as " 'the sum total of social conditions which allow people, either as groups or as individuals, to reach their fulfillment more fully and more easily.' The common good concerns the life of all. It calls for prudence from each, and even more from those who exercise the office of authority." *Catechism of the Catholic Church*, rev. ed. (Vatican City: Libreria Editrice Vaticana, 1997), § 1906 (quoting Second Vatican Council, *Gaudium et Spes*, § 26).
2 For a general introduction to Christian and Islamic ethics, including some attention to key similarities and differences, see Charles Mathewes, *Understanding Religious Ethics* (Malden, MA: Wiley-Blackwell, 2010).
3 Lisa Sowle Cahill, *Theological Bioethics: Participation, Justice, and Change* (Washington, DC: Georgetown University Press, 2005), 15. For further in-depth reflection from a Catholic perspective on the theological basis of bioethics, see David F. Kelly, Gerard Magill, and Henk ten Have, *Contemporary Catholic Health Care Ethics*, 2nd ed. (Washington, DC: Georgetown University Press, 2013), 3–45. The authors define theology as "our search for a greater understanding of . . . revelation and our response to it." Ibid., 4. They go on to articulate certain general theological principles that underlie a Christian (and specifically Catholic) approach to health care ethics, including human dignity

and integrity, the sanctity and quality of life, divine sovereignty over human life, and the purpose of suffering. The present essay will touch on some of these principles as they apply to the issue of HIV/AIDS.

4  Tom L. Beauchamp and James F. Childress, *Principles of Biomedical Ethics* (New York, NY: Oxford University Press, 1979). This work is currently in its seventh (2012) edition.

5  James F. Keenan, S.J., "Developments in Bioethics from the Perspective of HIV/AIDS," *Cambridge Quarterly of Healthcare Ethics* 14 no. 4 (2005): 417.

6  For similar concerns, see Cahill, *Theological Bioethics*, 17–18.

7  *Catechism of the Catholic Church*, § 1908.

8  Keenan, "Developments in Bioethics," 420.

9  Cahill, *Theological Bioethics*, 16. In Catholic social thought, the virtue that promotes the common good is justice, which "consists in the constant and firm will to give [one's] due to God and neighbor." *Catechism of the Catholic Church*, § 1807; see also ibid., § 1928 on social justice. As for the meaning of "the preferential option for the poor," it "denote[s] a solidarity with the poor that motivates affirmative action by the more privileged, with the aim of changing social structures." Cahill, *Theological Bioethics*, 258 n. 8; see also *Catechism of the Catholic Church*, § 2448.

10  Cahill, *Theological Bioethics*, 18–19.

11  Ibid., 39.

12  Hans Küng, "Towards a World Ethic of World Religions: Fundamental Questions of Present-Day Ethics in a Global Context," in *Concilium: The Ethics of World Religions and Human Rights*, eds. Hans Küng and Jürgen Moltmann (Philadelphia, PA: Trinity Press International, 1990), 102–119; Hans Küng, *Global Responsibility: In Search of a New World Ethic* (Eugene, OR: Wipf & Stock Publishers, 1991).

13  Küng, "Towards a World Ethic of World Religions," 107.

14  Ibid., 118.

15  Paul F. Knitter, *Introducing Theologies of Religions* (Maryknoll, NY: Orbis Books, 2002), 137.

16  Ibid.

17  Ibid., 136–142.

18  Though I have studied Muslim-Christian relations in sub-Saharan Africa for over a decade, the method adopted for this project involved conducting fieldwork during eight weeks over the summer of 2014, interviewing Sunni Muslim and Catholic leaders about their views regarding the HIV/AIDS epidemic in Kenya's capital city, Nairobi. This research was undertaken to help fill in the interstices between anthropological, sociological, and ethnographic accounts of this epidemic provided by other leading academics in their respective fields. My fieldwork produced interview data from Muslim and Catholic leaders living in and around Nairobi, data that suggests that religious practice can be located within a certain specific social context, while I also draw on the larger identity of the worldwide population of religiously faithful through the transcendence of theology. In the end, this work posits that religious patterns of belief, action, and organization among Muslims and Catholics in Nairobi are influenced by scripture and revelation as well as by society and culture. See Timothy James Carey, *Muslim and Catholic Responses to HIV and AIDS in Kenya* (Lanham, MD: Lexington Books, 2018), particularly xi–xii.

19  Regarding the early Muslims and their commitment to social justice, Karen Armstrong writes, "looking after the poor and needy, freeing slaves, performing small acts of kindness on a daily, hourly basis, the Muslims learned to cloak themselves in the virtue of compassion and would gradually acquire a responsible, caring spirit, which imitated the generosity of Allah himself. If they persevered, they

would purge their hearts of pride and selfishness and achieve a spiritual refinement." Karen Armstrong, *Muhammad: A Prophet for Our Time* (New York, NY: HarperOne, 2006), 53.

20 Abdulaziz Sachedina, *Islamic Biomedical Ethics* (New York, NY: Oxford University Press, 2009), 50.

21 Aasim Padela and Omar Qureshi write:

> Islam is divided into two major theological sects: Sunni and Shia, with approximately 85% of Muslims considering themselves to be Sunni. While Sunni and Shia theology share much in common, they differ on who they consider as authorities for scriptural transmission and interpretation as well as on the role of reason in determining moral obligations. Accordingly, each sect has its own distinctive moral theology (*uṣūl al-fiqh*). A *madhhab*, or a school of law, in the Islamic legal tradition consists of a body of legal opinions and hermeneutics developed by the eponymous founder of the school. The term applies to the founder's legal opinions as well as the opinion of jurists who subscribed to the hermeneutic of the school. . . . The four extant schools of law within Sunni Islam are Ḥanafī, Mālikī, Shafiʿī, and Ḥanbalī.

Aasim I. Padela and Omar Qureshi, "Islamic Perspectives on Clinical Intervention Near the End-of-Life: We Can but Must We?," *Medicine, Health Care and Philosophy: A European Journal* (e-published Sept. 9, 2016 ahead of print publication): 2–3.

22 Felicitas Opwis, *Maṣlaḥa and the Purpose of the Law: Islamic Discourse on Legal Change from the 4th/10th to 8th/14th Century* (Leiden, the Netherlands: Brill, 2010), 249.

23 Padela and Qureshi, "Islamic Perspectives on Clinical Intervention Near the End-of-Life," 2. The Arabic term *uṣūl al-fiqh*, generally translated as Islamic jurisprudence, is instead translated here as Islamic moral theology as per ibid. (citing Muhammad Fadel, "The True, the Good and the Reasonable: The Theological and Ethical Roots of Public Reason in Islamic Law," *Canadian Journal of Law and Jurisprudence* 21 no. 1 [2008]). This terminology has been adopted, in part, to clarify the theological basis of an Islamic bioethics grounded in certain ethico-legal traditions developed by Sunni jurists.

24 Ibid., 3.

25 Ahmad al-Raysuni, *Imam al-Shāṭibi's Theory of the Higher Objectives and Intents of Islamic Law*, trans. Nancy Roberts (Herndon, VA: The International Institute of Islamic Thought, 2005), 352; see also ibid., 394 n. 141 (where the translator explains that *maṣlaḥa* has been construed as "benefit," "source of benefit," or "interest"). For a brief overview of *maṣlaḥa* and al-Shāṭibi's own conception of it, see also Sachedina, *Islamic Biomedical Ethics*, 49–51 (which equates *maṣlaḥa* with "common good"). Although most of their respective discussions are out of the scope of the present essay, Felicitas Opwis and Muhammad Khalid Masud offer much more comprehensive analyses of al-Shāṭibi's understanding of *maṣlaḥa* in Opwis, *Maṣlaḥa and the Purpose of the Law*, 247–333; Muhammad Khalid Masud, *Shāṭibī's Philosophy of Islamic Law*, 2nd ed. (New Delhi, India: Kitab Bhavan, 2009), 151–162.

26 Al-Raysuni, *Imam al-Shāṭibi's Theory*, 137 (quoting *al-Muwāfaqāt*, 1:138). Along these lines, at one point al-Shāṭibi' formally defines *maṣlaḥa* as "that which concerns the subsistence of human life, the completion of man's livelihood, and the acquisition of what his emotional and intellectual qualities require of him, in an absolute sense." Masud, *Shāṭibī's Philosophy of Islamic Law*, 151 (quoting *al-Muwāfaqāt*, 2:25). Compare medieval Sunni Shafiʿī jurist Abū Ḥāmid al-Ghazālī: "*Maṣlaḥa* is actually an expression for bringing about benefit (*manfaʿa*) or forestalling harm (*maḍarra*) . . .. [W]e take *maṣlaḥa* in the meaning

of protecting the ends of the Revelation (*al-shar'*). The ends of the Revelation for the people are five: To protect for them (1) their religion, (2) their lives (*nufūs*), (3) their reason (*'uqūl*), (4) their lineage (*nasl*), and, (5) their property (*māl*). All that guarantees the protection of these five purposes is *maṣlaḥa* and all that undermines these purposes is *mafasada* (a source of detriment)." Sachedina, *Islamic Biomedical Ethics*, 50 (quoting Abū Ḥāmid Muḥammad bin Muḥammad al-Ghazālī, *Kitāb al-Mustasfā min 'ilm al-uṣūl* [Cairo, Egypt: Būlāq, 1904], 1:286–287). For more in-depth discussions of al-Ghazālī's notion of *maṣlaḥa*, see Opwis, *Maṣlaḥa and the Purpose of the Law*, 65–88; Masud, *Shāṭibī's Philosophy of Islamic Law*, 139–142.

27  Al-Raysuni, *Imam al-Shāṭibī's Theory*, 141. As Opwis indicates, al-Shāṭibī understands the word *maṣlaḥa* to concern both individual matters (including "the appetite for food and drink or the desire for a mate") and community affairs (such as "prayer and almsgiving"). Opwis, *Maṣlaḥa and the Purpose of the Law*, 270–271. Various other sources suggest that *maṣlaḥa* in general, and/ or al-Shāṭibī's conception of it in particular, contain utilitarian overtones. Masudul Alam Choudhury, *Comparative Economic Theory: Occidental and Islamic Perspectives* (New York, NY: Springer Science, 1999), 48; Wael B. Hallaq, *A History of Islamic Legal Theories: An Introduction to Sunni Uṣūl al-Fiqh* (New York, NY: Cambridge University Press, 1997), 214; Ebrahim Moosa, "Genetically Modified Foods and Muslim Ethics," in *Acceptable Genes? Religious Traditions and Genetically Modified Foods*, eds. Conrad Brunk and Harold Coward (Albany, NY: State University of New York Press, 2009), 141; Haluk Songur, "Fiqh, Modern Era," in *Muhammad in History, Thought, and Culture: An Encyclopedia of the Prophet of God*, eds. Coeli Fitzpatrick and Adam Hani Walker (Santa Barbara, CA: ABC-CLIO, 2014), 208.

28  Masud, *Shāṭibī's Philosophy of Islamic Law*, 135–136.

29  Translations of the Qur'an in this chapter are from *The Koran Interpreted: A Translation*, trans. A. J. Arberry (New York, NY: Touchstone, 1996).

30  Imām Abul Hussain Muslim Ibn al-Hajjaj, *English Translation of Sahih Muslim*, vol. 6, From Hadith No. 5646 to 6722, trans. Nasiruddin al-Khattab (Riyadh, Saudi Arabia: Darussalam, 2007), 437 (Book 45, Chapter 13, Number 6556). Sachiko Murata and William Chittick, two contemporary scholars of Islam at Stony Brook University, suggest that the notion of God's "slaves" extends to all humanity, "since there is no other ruler." Sachiko Murata and William C. Chittick, *The Vision of Islam* (St. Paul, MN: Paragon House, 1994), 125–126. Along these lines, the *Ṣaḥīḥ Muslim* continues, "There is no child who is not born in a state of Fitrah [the primordial state of being submitted to the will of God], then his parents make him a Jew or a Christian or a Magian, just as animals bring forth animals with their limbs intact, do you see any deformed one among them?" Imām Abul Hussain Muslim Ibn al-Hajjaj, *English Translation of Sahih Muslim*, vol. 7, From Hadith No. 6723 to 7563, trans. Nasiruddin al-Khattab (Riyadh, Saudi Arabia: Darussalam, 2007), 32 (Book 46, Chapter 6, Number 6755). See also Hamid Mavani, "Islam," in *World Religions for Healthcare Professionals*, 2nd ed., eds. Siroj Sorajjakool, Mark F. Carr and Ernest J. Bursey (New York, NY: Routledge, 2017), 147–148 (calling attention to one Qur'anic verse – "We have honored the children of Adam and carried them by land and sea" (17:71) – stating that it supports the idea of "universal human dignity," and noting that some jurists have accordingly concluded that "all life is equally precious and thus no distinctions ought to be made between the believers and unbelievers" in instances of autopsy and organ donation).

31  Much more could be said about different Islamic views on human moral responsibility and God's omnipotence. Two views prominent in early Islam were those of the Qadarites (libertarians who emphasized how the Qur'an spoke of the

former) and Jabarites (fatalists who highlighted Qur'anic verses about the latter). Later, Ash'arism, an early school within Sunni Islam, adopted a middle ground through its doctrine of *kasb* (acquisition). In this understanding, human beings freely "acquire" acts that only God is able to create; evil acts are permitted but not ordained by him. Accordingly, humans are morally responsible even in light of God's perfect power and goodness. Yasien Mohamed, "Fate," in *The Qur'an: An Encyclopedia*, ed. Oliver Leaman (New York, NY: Routledge, 2005), 204–206.

32 Joint United Nations Programme on HIV/AIDS (UNAIDS), *Global Report: UNAIDS Report on the Global AIDS Epidemic 2013* (Geneva, Switzerland: UNAIDS Secretariat, 2013), A7.

33 Hanjörg Dilger, "'We Are All Going to Die': Kinship, Belonging, and the Morality of HIV/AIDS-Related Illnesses and Deaths in Rural Tanzania," *Anthropological Quarterly* 81 no. 1 (2008): 209–211.

34 Ibid., 218–221.

35 Cahill has written on the social issues that have faced Catholic theologians in addressing the worldwide AIDS epidemic, including "effective means of preventing transmission (the debate about the use of condoms), the inequities of wealth and power that contribute to the spread of AIDS, the need of resource redistribution to treat all those with AIDS with antiretroviral drugs, and the obligation to care for communities afflicted by AIDS (especially AIDS orphans) as falling on the international community, especially its wealthiest members." Lisa Sowle Cahill, *Bioethics and the Common Good* (Milwaukee, WI: Marquette University Press, 2004), 67–68.

36 Michael J. Kelly, *HIV and AIDS: A Social Justice Perspective* (Nairobi, Kenya: Paulines Publications Africa, 2010), 225.

37 Peter Knox, *AIDS, Ancestors and Salvation: Local Beliefs in Christian Ministry to the Sick* (Nairobi, Kenya: Paulines Publications Africa, 2008), 79–81; Kelly, *HIV and AIDS*, 107–116.

38 Kenya Episcopal Conference, *This We Teach and Do: Catholic Church and AIDS in Kenya*, vol. 1 (Nairobi, Kenya: Paulines Publications Africa, 2006), 34–37.

39 Catholic Bishops of Kenya, "The Challenge of AIDS," in *Catholic Bishops of Africa and Madagascar Speak Out on HIV & AIDS: "Our Prayer is Always Full of Hope,"* 2nd ed. (Nairobi, Kenya: Paulines Publications Africa, 2006), 12 (quoting "[t]he first conference on AIDS in Britain under Catholic auspices, held in November 1986").

40 Kenya Episcopal Conference, *This We Teach and Do*, 29–30.

41 Agbonkhianmeghe E. Orobator, *From Crisis to Kairos: The Mission of the Church in the Time of HIV/AIDS, Refugees and Poverty* (Nairobi, Kenya: Paulines Publications Africa, 2005), 123.

42 Ibid., 123–128, 220–223, 229.

43 Much of the material in the last two paragraphs in the main text is adapted from Carey, *Muslim and Catholic Responses to HIV and AIDS in Kenya*, 6–7, 12.

44 Personal interview, Nairobi, Kenya (June 19, 2014).

45 See, e.g., Felicitas Becker and P. Wenzel Geissler, eds., *AIDS and Religious Practice in Africa* (Leiden, The Netherlands: E.J. Brill, 2009); Peter B. Gray, "HIV and Islam: Is HIV Prevalence Lower Among Muslims?," *Social Science and Medicine* 58 no. 9 (2004): 1751–1756; Jamal Nasir Khan, Sukhmeet Singh Panesar, Abdul Rashid Gatrad, and Aziz Sheikh, "The Cross, the Crescent, and the Contagion: Ecological Study of the Association Between Religious Affiliation to Christianity and Islam, and Adult Prevalence of HIV/AIDS in Africa," *Journal of the Islamic Medical Association of South Africa* 12 no. 1 (2005): 17–18; Domoko Lucinda Manda, "Comparative Ethics and HIV and AIDS: Interrogating the Gaps," in

*Religion and HIV and AIDS: Charting the Terrain*, ed. Beverley Haddad (Scotts-ville, South Africa: University of KwaZulu-Natal, 2011), 202–203. Of course, Christians have also been responsible for suggesting that the disease is a form of punishment for immorality. For a contrary perspective, see Isabel Apawo Phiri, "HIV/AIDS: An African Theological Response in Mission," *The Ecumenical Review* 56 no. 4 (2004): 422–431.

46  In particular, Islamic principles such as *tawhīd* (God's unicity) and *mustad'afun* (the marginalized and oppressed) summon Muslims "who aim[] to pursue Allah's call for unity, piety, and justice to stand in solidarity with those who are marginalized and oppressed by offering protection to the vulnerable," including those with HIV/AIDS. Manda, "Comparative Ethics and HIV and AIDS," 209.

47  For further reflection from an Islamic perspective on how suffering and illness should not generally be attributed to immorality but can actually serve some purpose, see also Mattson's chapter in this volume (77–79). Some additional relevant Qur'anic and biblical considerations can be found in John J. Fitzgerald, "Can Philosophy of Religion Be Pastoral? The Problem of Evil and the Ethics of Comforting the Sick," *Journal of Spirituality in Mental Health* 16 no. 4 (2014): 242–243 (citing Qur'an 21:35; Job; John 9; 2 Cor. 12:5–10).

48  Charles Nzioka, Allan Korongo, and Roseanne Njiru, *HIV and AIDS in Kenyan Teacher Colleges: Mitigating the Impact* (Paris, France: International Institute for Educational Planning, 2007), 24. The Supreme Council focuses its efforts on behalf of Sunni Muslims. Anne Cussac and Nathalie Gomes, "Muslims in Nai-robi: From a Feeling of Marginalisation to a Desire for Political Recognition," in *Nairobi Today: The Paradox of a Fragmented City*, ed. Deyssi Rodriguez-Torres (Dar es Salam, Tanzania: Mkuki na Nyota Publishers, 2006), 274–275.

49  Lilian Nduta, "Kenya: Faiths Agree on Strategy to Fight AIDS," June 13, 2002, http://allafrica.com/stories/200206120633.html (subscription only). There was some disagreement here on the matter of condoms; Sheikh al Haji Yusuf Murigu of SUPKEM argued that spouses could use them to prevent the transmission of the virus, whereas Catholic Archbishop John Onaiyekan objected. Ibid.

50  Catholic Information Service for Africa and the Catholic ICASA 2003 Task Force, "Kenya: Churches Asked to Vouch for People with HIV/AIDS," September 25, 2003, http://allafrica.com/stories/200309250944.html (subscription only).

51  National AIDS Control Council, "Faith Sector Response to HIV and AIDS in Kenya: Action Plan 2015/2016–2019/2020," n.d., http://nacc.or.ke/wp-content/uploads/2016/11/FAITH-ACTION-PLAN-2.pdf.

52  Regarding another possible practical application of *maṣlaḥa* in the context of HIV/AIDS, note that at least one author has suggested that the public interest calls for "HIV tests and mutual disclosure as mandatory conditions in legally valid Islamic marriages." Muhammad Khalid Sayed, "Challenges and Possibili-ties of Religious Health Assets: Charting an Islamic Response to the HIV and AIDS Pandemic," in *When Religion and Health Align: Mobilising Religious Health Assets for Transformation*, eds. James R. Cochrane, Barbara Schmid, and Teresa Cutts (Pietermaritzburg, South Africa: Cluster Publications, 2011), 114–115.

53  Al-Raysuni, *Imam al-Shāṭibi's Theory*, 227 (quoting *al-Muwāfaqāt*, 2:386). Cf. Opwis, *Maṣlaḥa and the Purpose of the Law*, 255 (showing that for al-Shāṭibī, universal principles are only safeguarded through particular legal decisions).

54  Cahill, *Theological Bioethics*, 8, 19, 130.

55  Francis, *Evangelii Gaudium: Apostolic Exhortation on the Proclamation of the Gospel in Today's World* (Vatican City: Libreria Editrice Vaticana, 2013), § 238.

56  While I have focused specifically on the notion of the common good in this essay, I would suggest that those who care for people with HIV/AIDS also manifest justice and the preferential love for the poor as defined above.

57  Cahill, *Theological Bioethics*, 164.

# Part III
# The body at the end of life

# 9 In the land of pain
## Why Daudet and Hitchens are still relevant

*Susan E. Zinner*

As long as pain and illness have existed, writers have attempted to capture the feelings they inspire. Two writers who lived a century apart and attempted this feat are the French writer Alphonse Daudet (1840–1897) and the English writer Christopher Hitchens (1949–2011). While religion played a significant role in the life of Daudet and virtually no role in the life of Hitchens, the similarities between the two are significant. They did their readers a great service in recording their responses to the pain and death that stalked them as their respective terminal illnesses eventually mastered them. This chapter will address how illness manifested itself in the writings of Daudet and Hitchens, the role of language in medical narratives, perceptions of the changing and dual natures of the sickest members of our society, the qualities and functions of medical narratives, and the implications for medical providers.

## Illness in the lives and writings of Daudet and Hitchens: an introduction

Daudet was a Provençal writer who wrote well-received novels of rural France and was a respected contemporary of Flaubert, Proust, and others. He wrote *La Doulou* (the Provençal word for "pain" or "suffering"), translated in English as *In the Land of Pain*,[1] to record his painful battle with tertiary syphilis.[2] He had plenty of company; it has been estimated that at least 15% of the Parisian population in nineteenth-century France was syphilitic.[3] Daudet himself claimed to have been sexually active since age twelve and that he had contracted syphilis from a woman of high social class. He was subjected to the now-discredited treatment involving traction therapy, a stretching of the spine that resulted in incredible pain for the patient.[4]

As for Hitchens, he is primarily remembered for his brilliant writing on politics, where he covered topics ranging from George Orwell to Thomas Paine, and remained an unapologetic atheist until his death. He was also known for his great love of life and enthusiasm for parties, drink, and talking for hours on a variety of subjects. He was diagnosed with esophageal cancer in 2010 and died the following year. Both writers left behind wives and children.

Beginning with Daudet, we see that he uses a series of metaphors to transmit to his reader the concept of the pain he experiences every day; he calls his illness an invasion,[5] and the pain that accompanies it in terms of an "impish little bird" that brings "wasps of pain."[6] This pain is preparing him for the larger pain of impending death and leaving behind his family. He anticipates this loss when he writes, "You have to die so many times before you die."[7] It is almost as if he cannot decide whether the pain and loss he experiences with his illness is a benevolent loss since they prepare him for the greater loss that will be his own death or whether the unanticipated death is a kinder loss.

Raised a Catholic, Daudet uses Christian imagery, perhaps as a way to bear the suffering he endures. He compares his pain to the Crucifixion of Christ and attempts to draw meaning from this suffering when he notes that "(p)ain leads to moral and intellectual growth. But only up to a certain point."[8] Even when he attempts to be brave and defiant, the pain stops him. He writes, "I only know one thing and that is to shout to my children, 'Long live Life!' But it's so hard to do, while I am ripped apart by pain."[9]

Hitchens uses many similar invasion and battle images,[10] but his are focused on both the agents fighting the disease as well as the disease itself. Chemotherapy provides as many surprises as his cancer. The random effects of the illness are unexpectedly challenging for Hitchens. He writes that "the disease serves me up with a teasing special of the day, or a flavor of the month. It might be random sores and ulcers, on the tongue or in the mouth. Or why not a touch of peripheral neuropathy, involving numb and chilly feet?"[11]

Unlike Daudet, however, he believes that the cross on the wall of his Texas hospital, while unobjectionable given its religious nature, nonetheless holds connotations for him that are different from those intended by the hospital. The images to which he refers are quite different than those employed by Daudet. He recalls Goya's paintings of individuals subjected to torture during the Inquisition, and he cannot help but compare his own chemotherapy to the torture these subjects received.[12]

He also acknowledges that taking on cancer has been a more frightening battle than he perhaps anticipated, since "I'm not fighting or battling cancer – it's fighting me!"[13] This imagery is consistent with Susan Sontag's notion of cancer as "an invasion of 'alien' or 'mutant' cells, stronger than normal cells." It is far scarier to find the unknown alien being inside oneself, wreaking unknown and unseen damage. In her groundbreaking work, *Illness as Metaphor*, Sontag notes the similarities between cancer and other unwanted growths in the patient's body and science fiction. Science fiction expands upon this idea of the unwanted invader in one group of films, such as *The Blob* and *The Thing*.[14]

As a confirmed atheist, Hitchens considers the notion of others praying for him to be cured or, at a minimum, praying for him to lose his atheism, disconcerting and somewhat amusing. When September 20, 2010 is designated "Everybody Pray for Christopher Hitchens Day," he can't resist asking "Praying for what?"[15] Where Daudet finds solace in Crucifixion imagery, Hitchens recalls only the torture images. Hitchens writes that he asks the cosmos, "Why me?" and the cosmos coldly replies, "Why not?"[16]

Drawing upon this coldness, Hitchens suggests that the friends and relatives of the terminally ill be issued a cancer etiquette manual to help them negotiate this new and perilous terrain. He states that comments by family members to those who survived an illness and to make light of a loss with ill-advised humor typically are not successful.[17] Prickly to the end, Hitchens suggests that sympathetic silence may be the best approach when words lose their power.

Both writers seek to cross the great divide of the page and reach out to the reader, present and future, to see whether it is possible to ascribe any meaning to their experiences. Howard Brody draws upon the work of Arthur Frank when he notes that story-telling possesses an inherent reciprocity that benefits both the teller and the recipient of the story; both are changed, and new selves are created after an encounter with a meaningful story.[18] When Daudet and Hitchens share their pain and anguish – physical and otherwise – with readers, benefits can accrue on both sides of the page.

## The role of language in the medical narratives of Daudet and Hitchens

The first issue to explore is the inadequacy of language in seeking to communicate pain. Writers typically resort to metaphor to accomplish this task, but it remains notoriously difficult. When successful, metaphors allow the reader to transcend the literal. Metaphor does not refer to a "simpleminded transfer of a word from one place to another like a rider who changes buses."[19] It is a more complex process. Metaphors allow us to "comprehend partially what cannot be comprehended totally: our feelings, aesthetic experiences, moral practices, and spiritual awareness."[20] Inventive writers like Hitchens and Daudet use metaphors to explain the heretofore unexplored territory of life-as-a-terminally-ill-person. The use of metaphor and imagery is startling and unique because their experiences are unique to them.

In addition to the fear engendered as a result of the creation of this new entity, experiencing life for the first time as a terminally ill person, a second fear can manifest itself with the concern that the self may become submerged in the illness. Daudet writes, "Am briefly humiliated by thinking of myself as a mere barometer glassed-in and marked-off."[21] His statement, which is quoted in full, even fails to begin with the "I" that is typical. The "I" that existed previously is threatened as illness begins to play an increasingly larger role in his life. What if the "I," Daudet-as-writer, is lost as Daudet-as-patient takes priority as his illness advances? Surely this must be one of the great fears of a writer.

Daudet is curiously objective about his pain at times, allowing the writer to take priority over the patient when necessary. Lucy Bending notes that he seems to both contemplate his own pain and externalize it to write about it.[22] Both Daudet and Hitchens are allowing readers to embark upon this experience of illness with them. The emotions are intensified as what is on the page is shared by the reader as it is experienced by the authors. In this way, the writers are serving their readers in a most profound way: moving from the theoretical to the personal so that the "I" may be experienced as "we."

What pain does Daudet experience? All types, he tells us. "Sometimes, on the sole of the foot, an incision, a thin one, hair-thin. Or a penknife stabbing away beneath the big toenail. The torture of 'the boot.' Rats gnawing at the toes with very sharp teeth. And amid all these woes, the sense of a rocket climbing, climbing up into your skull, and then exploding there as the climax to the show."[23]

For a reader with no direct experience of either cancer or syphilis, the writing of both Daudet and Hitchens can be a little frightening. They both experience extreme loneliness, fear, and anxiety. Both regret leaving behind wives and children. Daudet is the victim of "treatments" that are not only painful but have no medical value. Only morphine made life bearable for Daudet at the end.[24]

The pain that is at the heart of these memoirs, however, is notoriously difficult to capture. The challenge for the writer is that "pain resists language,"[25] but language is the only tool at the writer's disposal. Daudet is often able to capture his pain by making a direct connection to the reader. He writes, "[P]ain is always new to the sufferer, but loses its originality for those around him. Everyone will get used to it except me."[26] This passage is successful because the reader can easily see that it contains an inherent truth; the pain that may bore you when it is not your own becomes all you can think about when it is your own. Daudet, the writer/patient, not only risks suffering alone but risks boring others if this is his only topic of conversation.

Hitchens is less concerned with boring his reader and more concerned that even the warnings he received from his doctors prior to medical treatments with harsh side effects did not prepare him for the pain he encountered. "To say the rash hurt would be pointless. The struggle is to convey the way that it hurt *on the inside*. I lay for days on end, trying in vain to postpone the moment when I would have to swallow. Every time I did swallow, a hellish tide of pain would flow up my throat, culminating in what felt like a mule kick in the small of my back. . . . It's probably a merciful thing that pain is impossible to describe from memory. It's also impossible to warn against."[27] Hitchens feels that he has entered an alien land since his cancer diagnosis. Now living in what he calls Tumortown,[28] he acknowledges that he has left his old life behind and assumed a new identity as a cancer patient. The old rules no longer apply. He is a reluctant "citizen of the sick country . . . hopelessly clinging to [his] old domicile" in a new world.[29] Daudet also notes that his illness creates an alien landscape and that he is alone with pain in a foreign land.[30]

## Different dualities and growth through suffering

Susan Sontag, in *Illness as Metaphor*, begins by noting that we all "hold[] dual citizenship in the kingdom of the well and the kingdom of the sick,"[31] and we are all destined to spend time in both places. The lucky amongst us will spend little time in the kingdom of the sick. This duality haunts us because the presence of the sick reminds us that we can easily join them. We are all one unlucky mammogram, blood test, or screening test away from joining the denizens of the kingdom of the sick.

She later notes the inadequacy of limitations of language and finds that modern disease metaphors are cheap shots. Diseases such as cancer and AIDS are so complex that to use them as a metaphor for any other social phenomenon does a disservice to the patient. Social ills as varied as "the Jewish problem" in the 1930s, masturbation, Watergate, and other political challenges around the world have been deemed cancers. This metaphor minimizes the experience of the patient as a unique experience.[32]

For those dwelling in the kingdom of the sick, some may feel that the illness itself is taking over the body of the formerly well person. Sontag writes that "you are being replaced by the non-you,"[33] as the cancer or syphilis grabs hold of the patient in a very literal sense. This duality is consistent with modern notions of illness in many ways. Patients may feel friends, family, and the former life that they were able to lead – before illness forced them to accommodate a new schedule of chemotherapy, radiation, and multiple visits to specialists – are long gone. The patient has a new life comprised of medical visits and a new schedule and seldom sees those he or she saw previously. The patient is indeed a new person. Daudet's *Notes sur la vie* reflects this duality in its opening lines: *"Homo duplex, Homo duplex!"*[34]

Another duality is seen in the weakness of the patient in response to the strength of the enemy, cancer, or syphilis. However, today the stronger images may be of the chemotherapy fighting the disease itself. A battle is being fought and, whether it is illness versus the patient or chemotherapy versus the cancer, a victor must emerge at some point. Dualities seldom coexist peacefully for long.

In the midst of such challenging dualities, both Daudet and Hitchens maintain their desire to write. Daudet's son, Lucien, noted that he became determined to continue his writing, even at the cost of further physical pain, to provide some distraction from his pain. The process of writing and the knowledge that his death was imminent intensified Daudet's love for humanity.[35] There is a tenderness present in his writing. This has led one writer to comment that you can't separate Daudet from his writing; they explain each other.[36] In some ways, perhaps his attempt to communicate his pain allowed him to bridge the gap between reader and writer.

Hitchens also writes of the profound growth he experiences. He writes honestly of changes in long-held beliefs, although not necessarily religious beliefs. He notes that he lost faith in the value of the sentiment "whatever doesn't kill me makes me stronger,"[37] perhaps because he has moved closer to that which will ultimately kill him. He realizes that perhaps chance is at play here and that this sentiment is more correctly viewed as merely the notion of "there but for the grace of God go I" or, more honestly, "the grace of God has happily embraced me and skipped that unfortunate other man."[38] Through the illness he has randomly received, he is profoundly connected to others who are as vulnerable as he.

Daudet himself experiences such a connection, and accordingly finds temporary solace in books and the stories of others. He even refers to himself as a "poor old wounded Don Quixote."[39] This is a tribute to the power of literature to serve as a respite in the world of pain that these writers find themselves.

## The medical narrative: a closer look

Medical narratives, the records of medical and life experiences of patients such as Hitchens and Daudet, serve another vital function in this context. The medical narrative that is created when a patient becomes ill binds the physician and patient together in a unique relationship. The experience of illness will be a unique one because this patient and this physician (and the entire medical team) have never worked together previously and will see this illness together to its conclusion. They are forming a partnership with a specific goal in mind.

Narratives also bind writer and reader. For Daudet and Hitchens, the solitary act of writing serves the social act of creating a community, even a community of unknown future readers. For Daudet, the "social disease" he has (which is never named by his doctors) serves a social function of which even Daudet may not be totally aware. Each experience of illness calls for the reimagining of that person as a new person who has either survived or succumbed to an illness. The illness has resulted in the creation of a new social entity; the persons formerly known as Daudet and Hitchens have been so profoundly changed by their respective illnesses that society must now welcome the new persons they have become. How the patient navigates an illness will become a crucial component of his or her personal myth. This narrative will "illuminate the values of an individual life"[40] and is likely to become part of the story that the patient tells people that she or he meets. This becomes part of the story of the self that is being created by all of us as we navigate our way through the world. At the heart of that reimagining is the narrative itself.

Dan McAdams has said that a good personal narrative possesses six qualities: 1) coherence, 2) openness, 3) credibility, 4) differentiation, 5) reconciliation, and 6) generative integration.[41] Furthermore, "our own lives connect to other lives, our myths, to other myths."[42] The physician and patient compose a relationship that begins with two people and may ultimately expand to include many more.

The physician and patient together create a community of two people challenging the disease in a land of pain, new to the patient, where the final outcome is uncertain. Jan Marta has written that "[n]arrative identity interconnects the patient and physician and intertwines their moral and ethical concerns."[43] While the community will ultimately expand to include other providers and the patient's family members, the patient and physician are at the heart of this newly formed community. What will be learned, by both provider and patient, is still unknown, but it remains certain that there is something to be learned by both.

## Implications for providers

No two patients will experience the same illness in quite the same way. Daudet's syphilis and Hitchens's esophageal cancer were unique to each of them, and the way that each patient uses his or her available resources to face illness also will be unique. At the same time, patients desire to share their experience of illness with others. One important lesson for medical providers, then, is that each illness is a solo journey in need of a community, which includes family, friends, and providers. This is confirmed when one shares the experience of illness with another. As Arthur Frank notes, "Communities are formed out of stories; the story is the reflexive affirmation that a gathering of people *is* a community, or even that two people can become a community. The communal act of telling, hearing, and recognizing a story is how a group becomes a community. . . . The call to share stories is a call to the common work of *finding out what the experience we share might mean as an identity*."[44]

Second, each patient writes his or her own narrative. When the patient and provider do not share a worldview or causal explanation for the source of the illness or approach to treatment, the illness becomes more challenging. In *The Spirit Catches You and You Fall Down*, Los Angeles physicians could not convince Hmong immigrants that their daughter's epilepsy should be treated with prescribed medications and were therefore doomed to watch the girl face seizure after seizure. Author Anne Fadiman noted that if the providers had simply asked the question, "What do you think is wrong with your daughter?" the doctors would have made a great deal of headway into addressing the multiple communication failures inherent in this relationship.[45] Not only did they never ask the question, there were often simply no translators present to ask questions for the doctors. If the providers had learned that Hmong communities believed that an individual with epilepsy was in contact with the sacred during seizures and that those with this illness were very special people who should not be treated for this reason, then the child may not have been at risk for what turned out to be a forty-five-minute epileptic seizure, which left her severely brain damaged. The exercise of cultural competence and better communication might have saved this child. At a minimum, a frank conversation about the nature of the illness affecting their daughter, including Hmong spiritual beliefs and Western beliefs about the value of their medical treatments, would have resulted in a more thorough understanding of the nature of the girl's illness. From this understanding, a more respectful relationship could have blossomed that might have resulted in a better outcome for the child.

Third, there are advantages to reading other narratives. Just as readers experience intellectual growth from fiction, providers experience empathetic growth from medical narratives. The rapid growth in the number of medical schools offering literature and medicine classes reveals that the experiences of writers such as Henry James, Tolstoy, and others are valuable teaching tools. After all, "stories are less about facts and more about meanings."[46]

The final books of both Hitchens and Daudet reveal that insightful writers are insightful to the end, including about their impending deaths. While each was writing a century apart in time, both experienced the severe emotional pain that accompanied a terminal diagnosis and the knowledge that they were leaving behind beloved family members. The loss is tangible on the page to the reader today. For readers today, the emotional journey undertaken by reading Daudet and Hitchens is a true journey toward understanding the loss of the invaluable. While physically gone, Daudet and Hitchens live on.

## Notes

 1 Alphonse Daudet, *In the Land of Pain*, trans. Julian Barnes (New York, NY: Alfred A. Knopf, 2002).
 2 Macdonald Critchley, "Four Illustrious Neuroluetics," *Proceedings of the Royal Society of Medicine* 62 no. 7 (1969): 671.
 3 Michael Worton, "Of Sapho and Syphilis: Alphonse Daudet on and in Illness," *L'Esprit Créateur* 37 no. 3 (1997): 39.
 4 Critchley, "Four Illustrious Neuroluetics," 671–672.
 5 Daudet, *In the Land of Pain*, 6.
 6 Ibid., 28, 31.
 7 Ibid., 41.
 8 Ibid., 24–25, 43.
 9 Daudet, *In the Land of Pain*, 49.
10 Christopher Hitchens, *Mortality* (New York, NY: Twelve Books, 2012), 77–83.
11 Ibid., 46.
12 Ibid., 82.
13 Ibid., 67.
14 Susan Sontag, *Illness as Metaphor* (New York, NY: Farrar, Straus and Giroux, 1977), 68.
15 Hitchens, *Mortality*, 15.
16 Ibid., 6.
17 Ibid., 39–40.
18 Howard Brody, "Who Gets to Tell the Story? Narrative in Postmodern Bioethics," in *Stories and Their Limits: Narrative Approaches to Bioethics*, ed. Hilde Lindemann Nelson (New York, NY: Routledge, 1997), 20.
19 William H. Gass, *Life Sentences: Literary Judgments and Accounts* (New York, NY: Alfred A. Knopf, 2012), 267.
20 George Lakoff and Mark Johnson, *Metaphors We Live By* (Chicago, IL: University of Chicago Press, 1980), 193.
21 Daudet, *In the Land of Pain*, 17.

22 Lucy Bending, "Approximation, Suggestion, and Analogy: Translating Pain into Language," *The Yearbook of English Studies* 36 no. 1 (2006): 136.
23 Daudet, *In the Land of Pain*, 21.
24 A. Dickson Wright, "Venereal Disease and the Great," *British Journal of Venereal Diseases* 47 no. 4 (1971): 295.
25 Bending, "Approximation, Suggestion, and Analogy," 137.
26 Daudet, *In the Land of Pain*, 19.
27 Hitchens, *Mortality*, 67.
28 Ibid., 28.
29 Ibid., 3.
30 Daudet, *In the Land of Pain*, 42.
31 Sontag, *Illness as Metaphor*, 3.
32 Ibid., 83–85.
33 Ibid., 67.
34 Worton, "Of Sapho and Syphilis," 45.
35 Alphonse V. Roche, *Alphonse Daudet* (Boston, MA: Twayne Publishers, 1976), 80.
36 Ibid., 143.
37 Hitchens, *Mortality*, 59.
38 Ibid., 59–60.
39 Daudet, *In the Land of Pain*, 14.
40 Dan P. McAdams, *The Stories We Live By: Personal Myths and the Making of the Self* (New York, NY: Guilford Press, 1993), 34.
41 Ibid., 110.
42 Ibid., 113.
43 Jan Marta, "Toward a Bioethics for the Twenty-First Century: A Ricoeurian Poststructuralist Narrative Hermeneutic Approach to Informed Consent," in *Stories and Their Limits*, ed. Nelson, 202.
44 Arthur W. Frank, "Enacting Illness Stories: When, What, and Why," in *Stories and Their Limits*, ed. Nelson, 36–37.
45 Anne Fadiman, *The Spirit Catches You and You Fall Down: A Hmong Child, Her American Doctors, and the Collision of Two Cultures* (New York, NY: Farrar, Straus and Giroux, 1997), 260–261.
46 McAdams, *The Stories We Live By*, 28.

# 10 Suffering, death, and the significance of presence

*Autumn Alcott Ridenour*

Jeffrey Bishop's *The Anticipatory Corpse* disrupted the bioethical scene by asking whether the goals and practices of modern medicine are themselves corrupt. In a deconstructive diagnosis of modern medicine, he argues that not only do individualism and autonomous decision making reign supreme but also the goals that drive medicine, namely efficient and material causation, lack formal and final purposes to order medical practice. In other words, using Aristotelian reasoning, Bishop basically argues that unreflective, pragmatic control – and not larger goals associated with a good or meaningful life – determines the practices of medicine. Efficiency by way of "controlling matter" and biological processes becomes the primary focus of Western medicine in its desire to stave off disease, suffering, and death.[1] Ironically, however, the cadaver – or dead body – is valued as the central tool from which knowledge is transposed onto the living body. Bishop's provocative conclusion questions whether only theology might save medicine.[2] His analysis and conclusion implicitly ask medicine and theology about the nature of these suffering bodies we inhabit and the role of suffering and death in terms of human identity and meaning.

In an interesting response to Bishop, Brett McCarty offers a "second opinion" in which he describes Bishop's critique as incomplete given that "the purposes of life [and possibly of suffering and death] may be present and enduring, though perhaps hidden, in the modern practice of medicine."[3] Like McCarty, this chapter aims to respond to Bishop's thesis by turning to both the Christian tradition in its view of suffering, death, and the human body in its transience as well as those implicit or "hidden" purposes within the practice of medicine that care for the suffering body through presence at the end of life. In order to demonstrate Christian theology's and medicine's divergence and convergence through practice, I first explore the Christian tradition's understanding of suffering as an undesirable yet universal consequence of sin; second, I define the body in terms of transience or natural change and demonstrate how the notion that bodily change, suffering, and death are ubiquitous is shared by modern medicine; third, I consider how hope is imbedded in a Christian narrative in its desire for transformation beyond undesirable pain and our mechanistic aims at controlling transient nature; and finally, I return to the significance of grief and the practice of presence as an original goal of Christian love as well as the best of medicine's care in the face of suffering and death. Through these four steps, I hope to account for the tension of our existence, the hopeful solution found in our future destination, and the means for living in the tension of life's journey in the present moment in the meantime.

## The meaning, cause, and ubiquity of suffering

The Christian tradition is one of many approaches grappling with the profound mystery of suffering, pain, death, and their relation to our identities as individuals composed of bodies that both flourish and languish. For many, asking the question of suffering begins with the problem of evil and pain. While various attempts aim to respond in part through suggesting that there is a greater good or silver lining that emerges out of evil,[4] most answers leave readers dissatisfied and longing for more. This chapter is not an attempt to solve the puzzle of pain and suffering but an attempt to account for our experience of them as negative yet seemingly inevitable given our transience. To describe this phenomenon more explicitly, I offer a constructive Augustinian interpretation of the Christian narrative as one in which life involves suffering as undesirable pain.

Writing in the fourth and fifth centuries, St. Augustine of Hippo was well acquainted with suffering and pain through his own restless search for understanding the self, God, neighbor, and the meaning of life, as well as through his later experience as a bishop caring for parishioners enduring loss.[5] Much of Augustine's writing involved the interpretation of Genesis 1–3 through his *Confessions, City of God, On Genesis: A Refutation of the Manichees, Unfinished Literal Commentary on Genesis,* and *The Literal Meaning of Genesis.*[6] According to an Augustinian worldview, God creates space and time from freedom and love. Inhabiting the Garden of Eden are all forms of creation, including humans who are called to care for the Garden's inhabitants. The Garden represents an ideal world in which intimate knowledge of God and of one another exist in harmony. Human identity includes a union of soul and body as creatures made in the image of God who are also assigned value in that they are deemed "good."[7] God establishes all creation – including the material world – with purpose and meaning.

However, evil enters the scene through a deficient or unknown cause attributed to the serpent, whom C.S. Lewis describes as Satan or a "fallen angel."[8] Charles Mathewes calls the introduction of evil into a good world as "ontologically privational and hence intellectually incomprehensible."[9] Evil results from a defective will and is an indescribable phenomenon analogous to "seeing darkness" or "hearing silence."[10] Given the inability to see darkness or hear silence, evil appears more like an absence rather than substance, thereby affirming Augustine's view of evil as privation.[11] In other words, evil is an undoing of creation in its original purpose and final meaning.

While evil remains incomprehensible beyond Augustine's description as privation, the most direct experience of evil through human acts is through a phenomenon that Christians call "sin," understood as alienation from God, self, and other. Originally created good in the harmonious union of soul and body in the Garden, humans depend on God for ongoing sustenance and wisdom that conveys moral right and wrong.[12] However, because of pride and the human desire to love self and temporal goods above God, humans fell from their perfect, intimate relation with the Creator.[13] Falling from their source of wisdom that supplies purpose, morality, and even existence, humans are banished from the Garden and exiled as pilgrims on a journey fraught with life's mixture of grace and suffering. Death, too, is a part of universal human experience resulting from sin and disordered love of self above love of God.[14]

In other words, departing from his Pelagian opponents, Augustine's account of universal sin holds that humans no longer encounter the immediate presence of God personified through the Garden of Eden and aim to define moral right and wrong apart from divine purposes.[15] Accordingly, we might say that just as human beings have moved away from their spiritual purposes, their bodies have departed from their original purposes and experience the painful and undesirable realities of suffering and death. Diseases like cancer eat away at the human body. Interpreting Genesis in this way parallels Athanasius's description of human persons losing not only their inward purpose but also their outward physical or material existence in its movement toward death and decay.[16] To put it another way, outward physical loss points to inward spiritual loss of meaning and purpose made available through union with God.[17]

Augustine also departs from the mainstream Platonic, Manichaean, and Stoic philosophies of his day that prized the soul over the body and thereby welcomed death as natural rather than as unintended and lamentable.[18] Recognizing death as a result of sin and evil, Augustine affirms death as genuine loss and thereby establishes an ethics of compassion that includes grief rather than denying emotions.[19] Augustine finds himself departing from Stoic and Platonic philosophies by acknowledging the emotion of sorrow as an honest human experience in our reflection on the real loss encountered with disease, suffering, and death.[20] Here an Augustinian interpretation accounts for the pain and negative side of death and suffering. However, even though his theology includes death and suffering as evil, his theology also includes an account of transience as natural.

## Transience as natural

For an Augustinian worldview, bodies are originally intended to grow and change over time. In this sense, transience or "change" might be considered natural in the pre-fall Garden of Eden. Much like his later interpreter, St. Thomas Aquinas, Augustine saw creation and the material world as laden with potency and change. Time and seasons exist in the Garden, as seen through the advent of day and night, along with possibilities for growth and change. Rowan Williams says,

> The point could be better put by saying that God wills that there be reality quite other than God, and that this entails the positing of a reality that can change: if so, it entails also the dialectic of the possible and the actual, it entails a world of purposive fluidity, things becoming themselves, organizing themselves more successfully or economically over time. Possibilities are continually being realized, but realized in orderly and intelligible fashion. . . . [Thus] Creation is the constant process of realizing potential goods; and that is why the difference between God and creation cannot be elided.[21]

Augustine's allegorical interpretation of the Garden includes the idea that God simultaneously created all things at once – or as "possibility" (from Sir. 18:1) as well as in historical time.[22] Not unlike evolutionary biology or science, Augustine sees the material world as one of potency and actualization.

Interestingly, the idea of transience as natural is one consistent with the laws of nature espoused by science and physicians such as Bishop and Sherwin Nuland. Nuland describes the beauty of the various parts of the human body functioning together in single unity in the opening to his *Wisdom of the Body*. Enthralled by human nature and calling it "Revelation," Nuland is awestruck by "the infinite variety of processes by which we maintain that singular constancy and unity of moment-to-moment life."[23]

Accompanying Nuland's awe and reverence for the harmony of the body is his description of the body in terms of constant movement and change. Here he acknowledges instability as necessary for living organisms. Just as the body is one of perpetual motion (even while bodies rest or sleep), Nuland says, "A stable system is not a system that never changes. It is a system that constantly and instantly adjusts and readjusts in order to maintain such a state of being. . . . Stability demands change to compensate for changing circumstances. Ultimately, then, stability depends on instability." Whether metabolism or temperature, the human body is a self-regulating organism constantly moving, adapting, and changing according to our surrounding environment.[24] Nuland's medical diagnosis complements those philosophical and theological reflections on the experience of life as one of mutability, movement, and development. To exist as material bodies in time is to undergo aging in terms of continual adjustment and change.

Much like Nuland, Bishop affirms bodies as subject to continual change. Bishop says, "Life can be understood only as flux, not as death. Life is in flux; it is by definition a suffering, an undergoing of change."[25] Interestingly, Bishop's incisive critique of medicine is what he sees as the desire to control the uncontrollable. Life is flux, yet medicine ironically turns to "stasis" or a "controlled environment" in which time and space are captured in the cadaver or dead body. The dead body becomes the source for knowledge and wisdom pertaining to living bodies. While Bishop acknowledges the stark contrast between living and dead bodies, the cadaver, nonetheless, serves as the initial lab by which medical students learn the inner workings of the human body. Whether implicit within the practice of autopsy or conclusions derived from this practice, "control" and "decision" are what medicine aims for, according to Bishop.[26]

Under the scientist's gaze, efficient causes direct matter by way of ongoing processes that ignore larger questions of meaning and purpose. In search for control, Bishop says, "Death . . . is at the repressed core of medicine, and indeed much of contemporary society."[27] Interestingly, Bishop's diagnosis of medicine and society may not be entirely unlike Augustine's own critique of Rome and its political aspirations in his famous *City of God*. Robert Dodaro interprets the *City of God* as an analysis of pagan and competing philosophical responses to fearing death through various forms of false security.[28] Not unlike Ernest Becker's thesis in his famous *The Denial of Death*, civilization – including medicine – is another institution aimed at ignoring and controlling death.[29]

This aligns well with the argument made by bioethicist Daniel Callahan, who often finds irony in death's relation to medicine's goals. While finitude and death are a part of human life, medicine, he argues, tries to eliminate all forms of death and disease. Callahan says, "Although death may be inevitable, none of the medical causes of death need be accepted; all are in principle curable."[30] While the tension of death as undesirable and yet inevitable remains, Callahan argues that medicine ought to return to a sense of human nature composed of limits and to practices involving them.[31] Part of returning to limits begins with recognizing the body as one that involves transience. Rather than look for a point in time that might be ultimately controlled (as in the cadaver or dead body), instead the Christian narrative hopes for a future transformation beyond human control while seeking the practice of presence in this changing life toward death.

## Controlling nature? The hope of transformation and "the anticipatory corpse"

The etiological and moral stories we tell are important not only for communal identity but also for making meaning of the world and the bodies we inhabit. While the Christian narrative includes tension between created goodness and disordered reality, the story does not end with the negative portrayal of death as the final word. Instead, central to the Christian narrative is the image of a suffering and transient body that resurrects in the person of Christ. Here the full drama of negative and positive human experience transpires in the movement from cross to resurrection. In the cross, humanity sees "evil do its worst,"[32] while in the resurrection, the power of evil, along with suffering and death, is seemingly overcome. However, even in the victorious note that ends in resurrection, Christ is encountered by the disciples through a visible body – one recognized by his scars through suffering.[33]

Imbedded within the Christian narrative is a teleological vision of hope for future transformation in ways that depart from mechanistic aims at controlling nature. In Augustine's account of original creation, he describes humans as "ensouled bodies," with immaterial souls and material bodies made for and sustained through union with God and as a mean between angels and animals.[34] Through receiving a kind of sacrament symbolized by fruit from the Tree of Life in the Garden, humans maintained ongoing physical life.[35]

However, through sin and disordered loves, humans miss part of their original participation and are faced with the immediacy of material life that often overlooks spiritual wisdom and purpose for human existence. Yet, Augustine's understanding of humanity does not end with this post-lapsarian anthropology. Instead, he puts forth a teleological vision of humanity that involves "enspirited bodies" where persons are made incorruptible by ongoing union with God in eternity.[36] Unlike the ensouled bodies at creation, these new "enspirited" bodies gaze directly on the unchangeable substance of God (or wisdom), thereby making their existence better than the original.[37] He even accounts for ways the early disciples and later believers awaiting the eschatological vision might partially participate in "enspirited bodies" by "renewing the mind" in time.[38]

Christ becomes the new man for humanity both in wisdom and in existence. Christ's person remains in union with the Triune God as the divine logos and imparts such wisdom to humanity through union with his person.[39] The person of Christ also becomes the new way for life following his own death and resurrection.[40] Partaking of Christ as the new sacrament or new sustenance becomes the transformative vision for creaturely existence. Through receiving both wisdom and life from Christ, creatures hope not only for future transformation but also for spiritual renewal in this temporal existence. While the Christian narrative is realistic in its account of physical life as one enduring change as well as pain, it is optimistic about the inward renewal made available by union with the Spirit. As the second letter to the Corinthians says, "Even though our outer nature is wasting away, our inner nature is being renewed day by day."[41] By participating in the "mind of Christ," disciples renew their inward purpose for life while maintaining hope for their final resurrection that will leave their undesirable suffering/pain behind.

Jonathan Edwards nicely captures the teleological dimension of the material world by describing ways it points to our ultimate spiritual reality. His "Images or Shadows of Divine Things" explicitly describes the material world as a shadow of our spiritual existence. He says, "Thus I believe the grass and other vegetables growing and flourishing, looking green and pleasant as it were, ripening, blossoming, and bearing fruit from the influences of the heavens, the rain and wind and light and heat of the sun, to be on purpose to represent the dependence of our spiritual welfare upon God's gracious influences and the effusions of His holy spirit." Not only do the grass, vegetables, and fruits of the earth point to our spiritual dependence on God but so too do the thunder clouds and blue skies reflect God's majesty and love as does the silkworm pointing to Christ's righteousness that clothes sinners.[42] Even the sun's rising and setting includes a material and spiritual analogy that points to the death and resurrection of Christ. In other words, the physical world points to something greater. He concludes his examples by saying "the fruit is ripe . . . and easily gathered"[43] as is the saint ripe for heaven as one "transformed . . . from one degree of glory to another."[44] The saint, including her material body, is destined for something more.

In this way, the Christian narrative departs from a mechanistic or materialistic view of the human body alone. While science sees the cadaver as a dead body, Christianity sees an "anticipatory corpse." Bishop's title is appropriate not only in accounting for the Christian interpretation of nature as one destined for suffering, change, decay, and death resulting from evil but also for anticipating transformative renewal of these material bodies into something better. In the theological narrative, even the corpse is not devoid of "purpose"[45] but one intended for "perfection," also known as "glory" through the resurrection.[46]

This account of the suffering body departs from narratives that aim to manipulate or control nature. Ultimately, nature is something to receive, not manipulate. Unlike the premise that all forms of disease are somehow curable, instead, this vision aims to work with the body's capacity to both flourish and languish. Between the dialectic of flourish and languish, growth, and decay, disciples suffer change while groaning for something greater.[47] However, in the midst of the groaning that often composes the suffering of this dying life, Christ shows a way for disciples to imitate his compassion, namely through the expression of grief at loss and the practice of presence.

## The expression of grief and the practice of presence

The Christian narrative is one that is both optimistic about future transformation but also realistic about pain, suffering, and change in our temporal existence. Central to the tradition is the image of death and resurrection, holding together the dual tension of pain and joyful anticipation. St. Augustine was keenly aware of these dual realities and sympathetic to parishioners encountering death and loss in Rome.[48] His own preaching paused at the pain associated with death and legitimized sorrow in ways his philosophical peers, such as the Stoics and Manichaeans, discounted.

Citing Peter's tears of repentance and Christ's tears over the loss of Lazarus, Augustine recognizes both the legitimacy and strength in sorrowing over spiritual and physical loss.[49] Not coincidentally, perhaps, does Christ pause to mourn with Lazarus's family over his death shortly before resurrecting him from the dead with joyful reunion. Through this image, Christ does not sidestep pain, suffering, death, and their accompanied emotions but walks through this experience with faithfulness and honest lament.

Augustine recognizes Christ's further engagement with deep human emotions through his own anxiety expressed in the Garden of Gethsemane's prayer alongside his grief expressed on the cross at possible fear and abandonment.[50] Rowan Williams helpfully interprets Christ's cry to the Father, "My God, my God, why have you forsaken me?" as Christ's willingness to take on our suffering, pain, and sense of isolation from God and others.[51] For Augustine, it is Christ's compassionate solidarity with us in humanity as well as the cross that demonstrates his humility and glory.[52] Williams claims that Christ cries to God on our behalf not from sin or warring wills but from his desire to take on our sense of abandonment and align our emotions with his.[53] Sensing forsakenness from God, Christ demonstrates grief at the loss and isolation associated with death. His response opposes Stoic desires to repress emotions and is later personified through Augustine's own tears shed over the loss of his mother, Monica.[54] While initially Augustine tries to disguise his grief before his mentor Ambrose, he acknowledges the rest he finally felt in expressing his sorrow before God. He says, "I was glad to weep before you about her and for her, about myself and for myself. Now I let flow the tears, which I had held back so that they ran as freely as they wished. My heart rested upon them, and it reclined upon them because it was your ears that were there."[55] Resting his emotions before God, Augustine senses Christ's presence with him in his suffering.

Not only does Augustine legitimate grief when facing suffering and death, he also verifies the gift of presence of Christ and the significance of presence to one another in love. Dorothy Sayers recognizes the drama of a divine gift in that God took a dose of his own medicine by becoming "one of us," as Emmanuel.[56] Central to Christian identity is the doctrine of the Incarnation, affirming that God became flesh. Adam Neder interprets the hypostatic union of Christ's divine and human natures as central to Karl Barth's famous *Church Dogmatics*.[57] Building upon St. Athanasius, Barth says, "God becomes [human] in order that [humans] . . . come to God."[58] The Incarnation and hypostatic union are central for establishing not only our reconciliation with God but also Christ's presence with humanity in life and death.

Because of this presence, followers of Christ are called to remain present to one another through life and death. When considering the significance of religion for medicine, theologian Stanley Hauerwas appeals to Christian communities as those accustomed to practicing presence to one another over time.[59] Health care is another such community encountering human suffering and death. Here the practices of Christian community might assist the medical goal of healing as one that includes presence. He says, "Only a community that is pledged not to fear the stranger – and illness always makes us a stranger to ourselves and others – can welcome the continued presence of the ill in our midst. The hospital is, after all, first and foremost a house of hospitality along the way of our journey with finitude. It is our sign that we will not abandon those who have become ill simply because they currently are suffering the sign of that finitude."[60]

In other words, the practice of medicine ought to be a sign that the human community will not abandon those who are suffering and dying. We should not approach medical and hospital institutions as ones that separate the suffering from society; instead, they are to comfort the suffering through compassionate presence.[61] Physician Sherwin Nuland echoes this concern in his famous book *How We Die*, where he traces not only the various diseases from which we die but also his development as a physician. In his conclusion, Nuland describes how he went from initially training with the goal of serving others to striving to attain success in medicine by solving the "riddle" of disease.[62] Implicit within his desire to solve the riddle of disease is what Nuland describes as the "fantasy of controlling nature" that functions as the operative goal of medicine in its fear of death. Nuland says, "Medicine's humility in the face of nature's power has been lost, and with it has gone some of the moral authority of times past. With the vast increase in scientific knowledge has come a vast decrease in the acknowledgment that we still have control over far less than we would like."[63] Thus, fear of death and the desire for control often operate as motivations accompanying our beneficent desire to aid and assuage pain and suffering.

Instead, Nuland proposes that physicians and modern medicine recover their initial desire to mitigate suffering when facing death and disease rather than focus on the "quest to solve The Riddle [that] will sometimes be at odds with our best interests at the end of life."[64] Real hope, Nuland believes, comes not from a medical "cure" that involves remission and relief of temporary distress and disease but from the promise not to be abandoned in death, which itself helps reduce suffering.[65] Not abandoning the patient in death is medicine's primary human obligation for Nuland, one that complements well the Christian practice of presence in the face of suffering. Here, medicine and theology might intersect in "hidden ways" through loving presence as the appropriate response to human suffering and death.[66]

Theologian and ethicist Allen Verhey also recognizes the "hidden ways" medicine overlaps with Christian approaches to health care and the body through John Calvin's sense of common grace as operative within nature and the field of medicine.[67] Calvin recognizes grace present within the common spheres of life (beyond salvific grace), including politics, education, the arts, and medicine.[68] Verhey also acknowledges Bishop's critique of modern hospice as vulnerable to totalizing forms of "biopsychosocialspiritual" assessment or medicine that seemingly control every dimension of human life as quantifiable, including spirituality and grief. However, Verhey also argues we might reimagine medicine in the broader context of theological commitments currently operative within health care. One example he uses is to reimagine hospice care according to Dame Cicely Saunders's original vision "formed by Matthew 25, which privileges the sick and dying."[69] Here Jesus rewards his followers for feeding the hungry, clothing the naked, caring for the sick, visiting the imprisoned, and sheltering the homeless. By recognizing hospice care according to its original desire for spiritual and physical accompaniment in the face of suffering and death, physicians and health care workers might invoke the greater purpose of presence for animating their practices and daily care toward patients.

Along these lines, physician Daniel Sulmasy uncovers the significance of spiritual and physical care working together in *The Healer's Calling*. Invoking the use of the five senses in prayer and diagnosis, he finds union between the sensory and spiritual realms.[70] Uniting prayer and physical care for the patient is also important for entering the suffering of the patient with compassion. Sulmasy says, "Clinicians . . . can treat pain and disease and a few other medical conditions that cause suffering, but they cannot treat suffering itself. There are no pills to treat suffering. . . . They can only respond with human compassion toward those who are suffering."[71] Pills alone do not heal suffering, but compassion or "suffering with" reminds individuals they are not alone in their pain.

Acknowledging that not all suffering is caused by treatable pain, Sulmasy states that "feelings of fear, loneliness, embarrassment, helplessness, hopelessness, and abandonment are all aspects of suffering that morphine does not touch." Sulmasy challenges healthcare workers to not focus on treatment alone but see the spiritual calling of their practice through engaging patients with empathy and compassion. Sulmasy says, "Suffering is only healed through compassionate love. In imitating the healing work of Christ, Christian clinicians enter more deeply into the kingdom of God."[72] Rather than separate medicine and religion, we can appreciate that the two realms show hidden glimpses of union in care for the suffering other that is facilitated by common grace. Sulmasy opens *The Healer's Calling* by reminding physicians and medical professionals why they entered health care in the first place.[73] Appealing to their sense of original call, Sulmasy aims to unlock this spirit behind the various day-to-day activities that consume the practice of medicine.

Likewise, Bishop concludes his volume *The Anticipatory Corpse* by appealing to the physician's response to the suffering other. In an interesting move, Bishop recognizes the suffering other as the primordial call that initially beckons the health care professional into the field before forgetting his or her purpose of service in the broad apparatus that composes contemporary medicine.[74] The suffering other transforms the receiver into viewing the world differently. Bishop says, "In the suffering of the other, one is called into becoming – and thus into being – what the other needs. Both the other and the perceiver undergo a transformation of being. They both suffer. Though each suffers differently, and each undergoes a different kind of transformation, each suffers the loss of the way things were."[75] In other words, suffering contains the power to transform not only the perspective but also the identity of another who is compelled to respond. This embodied call shapes the receiving physician "more profoundly and deeply than the doctor's training and education."[76]

In this passage, Bishop acknowledges the "hidden way" the sacred response to suffering still impacts and transforms health care workers despite the contemporary medical apparatus in which they work. Physician Richard Selzer might agree with Bishop concerning this sacred vocation.

Selzer describes ways that the suffering other not only initially calls individuals into health care but also transforms the physician through ongoing engagement with that other. Writing eloquently of patients encountered on the surgical table, hospital bed, and ICU, Selzer's descriptive response to suffering is nothing short of transformational. He says,

> A surgeon does not slip from his mother's womb with compassion smeared upon him like the drippings of his birth. It is much later that it comes. No easy shaft of grace this, but the cumulative murmuring of the numberless wounds he has dressed, the incisions he has made, all the sores and ulcers and cavities he has touched in order to heal. In the beginning, it is barely audible, a whisper, as from many mouths. Slowly it gathers, rises from the streaming flesh until, at last, it is pure calling – an exclusive sound, like the cry of certain solitary birds – telling that out of the resonance between the sick man and the one who tends him there may spring that profound courtesy that the religious call Love.[77]

Herein lies the "hidden way" that medicine, despite its challenges and even failures born from good intentions, still maintains its sacred call. Laden within its practice – even seemingly deficient practice at times – remains the power of the suffering other and the transformed receiver.

## Notes

1 Jeffrey Bishop, *The Anticipatory Corpse: Medicine, Power, and the Care of the Dying* (Notre Dame, IN: University of Notre Dame Press, 2011), 20, 22.
2 Ibid., 313.
3 Brett McCarty, "Diagnosis and Therapy in *The Anticipatory Corpse*: A Second Opinion," *Journal of Medicine and Philosophy* 41 no. 6 (2016): 624.
4 See, e.g., C. S. Lewis, *The Problem of Pain* (New York, NY: HarperCollins, 1940), 111.
5 Autumn Ridenour, *Sabbath Rest as Vocation: Aging Toward Death* (London, UK: T&T Clark, 2018), 40; Eric Rebillard, "Interaction Between the Preacher and His Audience: The Case-Study of Augustine's Preaching on Death," *Studia Patristica* 31 (1997): 86.
6 Roland J. Teske, "Genesis Accounts of Creation," in *Augustine Through the Ages: An Encyclopedia*, ed. Allan D. Fitzgerald, O.S.A. (Grand Rapids, MI: Wm. B. Eerdmans, 2009), 379–381.
7 Augustine, *City of God*, trans. Henry Bettenson (London, UK: Penguin Books, 1984), 451–453, 502–503, 515.
8 C. S. Lewis, "Mere Christianity," in *The Complete C.S. Lewis Signature Classics* (New York, NY: HarperCollins, 2002), 45.
9 Charles T. Mathewes, "Augustinian Anthropology: Interior intimo meo," *Journal of Religious Ethics* 27 no. 2 (1999): 205.
10 Augustine, *City of God*, 480.
11 Ibid.
12 Augustine, *The Trinity*, trans. Edmund Hill (Hyde Park, NY: New City Press, 2012), 338, 366–369; Rowan Williams, "Sapientia and the Trinity: Reflections on *De Trinitate*," *Collectanea Augustiniana*, eds. Bernard Bruning, Mathijs

Lamberigts, and Jozef van Houtem (Leuven, Belgium: Leuven University Press, 1990), 317–332.

13 John C. Cavadini, "Pride," in *Augustine Through the Ages*, ed. Allan D. Fitzgerald, 679–680; see also Augustine, *On Christian Teaching*, trans. R. P. H. Green (Oxford, UK: Oxford University Press, 1997), 9–10.

14 Augustine, *Answer to the Pelagians III*, trans. Roland J. Teske, S.J. (Hyde Park, NY: New City Press, 1999), 696.

15 Ibid.

16 Athanasius, *On the Incarnation* (Crestwood, NY: St. Vladimir's Seminary Press, 1944).

17 Ridenour, *Sabbath Rest as Vocation*, 137.

18 John C. Cavadini, "Ambrose and Augustine: *De Bono Mortis*," in *The Limits of Ancient Christianity: Essays on Late Antique Thought and Culture in Honor of R.A. Markus*, eds. William E. Klingshirn and Mark Vessey (Ann Arbor, MI: The University of Michigan Press, 1999), 232–249.

19 Ridenour, *Sabbath Rest as Vocation*, 40–46.

20 Ibid., 54. See also Augustine, *City of God*, 561–564.

21 Rowan Williams, "Good for Nothing'? Augustine on Creation," *Augustinian Studies* 25 (1994): 17–19.

22 Teske, "Genesis Accounts of Creation," 381.

23 Sherwin B. Nuland, *Wisdom of the Body: Discovering the Human Spirit* (New York, NY: Knopf, 1997), xx.

24 Ibid., xix.

25 Bishop, *The Anticipatory Corpse*, 26. Bishop's understanding here of suffering as including mere change may seem like a surprisingly expansive one. However, one dictionary definition of suffering is to "undergo," "experience," or "change." "Suffer," *Dictionary.com Unabridged* (Random House, Inc., 2018). see also "Suffer," *Merriam-Webster.com* (Merriam-Webster, 2016). While I am sympathetic to such an understanding, defending it would involve a much larger philosophical exploration that I will save for a later date.

26 Bishop, *The Anticipatory Corpse*, 15, 21.

27 Ibid., 15.

28 Robert Dodaro, *Christ and the Just Society in the Thought of Augustine* (Cambridge, UK: Cambridge University Press, 2004), 27–31.

29 Ernest Becker, *The Denial of Death* (New York, NY: Simon & Schuster, 1973).

30 Daniel Callahan, *The Troubled Dream of Life: In Search of a Peaceful Death* (Washington, DC: Georgetown University Press, 2000), 72.

31 Ibid. See also Daniel Callahan, *What Kind of Life: The Limits of Medical Progress* (Washington, DC: Georgetown University Press, 1990).

32 Paul Dafydd Jones, "Karl Barth on Gethsemane," *International Journal of Systematic Theology* 9 no. 2 (2007): 168.

33 Augustine, *City of God*, 1061–1062.

34 Augustine, *On Genesis I/13*, trans. Edmund Hill (Hyde Park, NY: New City Press, 2002), 321–323.

35 Ibid.

36 Ibid., 505–506.

37 Ibid., 321.

38 Ibid.

39 Lewis Ayres, "The Christological Context of Augustine's *De trinitate* XIII," *Augustinian Studies* 29 no. 1 (1998): 111–139.

40 Augustine, *City of God*, 538–539.

41 2 Cor. 4:16–18. Bible quotations are from the New Revised Standard Version.

42 Jonathan Edwards, "Images or Shadows of Divine Things," in *Selected Writings of Jonathan Edwards*, 2nd ed., ed. Harold P. Simonson (Long Grove, IL: Waveland Press, 2004), 161–162.

43  Ibid., 164.
44  2 Cor. 3:18.
45  Allen Verhey, "Can Calvin Save Medicine? A Response to Jeff Bishop," *Christian Bioethics* 20 no. 1 (2014): 24, 35.
46  Augustine, *City of God*, 1060.
47  2 Cor. 5.1–10; Rom. 8.22.
48  Rebillard, "Interaction Between the Preacher and His Audience," 86.
49  Augustine, *City of God*, 562–564; see also John 11:1–44.
50  Augustine, *The Trinity*, 158.
51  Rowan Williams, "Augustine's Christology: Its Spirituality and Rhetoric," in *In the Shadow of the Incarnation: Essays on Jesus Christ in the Early Church in Honor of Brian E. Daley*, ed. Peter W. Martens (Notre Dame, IN: University of Notre Dame Press, 2008), 178–180; Rowan Williams, "Augustine and the Psalms," *Interpretation* 58 no. 1 (2004): 17–20.
52  John C. Cavadini, "Ambrose and Augustine: *De Bono Mortis*," 244–245.
53  Williams, "Augustine's Christology," 185–186.
54  Augustine, *Confessions*, trans. Henry Chadwick (Oxford, UK: Oxford University Press, 1991), 60.
55  Ibid., 176.
56  Dorothy Sayers, *Letters to a Diminished Church* (Nashville, TN: W. Publishing Group, 2004), 1–6.
57  Adam Neder, *Participation in Christ: An Entry into Karl Barth's Church Dogmatics* (Louisville, KY: Westminster John Knox Press, 2009), xi–xv.
58  Karl Barth, *Church Dogmatics* IV/2, trans. G. W. Bromiley (London, UK: T&T Clark, 2004), 106.
59  Stanley Hauerwas, *Suffering Presence: Theological Reflections on Medicine, the Mentally Handicapped, and the Church* (Notre Dame, IN: University of Notre Dame Press, 1986), 80–81.
60  Ibid., 81–82.
61  Ibid., 82.
62  Sherwin B. Nuland, *How We Die: Reflections on Life's Final Chapter* (New York, NY: Random House, 1995), 247.
63  Ibid., 259.
64  Ibid., 249.
65  Ibid., 257.
66  McCarty, "Diagnosis and Therapy," 624.
67  Verhey, "Can Calvin Save Medicine?," 30.
68  John Calvin, *Institutes of the Christian Religion*, trans. Ford Lewis Battles and ed. John T. McNeill (Louisville, KY: Westminster John Knox Press, 2006), bk. 2, ch. 2, §§ 14–17. Abraham Kuyper further elaborates on common grace operating in sovereign spheres of arts, science, politics, and culture. Richard J. Mouw, *The Challenges of Cultural Discipleship: Essays in the Line of Abraham Kuyper* (Grand Rapids, MI: Wm. B. Eerdmans, 2012).
69  Verhey, "Can Calvin Save Medicine?," 26.
70  Daniel P. Sulmasy, *The Healer's Calling: A Spirituality for Physicians and Other Health Care Professionals* (Mahwah, NJ: Paulist Press, 1997), 73–90.
71  Ibid., 104.
72  Ibid., 106.
73  Ibid., 18–19.
74  Bishop, *The Anticipatory Corpse*, 302.
75  Ibid., 301.
76  Ibid., 302.
77  Richard Selzer, *The Exact Location of the Soul: New and Selected Essays* (New York, NY: Picador, 2001), 80.

# 11 The dead body as an object of investigation, intrigue, and reverence

## D. Gareth Jones

For human anatomists, the dead human body is an object of investigation and analysis, providing them with material for study via dissection. The essence of the latter is to reduce the body to its component parts and from this to build up a picture of how the body functions in health, and by extension in disease. However, activities such as these exist to varying degrees on the edges of every society. While the scandalous and deeply unethical activities of anatomists two to three hundred years ago are well-known, the way anatomy as a profession responded to them is far less well-known.

The responses are interesting since they encompass not only scientific and ethical domains but also theological ones. They are far more relevant to the general public than generally appreciated. This is because they touch on issues of consent, respect for the dead (and living) body, the impact of cultural and religious perspectives on what is done with and to the dead body and body parts, and even the relationship between the mortal body and the resurrected body.

In this chapter, these themes are explored in terms of several specific issues, including the dissection of bodies without consent of the individual before death or of the family after death, the long-term retention of organs and body parts after post-mortem, and the preservation and display of dissected whole bodies using the technique of plastination. Each of these throws light onto fundamental values that are highly relevant to the way in which people are treated during life, not just after death. In view of the increasing uses to which human tissue is being put, it has become necessary to unpack the values underlying ethical imperatives such as those of informed consent. In doing this, acknowledgment of the many connections between living persons and the bodies of the deceased highlights the centrality of the human person in one's thinking and attitudes. This, in turn, highlights the role of theological input into what are generally seen as ethical discussions.

## Approaching the dead human body

For many centuries, there was widespread belief that dissection of the human body was an act of desecration, a belief prevalent even today in some circles.[1] In medieval times, the Roman Catholic Church and its popes had to interact with anatomists seeking to dissect the bodies of the recently deceased, and responses differed. Pope Boniface VIII (1235–1303) declared that whoever cut up a body or boiled it would fall under the ban of the Church,[2] whereas another pope, Clement VI (1291–1352), had an alternative view and approved of the autopsy of bubonic plague victims.[3]

In theological thinking today, one comes across considerable discussion of the body in its various manifestations: the spiritual or resurrection body against the natural or mortal body; the relationship between body, soul, and spirit; and the ways in which humans and their bodies image God, their creator. Important as are all such discussions, they provide few clues as to how we view the bodily remains of those who have died.

For many years, considerable store was placed not only on burial of the body but burial in consecrated ground. This was seen as a fit resting place for the mortal remains of a once-living person, a reminder of what that person was in life, and very often a reminder of the pain and anguish they had to bear during life. An appropriate burial place testified to their religious standing during life with its recognition that their mortal remains were intact and were laid to rest in "sacred" ground, frequently alongside their loved ones and family members. Moreover, their bodies were in a "fit state" to be raised at the last day.

However, considerations like these provide meager tools with which to answer questions about what can or cannot be done to dead bodies, or what relationship there is between the wishes of the now deceased regarding what is done to their body at death and those of living relatives. Neither do they throw light on the possibility of donating organs harvested from cadavers.

### Emerging attitudes toward the human body[4]

In Europe 300–400 years ago, there was intense interest in the largely hidden interior of the human body, in an era preceding by many years the advent of X-rays, let alone CT scans or MRIs. It was into this dark and perplexing territory that dissection began to shed some light. The culture, however, was far removed from the sterile scientific world of the twentieth and twenty-first centuries, since bodies were not routinely available for dissection, and the ones that did become available had come directly from the gallows. Not only this, the anatomy theaters were places where professor-centered performances took place, as much theatrical as educational.[5]

The criminals whose bodies were undergoing dissection, the executioners responsible for making the bodies available, and the anatomists whose profession depended upon this supply of bodies were united in "the culture of dissection." All were involved in an orchestrated series of events that existed on the edges of respectable society – barely accepted, dubious, and perhaps even taboo. Not surprisingly, the act of dissecting the bodies of criminals was talked about in the language of treason, treachery, duplicity, and secrecy, while the poets and writers outlined their dreams of dissecting their loved ones.[6] Strange as this sounds to contemporary ears, it represents a cultural environment in which dissection represented longings, sometimes erotic ones, alien to our world with its scientific and mechanistic horizons.

Anatomists, however, were viewed positively, as they were central to a quasi-spiritual event, since the dissected shell of the body provided a medium with which to understand the creative intent of God.[7] The interior of the body was regarded as a sacred temple, not merely the remains of a once-living person. Alongside this, the dead body was depicted as having an active role in the process of dissection, a model of self-dissection. This was accomplished by depicting the dead body in an upright pose, with the abdomen cut open to show the major abdominal organs. Examples are provided by artists such as Spigelius, Berrettini, and Petrioli in the seventeenth and early eighteenth centuries. Interestingly, the bodies depicted in apparently living stances were often those of females.[8]

This gave the impression that the dissected body (standing and sometimes provocatively posed) was alive, hinting that knowledge of the dead body was in reality knowledge of the living. By this means, dissection came to be depicted as a natural activity, even though the dissected bodies were frequently portrayed by anatomists like Vesalius as existing on the edges of living society: they constituted a new community of the dead. The take-home message was that anatomists were not disrupting the body as much as the body was willingly allowing them to assist a natural decaying process. This proved to be a useful way of justifying anatomy and dissection.[9]

Anatomy (and dissection in particular), now as then, transcends normal ethical boundaries. These considerations are also important within a religious perspective, where the integrity of the body is generally cherished and upheld. Anatomical investigations of the human body can only be justified if they throw light onto the structure and functioning of the body in health and disease. In these terms, the process of dissection aids in an understanding of the body as made in the image of God, both in the education of health professionals and as a basis for cellular and genetic research.

### Using bodies without consent[10]

The use of unclaimed bodies (where there has been no consent) has been one of the distinguishing features of the anatomy profession since the passing of nineteenth-century legislation aimed at solving the problem of grave robbing. Only in more recent years has the use of bequeathed bodies supplanted dependence upon unclaimed bodies in many (but not all) countries. The 1832 Anatomy Act in the United Kingdom provided anatomists with legal access to the unclaimed corpses of those who died in either workhouses or prison, in effect making poverty the sole criterion for dissection in Britain.[11] From these early beginnings, the utilization of unclaimed bodies has dominated anatomy for the greater part of its history as a scientific discipline and continues to this day in some jurisdictions. The availability of unclaimed bodies for anatomists to use as they see fit has had profound consequences for the practice of anatomy (and also pathology).

A great deal has been written about the episodes leading up to, and surrounding, the passing of the 1832 Anatomy Act in the United Kingdom.[12] While this was not the first legislation involving unclaimed bodies, it was one of the most pivotal. Ruth Richardson has argued in cogent fashion that the original decision in the 1820s and 1830s in the UK to use unclaimed rather than bequeathed bodies reflected negative social attitudes toward the poor and disadvantaged. Poverty, in effect, became the sole criterion for dissection since it was principally the poor who found themselves unable to protect their relatives dying in hospitals. However, even this Act did not end illegal activities, with many contraventions of it. These included deceiving mourners about the whereabouts of the body of the deceased, or even diverting a funeral so that the body could be delivered to the local anatomy department. Unfortunately, such deceptions were common.[13]

Running throughout these and other historical episodes was the prevalent use of unclaimed bodies, with its exploitation of those on the margins of society. This is illustrated in a number of ways. One legacy was the widespread use of the bodies of the mentally incapacitated in the early years of the twentieth century.[14] These subjects were not simply poor but were seriously disadvantaged because of their long-term impoverished mental state and, in many cases, their lack of competence to consent to dissection. In being (probably) poor and mentally incapacitated, they were doubly disadvantaged due to circumstances over which they had no control.

A second legacy in nineteenth-century North America was use of the bodies of African Americans alongside those of the urban poor, impoverished Irish and German immigrants, American Indians, and criminals. No matter how diverse these groups were, none of them was in a position to protect their dead. Additionally, their deaths in the eyes of some deserved no protection.[15] Slave owners, for their part, on the death of slaves sold their bodies to medical schools.[16]

The use of unclaimed bodies reached its moral nadir in Germany and its occupied territories under the National Socialist regime from 1933 to 1945.[17] The bodies of those sentenced to death and subsequently executed were made available to anatomy departments in Germany and Austria, and those ready to utilize them found themselves accepting a far greater number of bodies than in previous years and from a much wider variety of sources.

Lack of informed consent and the use of unclaimed bodies go hand in hand. Once it is accepted that informed consent on the part of the individual is not required, clear strictures on using unclaimed bodies disappear. This does not inevitably lead to the unfettered use of cadavers. After all, anatomists of integrity working in societies that place considerable value on human life make considerable efforts to trace relatives of the deceased before treating their bodies as unclaimed. Nevertheless, the door has been opened to a wide range of practices, including ethically dubious ones, depending on the moral climate, cultural practices, (in)equality, and political tenor of the societies in which the anatomists are functioning.

Why might the use of unclaimed bodies be ethically inferior to the use of those that have been bequeathed? A response starts from the basic assertion that cadavers, like the living, have intrinsic value, since people and their bodies are inseparable. Hence, there is a link between our treatment of the living and the dead. Additionally, cadavers have instrumental value since they serve as a source of memories and responses, particularly for those close to them, who are now grieving their death. Besides this, cadavers can either serve as a source of organs or provide opportunities for teaching and clinical practice.

It follows that we show disrespect to the deceased when we allow that person's body to be dissected after death in the absence of any consent on the person's part prior to death and/or in the absence of any close friends and relatives to protect his/her interests at the time of death. Consent, therefore, is central when contemplating the donation of organs, body parts, and whole bodies, in both clinical medicine and anatomy. Donation implies that the people concerned made a free and informed decision, prior to their death, to allow their own bodies to be used for transplantation or dissection. By acting like this, they are giving something closely identified with what they are and represent.

Autonomy lays stress on the values of the individual at the center of the decision-making process. This individual also has sets of relationships, and this brings into focus a second set of moral values: that of the interests of family members, who can override the wishes of the deceased, even when the latter has specified that his or her body is to be donated for teaching, research, or therapeutic purposes. While conflicts arise at this point, the dominant thrust is that of altruism, according to which it is better to give than to receive, and the good of others is better than self-interest. Central to this value is the notion of gift, according to which an opt-in scheme for organ donation is preferable to an opt-out scheme. Consent and altruism go hand in hand and constitute the basis for Christian thinking in this area.

### Elements of a Christian response[18]

In seeking clues for this response, examples of a high view of the dead body are to be found in both the Old and New Testaments. For instance, Amos specifically separated out for condemnation the crimes of one group of people who, after marauding, pillaging, and killing, unleashed their venom on the dead body of one of their enemies. Having killed the king of Edom, they burnt his bones to ash (Amos 2:1–3). By desecrating his dead body, they sought to undermine his integrity as an individual. Further insight is provided by Joseph's request that, upon his death in Egypt, his relatives were to take his bones with them to the land of Canaan (Gen. 50:22–26; Exod. 13:19). His wish that his mortal remains were not to be left in the land of captivity may have been symbolic, yet it underlines the importance of the dead body. In the New Testament, Jesus's followers tended his body after his death, while Joseph of Arimathea ensured that Jesus's body was laid in his own new tomb (Matt. 27:57–61; Mark 15:42–16:2). While their actions were culturally appropriate, they also recognized that the dead body is to be treated with respect.

There is no suggestion in the Bible that human beings can exist apart from the body, even in the future life after death. For instance, Paul stressed that the resurrection is a physical one (1 Cor. 15:42–52; 1 Thess. 4:13–18). There is no hint that human beings can exist apart from some bodily manifestation or form of expression.[19] The mortal body will be replaced by a resurrection body, which, while not identical to the former, will have sufficient similarities to warrant the term "body."

Respect for the dead body now foreshadows respect for the resurrection body in the future. Consequently, any willingness to desecrate or devalue the dead body shows a disregard for what that person may become, alongside a disregard for what that person has been. Inherent to this perspective is the notion that the prior wishes of the deceased are to be respected since our bodies constitute the one common strand between what we are now and what we may become.[20]

Hence, a Christian response contains within it a future orientation not found in general ethical stances, and this complements the more commonly encountered past orientation. The body is a reminder of the ongoing dimensions of human existence, as well as of our mortality. To value the dead body is to value the person and to see that person as one who mirrors God. To devalue the dead body is to devalue those still alive and also to question the purposes and intentions of God in creating people in his image.

The Christian emphasis upon humans as those who image God is generally discussed in relation to those still alive. Important as this is, it should not obscure the complementary perspective that those who have died were also made in the image of God, a reflection that does not disappear immediately at death (see "A modern eruption – plastination" below). If this is the case, the task confronting Christians is to translate this perspective into practice. At first take, it will include the general approaches outlined previously, namely respect for the body of the deceased, respect for their wishes expressed during life, and making every effort to translate these wishes into what is done to their bodies after death. These in turn will point to the ethical and theological significance of the donation of organs and body parts since removing these in the absence of consent points to an abrogation of the responsibility of the living to act as God's stewards. Stewardship of this order is enshrined within the image concept.

## Retention of bodies and body parts after post-mortem

Frequently, important issues arise from scandals and controversies, such as those in the 1960s through to the mid-1990s involving the retention of organs and body parts. The events became public knowledge toward the end of the 1990s and were accompanied by public outcries and media frenzy. In all the cases described, the relevant authorities took the events very seriously, and commissions of inquiry were created. Reports such as that of the BBC on January 29, 2001, reflect all too clearly the anguish of the parents affected and the inept manner in which hospitals dealt with the revelations (the parents in one case ended up with three funerals for their baby).[21] While the scandals varied in detail, they all revolved around the retention of organs, such as the heart and brain, following post-mortem so that the bodies returned to the family had one or more organs missing. This was not divulged to the family. The organs were retained for research purposes, rather than for an explanation of the cause of death. Not only had consent not been sought, but the relatives were left in the dark. It was only when inquiries were set up that family members were informed that organs of their loved ones had been retained. They were then faced with a decision on whether these organs should be buried, on some occasions many years after the death. The various working parties produced erudite reports mainly in 2001 and 2002. These contained detailed analyses of what had gone wrong, the fundamental ethical values that should direct the practice of post-mortem examinations and the subsequent retention of body parts and organs, plus explicit guidelines for the future.[22]

However, it must be acknowledged that these scandals played out against a background in which organs and body parts had been routinely removed at post-mortem for many years, with brains and hearts being kept for some weeks for further pathological analyses. Consent had not generally been sought from next of kin. This was seen as routine practice in an era when far less emphasis was placed on fully informed consent than has been the case over more recent years. This does not justify the practice since it was an illustration of unjustified paternalism. Perhaps even more problematic was the ethical environment it engendered whereby individual clinicians and pathologists felt able to retain organs and body parts well beyond the time necessary for carrying out essential pathological tests to ascertain the cause of death. Retention appears to have been regarded as a "right," whether the reason was for teaching or research, or, in extreme cases, for no good reason at all. In the UK, there was no statutory requirement for the consent of relatives to be sought prior to the 1961 Human Tissue Act.[23] This Act, like those drawn up in the 1960s in comparable societies, stressed "lack of objection" rather than "informed consent." However, they did not ignore informed consent.

The issues can be illustrated by reference to the most high-profile scandal, which occurred at the Royal Liverpool Children's Hospital (Alder Hey). In 1999, it was revealed that many organs had been retained from children's bodies after post-mortem. This elicited a considerable public outcry from parents, a protest that increased as the subsequent inquiry released its findings in 2001 and the extent of the scandal was revealed.[24] In fact, between the years 1988 and 1995, there had been systematic retention of almost every organ from every pediatric post-mortem case for the overriding purpose of research. Parents were not informed and had even been deliberately misled into thinking they were burying the bodies of their deceased children intact. The vast majority of the stockpiled organs were never used for medical education or research.

In the aftermath, a 2001 report from the Department of Health recommended changes to protect bereaved families, to show respect for the deceased, to provide clear explanations to patients and their families on the reasons for the removal and retention of organs and other tissues, and to ensure the families are actively involved in decision-making and in giving agreement for tissue removal and retention.[25] The Retained Organs Commission in 2002 highlighted the centrality of the following ethical values: adequate consent, respect for the post-mortem dignity of the human body, and respect for the preferences of the deceased and their closest relatives. In addition, the Commission contended that retention could be justified since it advanced public health, enabled effective diagnosis, and illuminated the probable causes of death. Later, in 2011, the Nuffield Council on Bioethics drew up an ethical framework based on the stewardship role of the state, the primacy of donation and the wishes of the donor, and the central role of altruism and the welfare of the donor. Attention was drawn to values such as trust and respect so that professionals would respect confidentiality and donated materials would be used for the purposes for which they were donated.[26]

These scandals served as a watershed for several countries, including Australia, New Zealand, and Scotland, as it became evident that unethical practice had been the order of the day. Although there was no evidence that medical professionals had acted in deliberately malevolent ways, their lack of awareness of essential ethical values had had a profoundly negative impact on their professionalism, with appalling repercussions for the parents and relatives of those whose body parts had been retained without their consent or even knowledge. The professionals involved had acted in a high-handed manner, paying little attention to the needs or feelings of those so badly wounded by their irresponsible behavior.

## Ethical considerations in light of the scandals[27]

In light of the above considerations, two models are relevant. The first is that of bequests. Whenever there is no consent for the use of body parts following a post-mortem, the potential exists for a double tragedy – the tragedy of the death itself plus the tragedy of the (unknown) retention of body parts. In the types of situation alluded to above, the impact of the two tragedies may have been separated by many years. While this played out most tragically in the death of children, it would also apply following the death of adults. The grief of the initial loss is compounded by the reawakened grief when it is revealed that organs have been retained unbeknownst to the relatives. In contrast, when consent is obtained, the death may to some extent be redeemed for the relatives by giving them the opportunity to bequeath body parts of the deceased to be used for good ends. This is akin to organ transplantation following a tragic death, on the condition that the body parts are freely willed by next of kin. The driving force in these instances is altruism, which is far preferable ethically to the double-tragedy alternative.

The second model is that of ethical awareness. It is not sufficient for health professionals to resort to perceived legal ambiguity or lack of clarity as justification for using human material without adequate informed consent. It would be sad if the medical profession gave the impression that it is incapable of acting ethically without legislative oversight.

It has been evident for many years that a society's allowance of uses for human material is relative to that society's moral values. Every use of such material requires justification, and the bounds are set by society since there is no automatic right to use human material for either research or teaching. Future uses of body parts depend on social acceptance and on convincing the public that the uses to which material will be put justify the public's support. Possible research benefits do not by themselves justify the use of human tissue; these must be viewed in the light of the values and constraints imposed by society.

## Christian considerations

The responses outlined above place considerable stress on the need to treat people with dignity and respect. Once this is appreciated, the role of informed consent follows automatically, as does a shift in emphasis from "taking" and "retaining" to "donation." These emphases fit in with Christian duties to treat others with care and due consideration for their standing as those created in the image of God (Gen. 1:26–27, 9:6; 1 Cor. 11:7; 2 Cor. 4:4; Col. 1:15; James 3:9). From here it is a short distance to focus on those on the outskirts of society – the poor, the mentally and culturally disadvantaged, the lonely, the weak, and those with no one to defend them or befriend them. In general, these are the vulnerable, those unable to defend themselves and their own interests, those who are in greatest need of protection.

God's care extends to all since all are his creations and all have been given the gift of life. We look to this principle often when confronted by the demands of modern technology,[28] yet it emerges here in a far more immediate form. Why do we treat the disadvantaged in ways in which we would not want others to treat us? Why do we expect to be able to provide consent for what others will do to us, albeit our bodies after death, but do not apply the same high set of expectations to those who have few financial resources and low status within society? Jesus's response to children rebukes our hard hearts (Matt. 19:14; Luke 18:16; Mark 10:13–16).

Allen Verhey reminds his readers that as they remember Jesus and his attitudes, they will respect people's freedom and identity, bear in mind the importance of community, and seek to uphold and look after the sick.[29] While the context within which he was writing was that of assessing the growing powers of medical technology, the values he was espousing are just as applicable to that of more general medical care. We are not even dealing with healing; we are addressing how to deal with those who can no longer be healed. This is a greater challenge because, as has become evident, it is easy to downplay the significance of body parts after death. Even a hint of this betrays an acknowledgment that those whose bodies are being used without adequate informed consent are regarded as of less value and have a lesser status than most other people. While many of these in many societies are derelicts, others are political and/or religious prisoners. Some may have been martyrs for their faith, those who have been faithful unto death. This brings into focus the horror of using their bodies, organs, or other body parts against their wishes and probably without their relatives knowing anything of their demise.

Neil Messer, in his book *Respecting Life: Theology and Bioethics*, asks several of what he terms "diagnostic questions." While he was looking at the power of modern technology in the health area, some of these questions are relevant more generally. These revolve around whether the technology is good news for the poor, whether it takes account of the welfare of the oppressed or marginalized, and the extent to which it will enhance or detract from our attitudes toward both our own bodies and those of our neighbors.[30] While the use of bodies and body parts after death elicits none of the bravado of biomedical technological approaches aimed at changing the human experience of life and health, our approach to body usage after death underlines our posture toward transforming bodies and people during life. It also reflects attitudes toward the poor, the powerless, and the marginalized. There is an intimate connection between what we do in life and how we treat the dead, one that should alert all those with religious perspectives to look beyond bodies as mere human material to be dissected and experimented upon at will.

## A modern eruption – plastination[31]

The dead human body, with its reminder of what everyone will one day become and the memories it enshrines of loved ones who are no longer with us, is inevitably an object of fascination. The dead human body invites attention, whether viewed as an object of veneration or pity, whether forbidding or macabre, whether an educational tool or a reminder of death.

How do people respond when presented with large exhibitions of dissected dead bodies as though they are still alive and communing with the living? This is where plastination and whole-body "plastinates" enter the picture. The major impetus behind these exhibitions is *Body Worlds*, the forerunner of a host of such exhibitions directed at the general public.[32] Cadavers are on general display in large exhibition spaces, surrounded by enormous publicity aimed at making the dead attractive.

In the process of plastination, human tissues are impregnated with plastics and silicone rubber. The resulting specimens are permanent, dry, and odorless. Tissues can also be molded, enabling body parts to be fixed in various positions. Therefore, some of these dead humans give the impression of walking, running, sitting, and playing all manner of sports. They appear life-like, but they also give the impression of being plastic models of the human body. They are not models; they are real (dead) people, who were once living, breathing, and thinking. It is this tension between life-likeness and a model that attracts some but appalls others.[33] Rarely have dead human bodies been seen like this before, although Egyptian mummies provide some pointers (although not even these are sitting upright). Thus, the questions arise: Are these uses transgressing important boundaries, and do they by their very nature demean our humanity? Is human dignity at stake?

### The ambiguity of plastinates[34]

Whole-body plastinates have an ambiguous ontological status in that they transgress the familiar categories with which we usually make sense of the world. Therefore, they raise a range of disconcerting questions: What is real and what is fake? Are they dead or alive? Are these bodies or persons? Are they like us or unlike us? Are they mortal or immortal?

The attraction for most exhibition-goers lies in what they perceive to be the reality of these exhibitions. These exhibitions also enable the public to approach the forbidden since this is territory they are normally unable to access. They experience a thrill, that of taboo-breaking and voyeurism. However, the plastination process itself has drastically reduced the amount of original human tissue in the plastinated body to a fraction of the whole. It makes fundamental changes to the composition of the bodies to ensure the presentability, structural integrity, and longevity of the plastinates.

Since these human remains are largely plastic, is their apparent reality deceptive? Plastics have replaced the 70% of tissue that was originally composed of water and lipids, yet much of the microscopic and macroscopic structure remains unchanged. Alongside the artificiality are substantial elements of the person's individuality.

In addition, physical modification, dissection, and artificial positioning of body parts create an artifact with traces of its original form, but a form that has been interpreted. The plastinates are often dissected and presented in highly theatrical ways: with their musculature splayed out behind them or in exaggerated poses, but never with intact skin. The plastinators have artificially modified the bodies to produce an exhibit that is made to appear life-like, through dying the tissues the color of living flesh and constructing animated poses. Yet these interventions distance the bodies from their natural state.

For some commentators, the bodies are chemically, surgically, and artistically modified to such a degree that the intrusion of the artificial makes them "hyper-real."[35] For others, it is not real bodies that are presented but representations of real bodies. The donated body has been manipulated and transformed in such a way that the end result is an artificial representation of perfected nature.[36]

Unnervingly, the bodies are both real and fake and are profoundly different from anything we normally encounter. They constitute a species of form that lies beyond our usual world. They are different from us, even though they are presented as being similar to us. While plastinates are dead (obviously), they give hints of being alive; they are part natural and part artificial. By modifying bodies in this way, the aim appears to be modification of natural bodies into artificial representations of the natural. The plastinated body is quite unlike the natural decomposing body.[37] The result is that visitors to these exhibitions experience plastinates as both real and unreal, dead and alive, welcoming and forbidding. Are they viewing a corpse, a statue, or something in between? Even though the public may go to *Body Worlds* looking for authentic bodies, they have not entered a world familiar to anatomists and health professionals but a make-believe world where the anatomical is best seen in the fine detail of the dissections.

### Do plastinates challenge our worldview?

Is there a worldview creeping through these exhibitions that is antagonistic to Christian thinking? The distinct impression is that there is since the process of plastination appears to be an attempt to transcend the limits of human mortality by suggesting that mortal bodies can become immortal through technology. Gunther von Hagens, the originator of the plastination technique and the founder of *Body Worlds*, considers that he has created a new category of body, neither fresh corpse nor decaying remains.[38] These plastinates are "frozen in time between death and decay," according to von Hagens,[39] and will never decompose. In a sense, they have achieved a form of immortality, namely, physical permanence. They are "post-mortal."[40]

However, more than this is being claimed. They are presented as though animated, as though capable of functioning, performing the sort of acts typical of those who are alive – from sitting and running to playing sports and chess, and even experiencing sexual intimacy. They give the impression of enjoying this new form of existence, just as much as the living enjoy their existence. But this is where problems become evident. The living do not enjoy every aspect of their existence; they have to cope with challenges and problems, with tensions and consternation, and they have to work and strive to be what they want to be. Plastinates, characterized – as they generally are – by serene expressions on their faces, seem to exist in a blissful world uncluttered by the niceties of mundane existence. And of course, this is the case; they are dead.

This secular, material form of immortality, with its impression of imparting biological life to these cadavers, is illusory and artificial. While the plastinates are posed to suggest movement or activity, they are in fact eternally static, merely mimicking vitality. This "post-biological existence" is no more than a synthetic afterlife; they may appear immortal, but they lack almost all identification with the person who once lived.[41] The trace that remains of those who were once alive is not of values, attitudes, or ideas. It is a static bodily remnant that itself is likely to bear little resemblance to the external bodily features by which the individual was known and by which he or she would usually be remembered.

Plastinates are metaphysical misfits, demonstrating a range of dichotomies, ambiguities, and contradictions. They are reminders of the medieval sketches of dissected cadavers living on the edge of society.[42] These exhibitions are doing the same but within a completely different cultural setting. There is no need any longer to justify anatomy and the dissection of cadavers. The motive now must be different, in that the earlier rationale has disappeared. What the motive today might be is open to speculation; to a degree the exhibitions are financially driven, but that is probably not a complete explanation. There appears to be a drive to secularize death and show that it no longer holds any fears. We can, it is asserted, live on as plastinates; death can even be attractive and welcoming. Heaven has been transformed into a plastinated, technological existence in the here and now, an existence open to all those willing to undergo plastination and dissection.

These bodies are exhibited in cultures that seek to ignore the reality of death and/or are committed to projects aimed at overcoming aging and mortality. The hint that we can live on as plastinates parallels the claims of transhumanists that it will shortly be possible to triumph over death. While the two projects have little in common technologically, they can both be contemplated within an environment in which the fear of death can only be overcome by eliminating it.[43] Having dispensed with any religiously based perspectives of death and of its place within a far broader worldview, all that remains is to construct a technologically based means of dealing with death, based upon science and human capabilities. Whatever we make of these efforts and the ideas behind them, if this is everlasting existence, it represents a very narrow form of eternal life; it is immortality within a mortal framework.

If everlasting (or long-term) existence has been achieved, this has been at the cost of a human core. When dead human tissue has been replaced with plastics, all that remains are plasticized remnants of what was once human, fascinating and yet perplexing, uplifting and yet troublesome. This is a new form of plastic existence, a troubling version of once-human existence. Unnervingly, at some point decisions will have to be made how to dispose of this imperishable material that is human and yet is only partially human. One observer comments that the absence of a personality, friends, family, and history leaves a gaping vacuum that is summed up by referring to these as "bodies with no soul."[44] This is indeed a disquieting version of what a future technological world might look like.

## Donation redefined[45]

What is the relation between the plastination of cadavers in anatomy departments for educational/research purposes and plastination for public display? The answer to this lies in the contrast between donating one's body to assist others through education and research and donating it principally to fulfill one's own desires. Whenever the latter is the case, the link between donation and altruism has been broken. There is no hint of donating one's body or organs to advance the medical profession or in gratitude for the contributions of the medical profession.

In the context of these public exhibitions, people are donating their bodies to achieve their own post-mortal desires or to contribute to the education and entertainment of those viewing the exhibition. But what if some donors were willing for their bodies to be plastinated but never displayed, being satisfied with the kind of physical immortality achieved? This would amount to a form of preservation, equivalent to plastinated mummies. This is not donation; it is plastinated afterlife.

Informed consent, while necessary, is not a sufficient ethical criterion to justify the use of dead bodies.[46] Each instance is to be assessed by society on merit, and this determination will involve social and other criteria regarding culturally acceptable ways of treating the dead, the burial of intact corpses, and the decision-making role of family members; these are often not explicitly ethical ones. These, in general, tend to regard organ donation with its positive repercussions for the quality of life of the recipients as of greatest importance, dissection with its educational and research values as of somewhat lesser importance, and entertainment as of very limited value.

The transformation of dead people into plasticized representations of living people can be viewed either as a stunning technological achievement or as a disturbing example of scientific and cultural reductionism. It probably elicits elements of both. Whole-body plastinates appear as they do because they have been "designed" by those who undertake the plastination process. This amounts to little more than a transformation from dead body to plastinated exhibit. In a real sense, the plastinator technicians are the creators of the final product.

## Theological overtones

Christian leaders have frequently opposed these displays based on their alleged failure to respect human dignity.[47] While one can appreciate this response, it fails to delve into what ways the dignity of the plastinated is being undermined, whose dignity is being infringed (the plastinated, the paying public, or humanity in general), and whether this would be the case if the plastinated bodies and body parts were not on public display. Neither is it clear what is the theological basis for these concerns.

Plastination, especially the production of plastinates, compels us to think more deeply about what can and cannot be done with and to dead human remains. The techniques at our disposal have the potential for displaying these remains in novel ways, giving them a hint of physical immortality, and forcing a reconsideration of the ethical underpinnings of body donation. Most of these considerations are of interest to those with no theological concerns.

Are there deeper theological questions raised by plastination? As we have seen, ideas on immortality have, surprisingly perhaps, been raised by some of the advocates of these major exhibitions, especially by von Hagens. These, in turn, confront theologians and others with questions about the resurrected body and life after death. In what ways might perceptions regarding the resurrected body throw light on how we treat the mortal body at death? Should these developments in plastination make us revisit the burial/cremation duopoly (as outlined in a recent article of mine)?[48] Might there ever be a place for plastinating a loved one or parts of a loved one at death, or are their ashes sufficient reminders of what they represented during life? While questions of this nature may have about them an aura of the grotesque and macabre, they stem from technologies that are currently applied in the biomedical sciences.

If the notion of the image of God carries with it functional and relational connotations and not simply physical ones, it is impossible to escape the query of the extent to which the dead are images of God. As explained earlier, they once were, and memories of what they were are carried over into the cadaver. In this sense, they continue to image God. What happens as the body decays? Does a point come when the remains of the once-vibrant human being no longer mirror what they once were? The answer for many appears to be in the affirmative since most Christians today in the Western world accept the legitimacy of cremation.

Where, then, does plastination (or, for that matter, any form of long-term fixation) fit in? The whole-body plastinates that feature so prominently in the public exhibitions are dissected and are only partially human material, yet they retain the marks of individuality that characterized the individual when alive. Are these still images of God, or should we classify them as once-but-no-longer images of God? Their family and loved ones would not recognize them; as time passes (remembering that plastinated material can be retained for many years), any link with those they loved and with whom they interacted will disappear.

This suggests that plastinates have few, if any, of the marks of humans as God's images. The theological challenge is not to ask how they are treated but whether it was appropriate to create them in the first place, and if so to what ends. Within a Christian context, this is to ask how best we act as stewards within God's world. As I have previously written, plastinates are "'immortal' specimens [that] have become what they are through the creativity of human beings," those responsible for their plastination. In achieving this end result, "they have been torn asunder from their human roots." They are no longer human beings with the gift of longevity but in part are human creations. Nevertheless, they remind visitors to public exhibitions of their own mortality and of the wonders of the human body, thereby offsetting to some degree the disquieting features of the exhibitions.[49]

## Notes

1 D. Gareth Jones, "The Human Cadaver: An Assessment of the Value We Place on the Dead Body," *Perspectives on Science and Christian Faith* 47 no. 1 (1995): 43–51, www.asa3.org/ASA/PSCF/1995/PSCF3-95Jones.html.ori.
2 Katharine Park, "The Life of the Corpse: Division and Dissection in Late Medieval Europe," *Journal of the History of Medicine and Allied Sciences* 50 no. 1 (1995): 111–132.
3 Charles B. Rodning, "'O Death, Where Is Thy Sting?' Historical Perspectives on the Relationship of Human Postmortem Anatomical Dissection to Medical Education and Care," *Clinical Anatomy* 2 no. 4 (1989): 277–292.
4 Much of this subsection is adapted with permission from D. Gareth Jones, "Anatomical Investigations and Their Ethical Dilemmas," *Clinical Anatomy* 25 no. 2 (2007): 338–343. Copyright © 2006 Wiley Publishing, Inc.
5 D. Gareth Jones and Maja I. Whitaker, *Speaking for the Dead: The Human Body in Biology and Medicine*, 2nd ed. (Farnham, UK: Ashgate, 2009), chs. 1–2.
6 Jonathan Sawday, *The Body Emblazoned: Dissection and the Human Body in Renaissance Culture* (London, UK: Routledge, 1995), 32–38, 43–53.
7 D. Gareth Jones, *Speaking for the Dead: Cadavers in Biology and Medicine* (Aldershot, UK: Ashgate, 2000), 2–7.
8 Sawday, *The Body Emblazoned*, plates 28, 30–32.
9 Ibid., 110–122.
10 Much of this subsection is adapted with permission from D. Gareth Jones, "Use of Bequeathed and Unclaimed Bodies in the Dissecting Room," *Clinical Anatomy* 7 no. 2 (1994): 246–254, and D. Gareth Jones and Maja I. Whitaker, "Anatomy's Use of Unclaimed Bodies: Reasons Against Continued Dependence on an Ethically Dubious Practice," *Clinical Anatomy* 25 no. 2 (2012): 246–254. Copyright © 1994, 2011 Wiley Publishing, Inc.
11 Ruth Richardson, *Death, Dissection and the Destitute*, 2nd ed. (London, UK: Phoenix Press, 2001), ch. 9.
12 Jones and Whitaker, *Speaking for the Dead*, 25–28; Richardson, *Death, Dissection and the Destitute*.
13 Helen MacDonald, *Human Remains: Episodes in Human Dissection* (Carlton, VIC: Melbourne University Press, 2005); Helen MacDonald, *Possessing the Dead: The Artful Science of Anatomy* (Carlton, VIC: Melbourne University Press, 2010).
14 D. Gareth Jones, "The Anatomy Museum and Mental Illness: The Centrality of Informed Consent," in *Exhibiting Madness in Museums: Remembering Psychiatry Through Collection and Display*, eds. Catharine Coleborne and Dolly MacKinnon (New York, NY: Routledge, 2011), 161–177.
15 Michael Sappol, *A Traffic of Dead Bodies: Anatomy and Embodied Social Identity in Nineteenth-Century America* (Princeton, NJ: Princeton University Press, 2002).
16 Todd L. Savitt, *Medicine and Slavery: The Diseases and Health Care of Blacks in Antebellum Virginia* (Urbana: University of Illinois Press, 1978).

17 Sabine Hildebrandt, "Anatomy in the Third Reich: An Outline, Part 1: National Socialist Politics, Anatomical Institutions, and Anatomists," *Clinical Anatomy* 22 no. 8 (2009): 883–893; Sabine Hildebrandt, "Anatomy in the Third Reich: An Outline, Part 2: Bodies for Anatomy and Related Medical Disciplines," *Clinical Anatomy* 22 no. 8 (2009): 894–905; Emily Bazelon, "The Nazi Anatomists," *Slate*, November 6, 2013, www.slate.com/articles/life/history/2013/11/nazi_anatomy_history_the_origins_of_conservatives_anti_abortion_claims_that. html; Sabine Hildebrandt, *The Anatomy of Murder: Ethical Transgressions and Anatomical Science During the Third Reich* (New York, NY: Berghahn, 2016).

18 Jones, "The Human Cadaver." Much of this subsection and some of the next are adapted from this article by permission from *Perspectives on Science and Christian Faith*.

19 B. O. Banwell, "Body," in *The Illustrated Bible Dictionary*, eds. J. D. Douglas and N. Hillyer (Leicester, UK: InterVarsity Press, 1980), 202–203.

20 See also D. Gareth Jones, "The Human Body: An Anatomist's Journey from Death to Life," in *A Tangled Web: Medicine and Theology in Dialogue*, eds. R. John Elford and D. Gareth Jones (Bern, Switzerland: Peter Lang, 2009), 105–121.

21 BBC News, "Organ Scandal Background," January 29, 2001, http://news.bbc. co.uk/2/hi/1136723.stm.

22 Bristol Royal Infirmary Inquiry, *Learning from Bristol: The Report of the Public Inquiry into Children's Heart Surgery at the Bristol Royal Infirmary 1984–1995* (Bristol, UK: Crown Copyright, 2001); UK Department of Health, *The Removal, Retention and Use of Human Organs and Tissue from Post-mortem Examination: Advice from the Chief Medical Officer* (London, UK: Her Majesty's Stationary Office, 2001); Retained Organs Commission, *A Consultation Document on Unclaimed and Unidentifiable Organs and Tissue: A Possible Regulatory Framework* (London, UK: National Health Service, 2002); The Royal Liverpool Children's Inquiry, *The Royal Liverpool Children's Inquiry Report* (London, UK: House of Commons, 2001).

23 Retained Organs Commission, *A Consultation Document*.

24 The Royal Liverpool Children's Inquiry, *The Royal Liverpool Children's Inquiry Report*.

25 UK Department of Health, *The Removal, Retention and Use of Human Organs and Tissue from Post-mortem Examination*.

26 Nuffield Council on Bioethics, *Human Bodies: Donation for Medicine and Research* (London, UK: Nuffield Council on Bioethics, 2011).

27 Much of this subsection and some of the next are adapted from D. Gareth Jones and Kerry A. Galvin, "Retention of Body Parts: Reflections from Anatomy," *New Zealand Medical Journal* 115 no. 1155 (2002): 267–269, by permission of the *New Zealand Medical Journal*.

28 D. Gareth Jones, *The Peril and Promise of Medical Technology* (Oxford, UK: Peter Lang, 2013), 231–233.

29 Allen Verhey, "What Makes Christian Bioethics Christian? Bible, Story, and Communal Discernment," *Christian Bioethics* 11 no. 3 (2005): 297–315.

30 Neil Messer, *Respecting Life: Theology and Bioethics* (London, UK: SCM Press, 2011), 105–147.

31 Some of this section is adapted with permission from David Gareth Jones, "The Public Display of Plastinates as a Challenge to the Integrity of Anatomy," *Clinical Anatomy* 29 no. 1 (2016): 46–54. Copyright © 2015 Wiley Publishing, Inc.

32 Gunther von Hagens and Angelina Whalley, *Prof. Gunther von Hagens' Anatomy Art: Fascination Beneath the Surface* (Heidelberg, Germany: Institute for Plastination, 2000).

33  D. Gareth Jones and Maja I. Whitaker, "Engaging with Plastination and the Body Worlds Phenomenon: A Cultural and Intellectual Challenge for Anatomists," *Clinical Anatomy* 22 no. 6 (2009): 770–776.

34  Mike R. King, Maja I. Whitaker, and D. Gareth Jones, "I See Dead People: Insights from the Humanities into the Nature of Plastinated Cadavers," *Journal of Medical Humanities* 35 no. 4 (2014): 361–376. Much of this subsection and some of the next are adapted from this article by permission from Springer Nature Customer Service Centre GmbH.

35  Megan Stern, "Dystopian Anxieties versus Utopian Ideals: Medicine from Frankenstein to The Visible Human Project and Body Worlds," *Science as Culture* 15 no. 1 (2006): 61–84; Jane Desmond, "Postmortem Exhibitions: Taxidermied Animals and Plastinated Corpses in the Theaters of the Dead," *Configurations* 16 no. 3 (2008): 347–378.

36  Iain Bamforth, "Bodyworlds," *London Review of Books* 22 no. 20 (2000): 34–35; Gianna Bouchard, "Bodyworlds and Theatricality: 'Seeing Death, Live,' " *Performance Research: A Journal of the Performing Arts* 15 no. 1 (2010): 58–65.

37  Von Hagens and Whalley, *Prof. Gunther von Hagens' Anatomy Art.*

38  Gunther von Hagens, "Gruselleichen, Gestaltplastinate und Bestattungszwang (On Gruesome Corpses, Gestalt Plastinates and Mandatory Interment)," in *Schöne Neue Körperwelten: Der Streit um die Ausstellung* (Brave New Body Worlds – The Question of the Exhibition), eds. Franz Josef Wetz and Brigette Tag (Stuttgart, Germany: Klett-Cotta, 2001), 260–282.

39  Linda Schulte-Sasse, "Advise and Consent: On the Americanization of Body Worlds," *BioSocieties* 1 no. 4 (2006): 369–384.

40  PR Newswire, "Anatomist Dr. Gunther von Hagens Reiterates His Mission of Public Health Education to Press Corps in Guben, Germany," November 30, 2006, www.prnewswire.co.uk/cgi/news/release?id=185453 (dead link).

41  Natalia Lizama, "Afterlife, But Not As We Know It: Melancholy, Post-Biological Ontology, and Plastinated Bodies," in *The Anatomy of Body Worlds: Critical Essays on the Plastinated Cadavers of Gunther von Hagens*, eds. T. Christine Jespersen, Alicita Rodríguez, and Joseph Starr (Jefferson, NC: McFarland & Co., 2009), 16–28.

42  Sawday, *The Body Emblazoned*, 113–115, and plates 12, 13, 24, 28, 30.

43  Jones, "The Human Body."

44  E. Henry Nicholls, "Selling Anatomy: The Role of the Soul," *Endeavour* 26 no. 2 (2002): 47.

45  Much of this subsection is adapted with permission from Jones and Whitaker, "Anatomy's Use of Unclaimed Bodies." Copyright © 2011 Wiley Publishing, Inc.

46  D. Gareth Jones, "Using and Respecting the Dead Human Body: An Anatomist's Perspective," *Clinical Anatomy* 27 no. 6 (2014): 839–843.

47  See the references in D. Gareth Jones, "The Artificial World of Plastination: A Challenge to Religious Perspectives on the Dead Human Body," *The New Bioethics: A Multidisciplinary Journal of Biotechnology and the Body* 22 no. 3 (2016): 237–252.

48  Ibid.

49  Ibid., 250.

# 12 Defining death in the context of Jewish, Christian, and Muslim perspectives

*Noam Stadlan*

Michael Broyde writes that the legal definition of death refers to when the person no longer has the rights and responsibilities assigned to a living human being.[1] The legal definition of death in a moral and just society can be expected to reflect some combination of scientific understanding and societal/philosophical concepts, as opposed to an arbitrary determination. For believers, religious texts and traditions provide an authoritative definition of death. Absent such an authoritative entity, the definition of death has no fixed reference point. Science can describe biological events, tests can determine the presence or absence of certain functions, but scientific inquiry cannot identify the characteristic that compels us to assign rights and responsibilities to a collection of tissue that we identify as a human being. The role of science, therefore, is to suggest options and, once the particular characteristic has been chosen, clarify the criteria and tests used to identify its presence or absence. One can also use logic to determine whether the various parts of a definition cohere with each other.

## Sources of authority

One possible consideration as a source of authority is history. For many years, the accepted definition of death has been the irreversible cessation of circulation and respiration. This, in fact, is still codified by the Uniform Determination of Death Act (UDDA) of 1981.[2] In the pre-modern era, the cessation of circulation and respiration implied that all functions of the body had ceased, and it was not necessary to establish which body function or part was essential for human life. With the advent of bypass pumps, dialysis, and organ donation, there is the potential for different parts of the body to cease function at different times. Therefore, the circulation/respiration definition is meaningless without an additional designation of which tissue has suffered the cessation of circulation and respiration. Additionally, a mechanical pump can be attached to a body, and circulation can be re-established, even hours or days after "death" has been declared.[3] If the standard of death is "the irreversible cessation of circulation and respiration" and this is literally applied,[4] death does not occur until the arteries and veins have degenerated in the body – days or weeks after the currently accepted determination. Therefore, it is not accurate to claim that the use of "irreversible cessation of circulation and respiration" as the definition of death in the modern era is just a continuation of the historical definition of death. Even though the UDDA uses this language, in practice this is not followed. Death is declared even when circulation could be restored with machines.

Two major schools of thought regarding the definition of death are currently represented in the literature: death is identified with cessation of neurological function or cessation of integrated function. Neither one can claim that it is the direct descendant of a longstanding and commonly recognized legal definition of death, and each must base its claim on internal logical validity, explanations of personal identity, and coherence with accepted situations.

## Internal validity

Stuart Youngner (following Bernat[5]) suggests that "a formulation of death must have three components" that are commonly referred to as tiers: Tier I: "*a concept* . . . of what it means to die"; Tier II: "operational *criteria* for determining that death has occurred"; and Tier III: "specific medical *tests* showing whether or not the criteria have been fulfilled." In addition, he notes that a problem with proposed definitions of death has been the lack of a "conceptual framework for answering the question, 'What quality is so essentially significant to a living entity that its loss constitutes the death of that entity?' "[6]

The definitions of "brain death" have frequently stated a complete three-part definition,[7] but those who define life as the presence of "integrated function" have not as a rule stated one. In this way, the debate has been a lopsided one. Only when all three tiers are filled can the approach be tested for internal validity. In other words, do the three tiers interact precisely and logically with each other? A definition with perfect internal validity would establish a Tier I concept, and the criteria would cohere perfectly with the concept. Furthermore, those determined to be dead via fulfillment of Tier III tests would also fulfill the philosophical standard established in Tier I.

Much of the critique of brain death has centered on the alleged lack of coherence between the philosophical concept and other tiers. If life is identified with the presence of brain function, it seems logical to conclude that any brain function should suffice for life to be considered present. Given this understanding of the term "brain function," even isolated EEG activity, or function of the hypothalamus, should be evidence for life. However, most guidelines for testing for brain death, including that of the American Academy of Neurology (AAN), do not mandate EEG testing; in fact, the AAN guidelines specifically state that the presence of EEG activity or hypothalamic activity are not inconsistent with a determination of death.[8] While some authors have advanced justifications and rationales for this seeming inconsistency,[9] many advocates for brain death have not adequately addressed the issue.

The advocates of "integrated function" have so far avoided similar critiques by providing – at best – vague Tier II criteria and none specific to integrated function. The closest statement of Tier II criteria for integrated function has probably been that of Alan Shewmon: "A probably valid criterion close to the moment of death might be something like: 'cessation of circulation of blood for a sufficient time (depending on body temperature) to produce irreversible damage to a critical number of organs and tissues throughout the body, so that an irrevocable process of disintegration has begun' ... I do not believe that the critical number of organs and tissues can be universally specified, as it will no doubt vary from case to case; surely the brain is included, but not *only* the brain."[10] The criteria to determine the cessation of life based on integrated function are not adequate for practical purposes and certainly not enough for an evaluation of internal validity.

Another critique of brain death has been that the rationales so far offered to justify the selection of neurological function as the defining concept of life and death have not always been logically coherent.[11] One possible justification is to define a person by the presence of his or her mental and/or brain function. Therefore, complete loss of that function would represent the death of that person. At any rate, a similar justification is lacking for the "integrated function" concept. A fully justified definition of death in terms of cessation of integrated function would require a statement of what exactly it is about integrated function that makes it define life, criteria to know that this specific amount/type of integrated function has been irreversibly lost, and a list of practical tests that can be done to make bedside determinations of the life-and-death status of the patient. I suggest that no matter how the integrated function is described, the understanding will be open to question as to why that level of integrated function was selected and not a bit more or a bit less, and the responses will not adequately answer the question. The advocates of integrated function have so far avoided these problems by avoiding precision.

## Personal identity

Precision is important not just theoretically but practically. Frequently a recipient receives several organs from one donor. If a heart, lung, and liver are providing integrated function in the donor, and they are all moved to a different set of tissue (usually termed the recipient – but under integrated function it may not be so clear) and still provide integrated function, why is the original life not still extant? The same integrated function is still present.

The above thought experiment leads to the issue of personal identity. Criteria are necessary to establish whether a collection of human tissue is one person or a different person. If we start with a person known as Jacob, the criteria for identity establish whether the collection of human tissue known as Jacob is still present or whether the identity of the collection of tissue has changed to that of a different person. It is frequently assumed that the identity covariates with the neurological function: the collection of human tissue that includes Jacob's brain is Jacob. For those who equate life with the presence of neurological function, the presence of factors necessary for personal identity are the same as those necessary for the presence of the human life. However, if life is identified with "integrated function" (which does not necessarily include neurological function), and the personal identity is identified with neurological function, then two new categories of functioning human tissue potentially have been created that require definition. There can be tissue that fulfills the requirements to be a particular person but does not qualify as a human life. There will also be tissue that will be identified as a live human being but will not have an identity. One or both of these situations is the inevitable result of separating the criteria for human life from the criteria for human identity. This is an issue that must be addressed by all those who do not define death using neurological criteria.

One alternative would be to redefine the basis for personal identity. Even if personal identity is defined as persistence over time, exactly what is persisting must be elucidated. Furthermore, identity would have to be defined as persistence of integrated function over time to avoid inconsistency with the definition of death. Ultimately, those who advocate integrated function have two options, neither of which appears to be palatable: define the rights and responsibilities of two novel forms of human life (and from a religious perspective, also define their standing in the religion and status of the soul) or attach personal identity to integrated function. This second option would mean that the source of personal identity would not be a thinking, talking human head/brain but the function of the heart/lungs/kidneys or whatever integrated function is defined to be.

### External validity

A related issue is that of accepted results. A scientific theory is graded by how well it explains known results and its accuracy in predicting future data.[12] There are some situations where the life-and-death status of collections of human tissue are essentially universally accepted. It is reasonable to expect that a definition of life and death will accurately predict the accepted results in these situations. For example, a child born with one body and two functioning heads is considered to be two people (conjoined twins) in Western cultures. Internal organs from the torso, when they are transplanted from one person to another, do not change the identity of the donor or the recipient. The definition of life as the presence of "integrated function" does not correctly predict that the child with two heads should be considered two separate lives. In addition, if organs from Jacob are now performing integrated function in the body of Esau, it stands to reason that the new combination should be Jacob, or at least a Jacob/Esau hybrid. This is not the accepted case. A review of similar situations reveals that our society associates human life with the presence of neurological function. This coherence with accepted results can be termed external validity. Defining life in terms of neurological function coheres well with established situations and therefore has excellent external validity. Defining life in terms of the presence of integrated function does not.

## Definitions of death based on religious texts

### Methodology

Religions supply a source of authority for the definition of life and death that the believer must utilize. The authoritative texts may be interpreted in various ways with diverse conclusions. Specific interpretations may supply a concept, criteria, tests, or some combination. If the interpretation supplies all three, or at least two of the three, some evaluation of the internal validity is possible. If all three are not supplied, the definition is incomplete, and those who advocate for it should be encouraged to provide the information to complete it. For example, a religious tradition may mandate that death involves the cessation of respiration, but this could have a number of different meanings. It could mean that respiration is the concept or fundamental essence of life – when it is present, life is present; when it is absent, life is absent. Respiration would be understood as both necessary and sufficient for a determination of life. But "death is defined as the cessation of respiration" could also mean that the cessation of respiration is the biological correlate of the essence of life. It could also mean that specific tests for the presence or absence of respiration need to be done to determine the presence or absence of life. In the second and third case, the concept of life is not necessarily respiration; rather, the absence of respiration is a means to determine that the actual concept of life, whatever it is, has irreversibly ceased. A religious text or interpretation of the text might not specify to which aspect of the definition it refers – whether it is stating a concept, biological correlate, or testing. However, in order to have a complete definition of death based on the religion, the modern authority not only has to identify to which tier the sources refer but fill in all the tiers.

One might wonder whether it is sufficient for religious sources to operate at the conceptual level (Tier I) without dealing with measurement science. While it may not be the role of certain ancient and broad-ranging religious texts (such as the Bible and Qur'an) to delve into specific criteria and testing for death, it is important that contemporary religious scholars address these matters when engaging in any extended analysis of the definition of death. If only a concept is supplied, the definition is difficult to apply in real-life situations. For example, if life is defined as the presence of brain function, how much or how little brain function has to be present in order to qualify as life? Does every brain cell have to be dead for the individual to be considered dead? A religiously based analysis that claims to operate in the practical realm must provide more than just a concept.[13] Indeed, while there is no singular understanding within any of the three major Abrahamic faiths regarding the relationship between religion and science, those working in each of these faith traditions have often looked to both fields for wisdom.[14]

Once all the tiers are completed, an understanding of death can then be applied to different situations as described above to assess for external validity. The application of the definition of death to these non-death situations will produce a particular result that may or may not cohere with societally accepted results and/or results mandated by the religious texts themselves. For example, as noted above, Western society defines dicephalus twins as two people. A religious tradition, separate from a position on the definition of death, may define dicephalus twins similarly or mandate that they are only one person. If the results from applying the definition of death concur with societally or religiously accepted results, then the definition would have high external validity. On the other hand, if the application of the definition of death does not produce the societally accepted result, the definition has poor external validity, or the religion can reject the societal determination – a course that would put it in conflict with society. If the application of the definition of death also does not concur with the religiously mandated determination, then not only is the external validity poor, but this poses a severe problem for the advocate of that definition. A religion can be expected to be consistent with itself, and the lack of consistency can cast doubt on the correctness of one or both of the determinations.

Religious sources in general can be interpreted literally or non-literally. A religious authority would be expected to have a consistent approach to sources. Insisting on a literal interpretation of some sources and using a non-literal interpretation of other sources, without an underlying methodological or religiously acceptable rationale, implies that the authority is imparting its own views on the sources, perhaps illegitimately. For example, some authorities claim that Jewish tradition mandates that every word in the Jewish Bible is literally true. The lack of scientific evidence of a great flood (mentioned in Genesis) is problematic for this point of view and leads some of its advocates to reject the value or validity of science. Other Orthodox traditions allow that the narrative sections do not necessarily reflect literal truth but can be understood as metaphors or as a moral lesson.[15] A tradition can have different rules for different types of sources and still maintain consistency if those rules are followed. Inconsistency in following the rules of interpretation raises the question of illegitimate interpretations or perhaps an incorrect approach.

Most, if not all, religious authorities writing on the definition of death have not addressed the topic in the comprehensive fashion outlined above. With few exceptions, the three parts of the definition of death have not been delineated, and writers frequently do not address the broader implications of their definitions of death. In the following subsections, the definitions of death of several authors representing the three Abrahamic religions are analyzed with attention to internal validity, external validity, personal identity, and approach to sources. While there are some common themes, the source material for each faith is different enough so that each discussion has some unique aspects. Note that the following discussion is not meant to be exhaustive or address every stream within each religion. Rather, examples have been chosen based on the amount of material available and on the unique issues that pertain to the particular religion. Streams of religions that do not claim to be rigorously bound by received texts and traditions have not been included since part of the analysis includes how a religion interprets its texts. Also, while I focus on English-language sources, I point toward key non-English sources discussed therein.[16]

## Islam

The physician Faroque Khan notes that the Qur'an does not contain an exact definition of death. However, the author reasons that the components of a person mentioned in the Qur'an all coincide with the functions of the brain alone, and therefore accepting brain death does not violate any Islamic principles.[17] Other authors have concluded similarly.[18] A number of Islamic juridical councils have also addressed the issue of brain death, with many, but not all, endorsing brain death as legal death (an opinion from those councils opposing brain death will be discussed shortly).[19] As noted previously, neurologically based definitions of death have high external validity because societal ideas of death are most frequently based on neurological function. With regard to internal validity, most of those writing in the juridical councils address brain death as a concept and do not appear to specify a set of criteria. The issues with internal validity with this approach are therefore similar to those identified for certain secular neurologically based definitions of death.

Significant opposition to brain death also exists in Islam, and at least some appears to be due to a literal interpretation of the Qur'an. Mohamed Rady and Joseph Verheijde contend that "[t]he moment of death is the time when all the signs of life have ceased irreversibly and the soul has departed the body." They do not specify exact signs of life, but note that "the Quran describes that the signs of life are present as long as either the brain and/or the heart are capable of functioning" (citing Qur'an 32:9). In other words, a potentially functional heart is adequate for human life.[20] Another approach maintains that the movement of air, even via machine, is proof enough that death has not occurred, according to Islamic teaching.[21]

Unfortunately, the various tiers of a definition of death are not filled out by the authors, so internal validity is impossible to assess. But these definitions, which identify life with movement of air even via a machine or just a beating heart, suffer from extremely poor external validity. In fact, these definitions become nonsensical in the era of modern medicine. If the heart is supported by itself, outside the rest of the body, is the person still alive? What if it is placed in a different body? Is the body alive as long as a machine is pushing air into the lungs? What happens if the lungs are transplanted? While the authors obviously concentrate on determining the line between life and death, it does not appear that they consider the implications of their approach when applied to transplants or isolated organs.

The above opinions opposed to brain death are based, at least in part, on a literal understanding of sources, which were created under specific societal and/or scientific assumptions. Islamic studies professor Ebrahim Moosa has written extensively on whether and how religious opinions on death should change when there are changes in those assumptions. He identifies one approach as "neo-revivalist" and states that it makes constant references to the primary sources of the Qur'an and Sunna. He writes that this approach "tends to avoid the inherited juridical legacy if it can, claiming the right to interpret the sources. The appropriation of the revealed sources, however, has a semblance of providing a justification for existing practices."[22] Essentially, this approach understands the sources very literally. One example identified with this approach is that of Tawfiq al-Wā'ī, who wrote a detailed opposition to brain death at the meeting of the Academy of Islamic Jurisprudence in 1986 (under the auspices of the Organization of Islamic Conferences). Moosa notes that the opinion draws evidence mainly from the Qur'an and that from the Qur'an the author derives the fact that the stoppage of the heart is a sign of death. Even further, the opinion states that all life in the human body, whether it is cell life or motor movement, deserves to be recognized as part of the divine miracle and mystery of life.[23] This opinion is similar to that of Rady and Verheijde and suffers from the same shortcomings when examined for internal and external consistency.[24]

Islamic religious edicts or scholarly sources that explicitly address the personhood of conjoined twins are very difficult to find. In 2000, Ebraham Desai, a South African Grand Mufti associated with the Deobandi movement within Sunni Islam, issued a fatwa in response to the question, "What does Islam say about the killing of the weaker Siamese twin in order to save the stronger one?" He responded that "Allah . . . has endowed the [weaker] child with life," and that therefore killing that child was always impermissible.[25] Also of interest here is the case of the Egyptian twins Manar and Islaam Maged, who were born joined at the heads and with only one heart (Islaam lacked a torso and limbs but was capable of facial expressions) but given two separate names.[26] If from an Islamic perspective, a newborn with two heads is considered two people (even in the presence of only one heart), then this obviously creates a significant problem for Islamic non-neurological definitions of life and death. Those who define life by heart function or lung function would find it difficult to reconcile their definition of death with such realities. They also do not appear to have addressed the definition of personal identity and how it is determined. If any Islamic scholars were to hold that a child with two functioning heads and one heart is actually only one person – and to be clear, I have not found any willing to take this step – they would need to explain how that determination was made and how it cohered with their definition of life and death and with notions of personal responsibility and personal identity.

Overall, the literal approach to the Qur'an and Islamic sources appears to result in discordance with what are widely accepted results. It also appears that the authors who support this approach continue to rely on outdated and incorrect assumptions. Thus far, the authors have not addressed these issues in a systematic fashion.

## Catholic Christianity

Perhaps the most important text for Catholics in the discussion of the definition of death comes from the Council of Vienne in 1311–1312:

> We reject as erroneous and contrary to the truth of the catholic faith every doctrine or proposition rashly asserting that the substance of the rational or intellectual soul is not of itself and essentially the form of the human body, or casting doubt on this matter. In order that all may know the truth of the faith in its purity and all error may be excluded, we define that anyone who presumes henceforth to assert, defend or hold stubbornly that the rational or intellectual soul is not the form of the human body of itself and essentially, is to be considered a heretic.[27]

This has usually been interpreted as a position that the soul is present as long as there is integration or unity in the body. Pope John Paul II states, "The death of the person is a single event, consisting in the total disintegration of that unitary and integrated whole that is the personal self. It results from the separation of the life-principle (or soul) from the corporal reality of the person. The death of the person, understood in this primary sense, is an event which no scientific technique or empirical method can identify directly."[28]

As Nicholas Tonti-Filippini points out, this linkage of integration and life from a religious point of view makes the 1981 U.S. President's Commission for the Study of Ethical Problems in Medicine and Biomedical and Behavioral Research statement of crucial importance. The Commission states that brain death is indeed death because loss of brain function means loss of integration in the body.[29] Therefore, loss of brain function could be accepted as fulfilling the religious definition equating death with loss of integrated function in the body. Subsequently, it was realized and publicized that the bodies of brain-dead patients have been supported for extended periods of time, refuting the premise that loss of brain function results in the loss of bodily integration.[30] This not only led to the re-evaluation of the concept of death by the U.S. President's Council on Bioethics in 2008[31] but re-evaluation by some in the Church as to whether brain-death criteria were religiously acceptable.

In other words, the basis for the Catholic acceptance of brain death was the scientific belief that the body of a patient fulfilling brain-death criteria no longer contained integrated function. This loss of integrated function was "proven" by the inability to sustain the body for a significant period. But today, at least for some, the capacity for the body to be sustained for a period of time or to gestate a fetus is a sign of integrated function in the body. According to that position, fulfilling brain-death criteria no longer qualifies as death. Tonti-Filippini himself appears to agree with that position. However, another crucial factor is that the most commonly utilized criteria for brain death do not mandate cessation of function of every cell or in fact every function. Tonti-Filippini does state that "if adequate tests that positively exclude the possibility that some brain function may continue have been undertaken, then it is morally acceptable to diagnose death by the loss of all function of the brain."[32] It is not entirely clear, but it appears that he is under the impression that loss of all function of the brain (as opposed to the loss of functions covered by brain-death criteria) would result in the loss of integrated function in the body as manifested by failure to support a body for any significant period of time. But if a body could be supported even with complete destruction of the brain, and that supported body was considered a sign of integration and therefore life, then cessation solely of brain function should not be a definition of death according to the standards of Tonti-Filippini and anyone else who interprets the Council of Vienne in a specific literal fashion. The persistence of integrated function in the body would make the presence or absence of neurological function a moot point.[33]

Others, such as John Haas, may disagree with that last point. Haas references a different part of Pope John Paul II's address: "It is a well-known fact that for some time certain scientific approaches to ascertaining death *have shifted the emphasis . . . to the so-called 'neurological' criterion.* Specifically, this consists in establishing . . . the complete and irreversible cessation of all brain activity. This is then considered the sign that the individual organism has lost its integrative capacity."[34] Haas seems to interpret the Pope as making the cessation of brain activity a sign of the loss of integrative function, regardless of what function persists in the body. It should be kept in mind that at the time of the Pope's pronouncement, it was widely assumed that cessation of integrated function in the body coincided with brain death. What Haas does not address is whether a change in the medical understanding of the relationship between cessation of neurological function and integrated function affects the Catholic understanding. If his position is that the presence of neurological activity is the key in labeling function "integrated" (and that the actual function of the rest of the body is not of importance), then his understanding of the Pope's position theoretically would not be affected by whether a body can be supported in the absence of neurological function. Thus far, official Catholic doctrine does not seem to have specifically addressed the possible severing of the link (assumed present in 1981 but subsequently questioned) between brain function and "integrated function in the body." In other words, there does not appear to have been any publicized change in official Catholic teaching.

Those Catholics such as Haas (if he has been understood correctly) and Tonti-Filippini (under his scientific assumptions that, as demonstrated, may or may not be correct) who agree with neurological criteria for death appear to have a three-part definition of death. The concept is that death is the cessation of integrated function, the biological correlate (criterion) is the cessation of brain function, and the tests are possibly the usual non-maximal tests for brain death (in the case of Haas) or tests for the cessation of *all* brain function (in the case of Tonti-Filippini). Those who disagree with this approach could point out a problem with internal validity, maintaining that the cessation of neurological function does not result in the cessation of integrated function as they define it.[35] If there is to be a resolution, it will be necessary to define, from a Catholic point of view, more precisely what integrated function means in biological terms. In other words, what exact biological functions or interactions are meant when the religion utilizes the term "integrated function"? Only then will it be possible to determine if cessation of neurological function fulfills the demands of the concept.

The Catholic opponents of brain death have so far failed to provide a biological correlate of integrated function except to say that it is not the cessation of neurological function. They also have failed to provide tests to distinguish a dead body from a live one. While the position of the Catholic brain-death advocates suffers from a possible problem with internal validity, those opposed to brain death have yet to supply enough parts of the definition to even test for validity. As for external validity, again, the neurological formulations of death will cohere with societal concepts of life and death, and the non-neurological understandings of death will suffer from poor external validity from a societal point of view.

Paul Byrne, former President of the Catholic Medical Association, takes a different approach. He endorses legal language stating that "No one shall be declared dead unless respiratory and circulatory systems and the entire brain have been destroyed. Such destruction shall be determined in accord with universally accepted medical standards."[36] What is identified here is a biological state. The stated concept of life and death remains unclear. There is no explanation as to why three systems were selected and not a different number. Missing as well are specific tests for the determinations sought. In sum, there is no specific justification, neither religious nor societal, for the chosen criteria, and the definition itself is incomplete.

Finally, Byrne's notion of death suffers from a severe lack of external validity. He believes that "the soul is the life of the body, and as such, it is whole and entire in the whole body and whole and entire in each part."[37] Taking this at face value, if every organ were separated and kept functioning with artificial blood flow, each organ would be a whole and complete soul. Furthermore, if a kidney was to be united with another body (usually understood as transplantation), the body would contain two souls, one associated with the kidney and another with the rest of the body. Byrne and other opponents of brain death are trying to provide a conceptual basis for their opposition, and their positions may appear to make sense when the body is considered an indivisible whole. However, such opponents fail to account for how their definition of death confers the title of "alive" or "containing a soul" to collections of tissue that they probably would not want to recognize as alive or containing a soul.

## *Judaism*

The Jewish legal tradition contains many sources that touch upon human life and death. Some, perhaps many, are potentially contradictory when taken literally and without attending to the historical and scientific context of the pronouncement. Many who oppose brain death have focused upon the statements of the great medieval Talmudic commentator Rashi and also those of the nineteenth-century halachic authority R. Moshe Sofer (known as the Hatam Sofer after the title of his compendium of responsa). Statements by these two authorities can be interpreted as defining a beating heart as a sign of life.[38] The opponents of brain death therefore interpret them as denying brain death and declare them as authoritative, to the exclusion of other interpretations of these opinions and the exclusion of the opinions of other authorities that can be interpreted as accepting brain death.[39] Many of the opponents of brain death conclude that death is the cessation of heartbeat and respiration.[40] However, defining life as the unqualified presence of heartbeat in the modern era, as previously discussed, produces implications that would be hard to accept.

One response to this quandary has been to transform cardiac function into something else, while still maintaining the authority of the above opinions. In other words, cardiac function is changed to be indicative of life only when it supports something else. While cardiac function is still given a place of primary importance, it by itself is no longer sufficient for the determination of life. Rabbi J. David Bleich has written extensively on many aspects of Jewish law, including bioethics. He defines life as the presence of "vital motion," and death therefore as the irreversible cessation of vital motion.[41] He then goes back and reinterprets Rashi and others as incorporating the concept of "vital motion" in their work, even though neither the exact words nor the concept are actually found there. For example, Rashi's statement regarding heartbeat is understood to mean that heartbeat indicates life only when it supports vital motion. In addition to the obvious methodological problems, Bleich has not defined the criteria or testing needed to establish the presence or absence of vital motion and, in fact, has not defined vital motion in a rigorous fashion.[42] Therefore, his definition of death cannot even be tested for internal validity due to the absence of tests and criteria.

Bleich has also written about conjoined twins and notes that Jewish law identifies a body with two functioning heads as two people.[43] Since his notion of vital motion does not include neurological function, this finding does not cohere with his definition of death/life. Whether a body has one or two heads does not seem to impact the amount of vital motion. This illustrates a lack of external validity that has not been addressed.

The Chief Rabbinate of Israel in 1987 produced a rather complete definition of death.[44] It has been expanded recently by Rabbi Avraham Steinberg, one of the authors of the original opinion. Death, according to Steinberg, is the cessation of respiration caused by overwhelming brain damage sufficient to eliminate brainstem function, including the areas responsible for triggering respiration.[45] Cessation of respiration as a definition of death is found in the Talmud and other sources.[46] The addition of the context of brain damage has been criticized for lacking appropriate textual support.[47] This critique can be answered in a number of ways.[48] The Talmud (*Gittin* 70a) states that a person who is on the verge of certain death can validly divorce his wife, thus indicating that as long as he is conscious, he is considered alive. Steinberg notes that some authorities mandate unconsciousness as part of a definition of death.[49] It is reasonable based on sources to mandate destruction of at least part of the brain as a basis for a determination of death.

The respiratory-brain definition of death is a complete definition that includes a concept, criteria, and specific tests and results. Steinberg fills out the tiers as follows. The Tier I concept is that the neurologically based ability to breathe is the essence of life. With regard to Tier II, he says, "When it is medically obvious that a person has no spontaneous respiration at all and is lying motionless like a stone without any consciousness and no movements or reactions (to stimuli), and if there is clear evidence from the medical testing which is reliable and unanimous in proving complete and irreversible cessation of the functioning of the brain and especially the brain-stem, which is the central control of respiration, one has established the condition known as 'respiratory-brain death,' and this is the Halakhic [legal] moment of death of a human being." Tier III includes specific tests (outlined in his book and in Israel's Brain-Respiratory Death Law). A patient who fulfills all the tests is dead. They include documenting apnea and loss of brainstem reflexes, specific confirmatory tests such as blood flow tests, and ruling out conditions that might be reversible but mimic the loss of function.[50] Furthermore, this definition of life and death has good external and internal validity, both with societally accepted results and, more importantly, with religiously mandated results. For example, it correctly identifies a baby with two heads as two people. Furthermore, it aligns the definition of death with personal identity.

The approach of the Chief Rabbinate to the sources is traditional. However, unlike the other authorities, they did not accept any one source or interpretation as set in stone and were more willing to look at sources in historical and scientific context.

### Some additional challenges to religiously based integrated-function views

Abrahamic religions have various doctrines of free will and reward and punishment. The functioning human brain is the source of human decision-making. Imagine a human being where the head has been separated from the body, but the functions of both have been preserved via circulation pumps.[51] Which part is the human being? The head that is still capable of making decisions, thinking, communicating, perhaps controlling movement (via EEG control of mechanical or biological arms/legs)? Or the body that contains integrated function of heart, lungs, kidneys, and intestines but is not capable of thought and decision-making? Can a head containing a functioning brain, which is a collection of human tissue capable of divinely given free will and capable of incurring divine reward and punishment for those choices, not be a human being? Those who equate death with the cessation of integrated function appear to have no choice but to embrace this counterintuitive position.

The equation of life with "integrated function" is also problematic from another point of view. There is no fundamental difference between the integrated function in one person and that in another person.[52] In fact, this is the basis for the success of transplants. The definitions based on integrated function fail to distinguish between one person and another. Furthermore, the definition does not adequately differentiate between humans and animals since animals' vital organs can be substituted for human ones. It would be possible to start with a human being and exchange all the organs (except for the brain) one by one with animal organs so that, ultimately, there would be animal organs supplying the vital function in the body. If the head were to be removed, there would be nothing human about what was left except for the seemingly insignificant torso, but those who equate integrated function with life would claim that the human soul was still present. It was essentially present at the beginning, and none of the individual organ substitutions affected the presence of the soul, so it would have to be present at the end as well, even when no human organs were involved in the production of "integrated function." This is all the more ironic because those who use "integrated function" usually interpret their texts in a more literal fashion and are probably even more opposed to concepts of equivalence between man and animal than those who define life by neurological function.[53]

## Conclusion

I have attempted to illustrate how non-neurological definitions of death focus narrowly on opposition to "brain death," are usually stated only as concepts, and frequently are not actual functioning definitions of death at all – none could be used on a practical basis to distinguish between a live person and a dead person. Some correlate a biological state with death but still do not contain specific tests for death. These formulations are not only incomplete but are incompatible with the wider context that requires a definition of life and death. Admittedly, it has been difficult for brain-death advocates to state why a certain amount of brain function is death and a certain amount is not, but this is also an unrecognized problem for anyone attempting to define death on any conceptual basis, neurological or not. The brain-based definitions of death have been more complete and cohere with the wider universe of situations where life-and-death determinations are needed, including personal identity.

Non-neurological definitions of death from a religious perspective have also suffered from the same problems. Again, while the ways in which different religions and different streams within religions incorporate scientific data into argument may be distinct, attention to such data is important if one's definition of death is to operate in the practical realm and consistent with those religious streams that have looked to science for guidance. The fundamental, traditional religious sources for the definition of life and death come from the pre-modern era of medicine, where the cessation of heartbeat and/or breathing was assumed to not only be irreversible but mark the cessation of all function in the body. Religious authorities face the challenge of applying these sources to a very different scientific reality. Those authorities – who take a literal approach to the sources, refuse to take into account the differing scientific circumstances, and/or set into stone specific opinions that are based on that previous reality – will have difficulty arriving at a cogent complete definition of death that is not only internally but externally valid and compatible with the definition of personal identity. In fact, it may be an impossible task with those specific approaches. I have illustrated how a more flexible but still traditional approach (within Orthodox Judaism) taken by the Chief Rabbinate of Israel is able to surmount the difficulties. The definition of death of the Chief Rabbinate still faces serious and significant opposition from those who insist that the older sources are sacrosanct, but those opponents have failed to provide a functional definition of death, and those concepts that have been proposed have very poor external validity and conflict with personal identity. The less literal approaches to Islam and Christianity also produce more coherent (although still incomplete as of now) definitions of death than the approaches that mandate a more literal understanding.

Scientific understanding and societal norms have changed over the years. There are many current issues that require the application of older sources to new situations. In many situations, a specific determination on a particular topic does not have any implications for other situations. There is no way to "prove" that the approach that rejects taking changing circumstances into account is right or wrong. There is no way to "prove" that codifying a specific opinion is a right or wrong approach. On the other hand, the definition of death is perhaps unique in that it applies not only to a specific determination of life/death but also to situations such as organ transplantation, dicephalus twins and other situations of children born with duplicated organs, and personal identity. A specific approach to sources results in a particular definition of death, and that definition of death can be tested for internal and external validity as well as coherence with personal identity. I suggest that thus far, the analysis has shown that rigid approaches to sources result in incoherence. They cannot even provide a set of specific tests to determine whether a person is dead or not. They cannot account for why a two-headed baby is considered two human beings. They cannot explain why, if all of the abdominal organs were taken out of Jacob and placed into Esau, the resulting combination is considered Esau and not Jacob, despite the integrated function provided by Jacob's organs. Consistency of approach is a necessary part of a religious legal system. One cannot legitimately take change of fact and/or circumstance into account in one situation and then state categorically that these cannot be taken into account in a different but similar situation. Those taking one of the rigid approaches to pre-modern sources need to be able to provide a definition of death that is valid and coherent within their chosen approach to sources. If they are not able to do so, I suggest that this is sufficient "proof" that the rigid approach is inferior to the more flexible one.

Furthermore, if a more flexible approach is adapted in the determination of life and death, this same flexibility should be adapted in all similar circumstances where science and society have changed. This potentially could have widespread ramifications. There are fields where societal and scientific assumptions have changed – perhaps most prominently regarding gender. To reiterate, the failure to establish a coherent definition of death using a literal approach to sources implies that that literal approach is not the "best" approach to religious sources. If a religion values coherence, and the degree of coherence is considered a valid method of evaluation, then the more contextual approach is the more religiously desirable and should be employed not just in the isolated area of the definition of death but in all areas where changes of context have occurred.

## Notes

1 Michael J. Broyde, "Letter to the Editor: The Diagnosis of Brain Death," *The New England Journal of Medicine* 345 no. 8 (2001): 616.
2 In the United States, the definition of death is established by each state. However, all, either by law or court precedent, are based on the UDDA, a copy of which is available here: www.uniformlaws.org/shared/docs/determination%20 of%20death/udda80.pdf. The UDDA also states that "[a]n individual who has sustained . . . irreversible cessation of all functions of the entire brain, including the brain stem, is dead." Ibid.
3 Respiration can be defined either as air being pumped in and out of the lungs or by the gas exchange (oxygen for carbon dioxide) that occurs in the lungs themselves. Mechanical ventilators are commonly used in intensive care units for patients who are unable to move air adequately for themselves. The gas exchange can be mimicked by special machines, but for simplicity, this section has concentrated on circulation.
4 The philosophical discussion of the meaning of "irreversible" and "potential" is relevant but beyond the scope of this paper. John P. Lizza, "Potentiality, Irreversibility, and Death," *Journal of Medicine and Philosophy* 30 no. 1 (2005): 45–64.
5 James L. Bernat, "A Defense of the Whole-Brain Concept of Death," *Hastings Center Report* 28 no. 2 (1998): 14–23.

6  Stuart J. Youngner, "Defining Death: A Superficial and Fragile Consensus," *Archives of Neurology* 49 no. 5 (1992): 570–572 (the emphasis within quotation marks is mine).

7  See, e.g., Eelco F. M. Wijdicks, Panayiotis N. Varelas, Gary S. Gronseth, and David M. Greer, "Evidence-Based Guideline Update: Determining Brain Death in Adults: Report of the Quality Standards Subcommittee of the American Academy of Neurology," *Neurology* 74 no. 23 (2010): 1911–1918.

8  The American Academy of Neurology published guidelines in 1995 and updated them in 2010. Wijdicks et al., "Evidence-Based Guideline Update"; The Quality Standards Subcommittee of the American Academy of Neurology, "Practice Parameters for Determining Brain Death in Adults (Summary Statement)," *Neurology* 45 no. 5 (1995): 1012–1014.

9  For example, see Samuel H. LiPuma and Joseph P. DeMarco, "Reviving Brain Death: A Functionalist View," *Journal of Bioethical Inquiry* 10 no. 3 (2013): 383–392. I have also addressed the issue in Noam Stadlan, "Neurological Death: A Twenty-First-Century Definition," in *Halakhic Realities: Collected Essays on Brain Death*, ed. Zev Farber (Jerusalem, Israel: Koren, 2015), 33–79.

10  D. Alan Shewmon, "Mental Disconnect: 'Physiological Decapitation' as a Heuristic for Understanding 'Brain Death,'" in *The Signs of Death: The Proceedings of the Working Group 11–12 September 2006*, ed. Marcelo Sánchez Sorondo (Vatican City: Pontifical Academy of Sciences, 2007), 292–333. Shewmon previously wrote in more detail on the concept of integrated function and provided a preliminary outline of criteria in D. Alan Shewmon, "The Brain and Somatic Integration: Insights Into the Standard Biological Rationale for Equating 'Brain Death' with Death," *Journal of Medicine and Philosophy* 26 no. 5 (2001): 457–478.

11  Ari R. Joffe, "Are Recent Defences of the Brain Death Concept Adequate?," *Bioethics* 24 no. 2 (2010): 47–53.

12  In this situation, predicting future results is not a feasible criterion, as accepted determinations of life-and-death status are exactly that – accepted – and therefore the result is not foreordained until a societal consensus has coalesced. In this way, the determination of death differs from scientific theories, but we should still expect it to predict known results well. The advocates of a particular approach need to accept the results of their approach in all situations. For example, if circulation is considered sufficient for life, then even a heart with a few blood vessels would qualify as life. One alternative is to suggest that different criteria could be used for different stages of death, but there needs to be adequate justification for the various criteria chosen for the various stages. An example of how to divide death into stages and assign different rights/obligations to each stage is here: Amir Halevy and Baruch Brody, "Brain Death: Reconciling Definitions, Criteria, and Tests," *Annals of Internal Medicine* 119 no. 6 (1993): 519–525. In brief, this approach would be rejected by those who believe in a unitary definition of death, but could have appeal to those who are not wedded to that concept. From a religious point of view, the various stages of death would have to be justified by sources from the religious tradition.

13  In other words, religion provides the rules that the believer obligates him/herself to live by. Fundamentalists may claim that the rules never change. Other traditionalists may believe that the rules are reinterpreted in each age to a greater or lesser extent. But whether it is applying ancient rules to new situations or deciding whether there are changes in the rules, religious scholars have to interpret the concepts *and* provide the specifics of the rules (and in the case of defining death, these specifics include criteria and tests for death). If the religion provides only a concept, then the interpretation is open to everyone, even those who are not the acknowledged leaders/experts of the religion. The religion must provide specific rules, or else the concept is of minimal use and there is no guidance. This is especially true of Judaism and Islam, which have highly developed and specific rules for essentially all activity. In this situation, it is also true of Catholicism.

For example, as indicated below, some claim that Pope John Paul II's use of "integrated function" as a sign of the presence of the soul means that brain death is not death. As illustrated in this chapter, just defining life as the concept of integrated function does not provide authoritative guidance. Some are going to interpret integrated function as one thing and some as something else. It is the duty of the religious scholars to interpret, and the duty of the faithful to follow those interpretations.

In order to determine the appropriate rules and specifics, religious scholars ideally need to understand the relevant facts. Since it is not reasonable to expect every religious authority to be proficient in all aspects of knowledge that pertain to a particular issue, those who are conscientious will consult with appropriate experts. However, the ultimate responsibility for determining the religious law devolves upon the religious scholars. Even if they defer to the conclusions of a scientific expert or panel, that deference imparts the imprimatur of religious authority on those conclusions. An example of the interaction of law and science can be seen in recent discussions regarding the life-and-death status of Jahi McMath and other legal aspects of brain death. In mid-2017, a judge gave an opinion as to whether Jahi McMath was alive or dead; he took into account the opinions of the scientists, but ultimately the judge made the decision. Around the same time, lawmakers in Nevada voted on a new law defining brain death. The law in New Jersey regarding brain death contains specific tests that must be done in order to qualify as brain dead. In all these situations and more, the legal scholars have the task of making the final decision and determination. None of them are scientists. However, they do need to understand the science, depend on input from the scientists, and then base the law on the scientific facts. In such an instance, the conclusions of that scientific body have legal force.

Perhaps the most complete archive of medical and legal information as well as commentary on the Jahi McMath case has been complied by a lawyer, Thaddeus Pope, and is available here: http://thaddeuspope.com/jahimcmath.html. His blog (referenced at the bottom of this page) contains references and in-depth discussions of the issues at hand. For reference to the Nevada law, see Sandra Chereb, "Nevada Adopts National Brain Death Guidelines under Bill," *Las Vegas Review-Journal*, May 8, 2017, www.reviewjournal.com/news/2017-legislature/nevada-adopts-national-brain-death-guidelines-under-bill. For an analysis of the New Jersey law on brain death and recent suggestions for modifications, see New Jersey Law Revision Commission, "Final Report Relating to New Jersey Declaration of Death Act," January 18, 2013, www.lawrev.state.nj.us/UDDA/njddaFR011813.pdf.

14 For further discussion of the relationship between religion and science in the Jewish, Christian, and Islamic traditions, see, e.g., Rabbi Jonathan Sacks, *The Great Partnership: Science, Religion, and the Search for Meaning* (New York, NY: Schocken, 2011); David Marshall, ed., *Science and Religion: Christian and Muslim Perspectives* (Washington, DC: Georgetown University Press, 2012).

15 For an extended analysis of this topic in the Jewish tradition, see Joshua L. Golding, "On the Limits of Non-Literal Interpretation of Scripture from an Orthodox Perspective," *The Torah u-Madda Journal* 10 (2001): 37–59, www.yutorah.org/_shiurim/Joshua%20L.%20Golding%20-%20On%20the%20Limits%20of%20Non-Literal%20Interpretation%20of%20Scripture%20From%20An%20Orthodox%20Perspective%20(1-1-2001).pdf. For sources on non-literal interpretations of the flood story, see Natan Slifkin, "Dealing with the Deluge," October 3, 2010, www.rationalistjudaism.com/2010/10/dealing-with-deluge.html.

16 Fortunately, many sources for Christianity and Judaism are written or translated into English. In addition, since I am fluent in Hebrew and a practicing Jew,

Judaic sources were readily accessible, although all such sources I cite in the present chapter are in English. I searched PubMed for all papers on Islam and brain death, and, as best as I can determine, read them all.

17 Faroque A. Khan, "The Definition of Death in Islam: Can Brain Death Be Used as a Criteria of Death in Islam?," *The Journal of the Islamic Medical Association* 18 no. 1 (1986): 18–21.

18 Yousef Boobes and Nada Al Daker, "What It Means to Die in Islam and Modern Medicine," *Saudi Journal of Kidney Diseases and Transplantation* 7 no. 2 (1996): 121–127. Ebrahim Moosa seems to be cautiously in favor of brain death as well. Ebrahim Moosa, "Brain Death and Organ Transplantation – An Islamic Opinion," *South African Medical Journal* 83 no. 6 (1993): 385–386.

19 See the summary table in Aasim I. Padela, Ahsan Arozullah, and Ebrahim Moosa, "Brain Death in Islamic Ethico-Legal Deliberation: Challenges for Applied Islamic Bioethics," *Bioethics* 27 no. 3 (2013): 134. The table includes those who disagree with brain death as well. The basis for the disagreement will be discussed in more detail.

20 Mohamed Y. Rady and Joseph L. Verheijde, "Brain-Dead Patients Are Not Cadavers: The Need to Revise the Definition of Death in Muslim Communities," *HEC Forum* 25 no. 1 (2013): 25–45. As quoted in the article, Qur'an 32:9 states, "Then He fashioned him in due proportion, and breathed into him the soul and He gave you hearing, sight and hearts." The authors conclude, "The definition of death in Islam should reaffirm the singularity of human death as revealed in the Quran 14 centuries ago." Ibid., 37, 41.

21 Ahmet Bedir and Şahin Aksoy, "Brain Death Revisited: It Is Not 'Complete Death' According to Islamic Sources," *Journal of Medical Ethics* 37 no. 5 (2011): 290–294.

22 Ebrahim Moosa, "Languages of Change in Islamic Law: Redefining Death in Modernity," *Islamic Studies* 38 no. 3 (1999): 309–312.

23 Ibid., 321–325 (citing Tawfiq al-Wā'ī, "Ḥaqīqat al'Mawt wa 'l-Hayāh fi 'l-Qur'ān wa 'l-Aḥkām al-Shar'iyyah," *Majallat Majma' al-Fiqh al-Islāmī* 3 no. 2: 695–718).

24 Moosa also analyzes the opinion of Muḥammad Na'īm Yāsīn, who notes that there is no revealed text to determine the end of human life and therefore it is necessary for the jurists to develop legal norms from the texts. Furthermore, Yāsīn holds, it is necessary for jurists to collaborate with medical specialists, and that "in the final instance . . . the observations and research findings of medical specialists will prevail." Ibid., 316–320 (quoting Muḥammad Na'īm Yāsīn, "Nihāyat al-Ḥayāt al-Insāniyyah fī ḍaw Ijtihādāt al-'Ulamā' al-Muslimīn wa 'l-Mu'tayāt al Ṭibbiyyah," *Majallat Majma' al-Fiqh al-Islāmī* 3 no. 2: 635–660).

25 Ebrahim Desai, "What Does Islam Say About the Killing of the Weaker Siamese Twin in Order to Save the Stronger One?," September 12, 2000, http://askimam. org/public/question_detail/848.html. I am indebted to an anonymous, helpful Islamic reviewer for calling my attention to this fatwa. This reviewer adds that Islamic ethical debates over conjoined twins appear to not be about whether they are two persons but about whether it is ethical to operate on the twins when there is the risk of harming one of them and that the tacit assumption seems to be that where there are separate mental faculties there are two people.

26 Subsequent to the detachment of Islaam, Manar and her mother appeared on The Oprah Winfrey Show, although Manar died shortly thereafter. Pamela Prindle Fierro, "Craniopagus Parasiticus and the Unformed Conjoined Twin: Rare Cases of a Two-Headed Twin With One Body," *Verywell Family*, August 16, 2018, www.verywellfamily.com/parasitic-twin-profile-manar-maged-2446993.

27 Nicholas Tonti-Filippini, "Religious and Secular Death: A Parting of the Ways," *Bioethics* 26 no. 8 (2012): 415.

28  Ibid., 411 (quoting John Paul II, "Address at the 18th International Congress of the Transplantation Society" [2000]).

29  Ibid., 410. The original statement, *Defining Death: A Report on the Medical, Legal and Ethical Issues in the Determination of Death* (Washington, DC: U.S. Government Printing Office, 1984), https://repository.library.georgetown.edu/bitstream/handle/10822/559345/defining_death.pdf.

30  Shewmon reports on a brain-dead pediatric patient, TK, whose body was supported for many years. D. Alan Shewmon, "Chronic Brain Death: Meta-Analysis and Conceptual Consequences," *Neurology* 51 no. 6 (1998): 1538–1545.

31  The President's Council on Bioethics, "Controversies in the Determination of Death: A White Paper by the President's Council on Bioethics," December 2008, https://bioethicsarchive.georgetown.edu/pcbe/reports/death.

32  Tonti-Filippini, "Religious and Secular Death," 421.

33  It should be noted that the autopsy of TK failed to reveal even one neuron. Tonti-Filippini's paper mentions TK but does not reference the autopsy article, and it is not clear if he is aware of it. The report of the autopsy of patient TK is here: Susan Repertinger, William P. Fitzgibbons, Mathew F. Omojola, and Roger A. Brumback, "Long Survival Following Bacterial Meningitis-Associated Brain Destruction," *Journal of Child Neurology* 21 no. 7 (2006): 591–595.

34  John M. Haas, "Catholic Teaching regarding the Legitimacy of Neurological Criteria for the Determination of Death," *National Catholic Bioethics Quarterly* 11 no. 2 (2011): 286. Despite the word "complete" in this excerpt from the papal address, Haas appears to support non-maximal tests for brain death. Ibid., 282–283.

35  For examples of Catholic opposition to brain death, see Doyen Nguyen, "Pope John Paul II and the Neurological Standard for the Determination of Death: A Critical Analysis of His Address to the Transplantation Society," *Linacre Quarterly* 84 no. 2 (2017): 155–186; Robert Spaemann, "Is Brain Death the Death of the Human Being? On the Current State of the Debate," in *The Signs of Death*, ed. Sorondo, 130–141.

36  Paul A. Byrne, Sean O'Reilly, Paul M. Quay, and Peter W. Salsich, Jr., "Brain Death – The Patient, the Physician, and Society," in *Beyond Brain Death: The Case Against Brain Based Criteria for Human Death*, eds. Michael Potts, Paul A. Byrne, and Richard G. Nilges (Boston, MA: Kluwer Academic Publishers, 2000), 72.

37  Michael Potts, Paul A. Byrne, and Richard G. Nilges, "Introduction: Beyond Brain Death," in *Beyond Brain Death*, eds. Potts, Byrne, and Nilges, 3.

38  In the Talmud, Rabbi Shlomo Yitzchaki (1040–1105), known by the acronym Rashi, comments: "For one says: in his heart one can discern if there is life, since his *neshamah* [breathing, but also the word for soul – both are reasonable understandings] beats there; and the other says: [we examine] until his heart, for sometimes life is not discernible at the heart, but is discernible at the nose." This statement has been understood as mandating that heartbeat is sufficient for life. Taken literally, this eliminates the religious acceptance of neurological criteria for death since the heart continues to beat under those circumstances. For further discussion, see Daniel Reifman, "The Brain Death Debate: A Methodological Analysis – Part 1 (Yoma Passage)," January 16, 2011, http://text.rcarabbis.org/the-brain-death-debate-a-methodological-analysis-part-1-yoma-passage-by-daniel-reifman. There are other interpretations of Rashi that are consonant with neurological definitions of death. For example, see Avraham Steinberg, *Respiratory-Brain Death*, trans. Fred Rosner (Jerusalem, Israel: Merhavim-Torah Center for Judaism and Education, 2012).

    Rabbi Moshe Sofer's responsum addressing the determination of death is quite lengthy and complex. The opponents of brain death emphasize one particular portion: "But as long as he lies like an inanimate stone and has no pulse, if afterward breathing ceases, we have only the words of our holy Torah [to rely on and determine] that he is dead . . .." Daniel Reifman, "The Brain Death Debate: A Methodological Analysis – Part 2 (Hatam Sofer)," March 28, 2011, http:// text.rcarabbis.org/the-brain-death-debate-a-methodological-analysis-part-2-hatam-sofer (quoting Rabbi Moshe Schreiber [Sofer], *Responsum Hatam Sofer Yoreh Deah* #338). This is understood by the opponents of brain death as saying that a person is dead only when he or she is not moving – the heart has stopped, and respiration has stopped. Similar to the above, under this understanding, the continued beating of the heart would negate any determination of death. For other interpretations and analysis, see Reifman, "The Brain Death Debate: A Methodological Analysis – Part 2 (Hatam Sofer)."

39 This is a not-uncommon approach by some in the Orthodox world to contemporary issues – selecting one opinion or approach and declaring it authoritative, perhaps without regard to the historical and factual context.

40 See also David Shabtai, *Defining the Moment: Understanding Brain Death in Halakhah* (New York, NY: Shoresh Press, 2012), 345–366.

41 J. David Bleich, "Of Cerebral, Respiratory and Cardiac Death," *Tradition: A Journal of Orthodox Jewish Thought* 24 no. 3 (1989): 44–66.

42 For further analysis, see Noam Stadlan, "Is the Concept of Vital Motion a Halakhic Definition of Death?," *Ḥakirah: The Flatbush Journal of Jewish Law and Thought* 18 (2014): 91–106.

43 J. David Bleich, "Conjoined Twins," *Tradition: A Journal of Orthodox Jewish Thought* 31 no. 1 (1996): 92–125.

44 "[Brain Death and] Heart Transplants: The [Israeli] Chief Rabbinate's Directives," trans. Yoel Jakobovits, *Tradition: A Journal of Orthodox Jewish Thought* 24 no. 4 (1989): 1–14.

45 Steinberg, *Respiratory-Brain Death*.

46 See ibid. for a detailed citation and discussion of sources supporting the use of respiration/brain function as the definition of death based on traditional Jewish sources.

47 See, e.g., Shabtai, *Defining the Moment*, 367.

48 For further discussion, see Noam Stadlan, "Review Essay: New Books and Points of Discussion in the Definition of Death: *Respiratory-Brain Death* by Avraham Steinberg, and *Defining the Moment – Understanding Brain Death in Halakhah* by David Shabtai," *Meorot: A Forum of Modern Orthodox Discourse* 10 (2012): 1–30, https://library.yctorah.org/files/2016/07/5-stadlan.pdf.

49 Steinberg, *Respiratory-Brain Death*, 46.

50 This overview of Steinberg's views is adapted mostly word-for-word from my "Is the Concept of Vital Motion a Halakhic Definition of Death?," 94 (quoting Steinberg, *Respiratory-Brain Death*, 14).

51 This is something that is not only technologically feasible but was done in primates in the 1970s by Robert White. Robert J. White, Lee R. Wolin, Leo C. Massopust, Jr., Norman Taslitz, and Javier Verdura, "Primate Cephalic Transplantation: Neurogenic Separation, Vascular Association," *Transplantation Proceedings* 3 no. 1 (1971): 602–604; Robert J. White, Lee R. Wolin, Leo C. Massopust, Jr., Norman Taslitz, and Javier Verdura, "Cephalic Exchange Transplantation in the Monkey," *Surgery* 70 no. 1 (1971): 135–139.

52 A good analogy here is a computer. Certainly, one computer functions the same as any other computer. However, a computer with specific programs and memory is very different from the same computer with different programs and stored memory. They are not interchangeable. On the other hand, peripherals such as printers, monitors, mice, keyboards, and even power cords are frequently interchangeable.

53 Some would attempt to counter this by suggesting that a similar thought experiment could be done but substituting neurological function (instead of organs) from animals. For example, consider a situation where animal cells were transferred to a human brain; at some point, the entire brain was made up of animal cells, not human cells. If identity is dependent on brain function, it might be possible to have a brain that functions like a human brain but is made up of animal cells, and perhaps the brain-death advocate would have to acknowledge that the resulting being with an animal brain was still human. However, this is not anatomically/technically possible. Even with today's current advanced biotechnology, one cannot connect parts of one brain to another brain, so one cannot substitute an animal brain, or a part of an animal brain, for a human brain. A similar (and to my mind incorrect) counterargument was presented here: D. Alan Shewmon, "Constructing the Death Elephant: A Synthetic Paradigm Shift for the Definition, Criteria, and Tests for Death," *Journal of Medicine and Philosophy* 35 no. 3 (2010): 256–298. I suggest that even if it were technically possible for a brain made up of cells with animal DNA to function like a human brain, it is not problematic for those who define life and identity by neurological function. The key is function. If a brain functions as a human brain – producing consciousness, emotion, and human qualities – it should be classified as a human brain, regardless of its provenance.

One additional counterargument against brain-death advocates such as myself could be made regarding patients with brain damage who cannot think. In other words, if consciousness is the dividing line between life and death, then those who are permanently unconscious or anencephalic would be labeled dead, which would be an undesirable conclusion. In response, the point here is to establish that if a particular function such as consciousness is present, that very presence mandates the label of human life, so consciousness by itself is sufficient for a determination of life, but it does not have to be a necessary component of life. Someone who is unconscious but retains certain brain function can still be classified as alive, and that determination does not contradict the idea that all who are conscious are alive.

# Index